WOUND HEALING - CURRENT PERSPECTIVES

Edited by **Kamil Hakan Dogan**

Wound Healing - Current Perspectives
http://dx.doi.org/10.5772/intechopen.73808
Edited by Kamil Hakan Dogan

Contributors

Christian Agyare, Yaw Duah Boakye, Newman Osafo, Mohammadreza Farahpour, Rafael Mendoza, Robert Galiano, Ji-Cheng Hsieh, Claudia Pellizzon, Fernando Beserra, Peter A. Everts, Diego Caicedo Valdes, Jesús Devesa, Raffaele Capoano, Manuel Cadena, Girish Kotwal, Rebekah Amarini, Sufan Chien, Emanuele Salvatore Aragona, Juin-Hong Cherng, Yan Wang, Wenjing Wu, Victor Y. A. Barku, Kamil Hakan Dogan

First published in London, United Kingdom, 2019 by IntechOpen
IntechOpen is the global imprint of INTECHOPEN LIMITED, registered in England and Wales, registration number: 11086078, The Shard, 25th floor, 32 London Bridge Street
London, SE19SG – United Kingdom
Printed in Croatia

British Library Cataloguing-in-Publication Data
A catalogue record for this book is available from the British Library

Additional hard and PDF copies can be obtained from orders@intechopen.com

Wound Healing - Current Perspectives, Edited by Kamil Hakan Dogan
p. cm.
Print ISBN 978-1-78985-537-1
Online ISBN 978-1-78985-538-8
eBook (PDF) ISBN 978-1-83880-645-3

For EU product safety concerns:
IN TECH d.o.o., Prolaz Marije Krucifikse Kozulić 3, 51000 Rijeka, Croatia,
info@intechopen.com or visit our website at intechopen.com.

Meet the editor

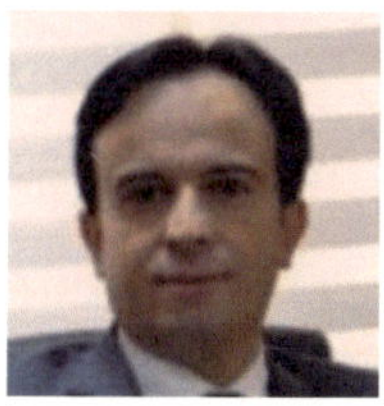

Kamil Hakan Dogan MD, PhD is a full professor and chair in the Department of Forensic Medicine at Selcuk University Faculty of Medicine in Turkey. Dr. Dogan received his MD from Gazi University Faculty of Medicine in 2000. After his extensive research in the field of forensic medicine, he received his PhD in Biochemistry in 2012. He gives lectures on forensic medicine and medical ethics to medical students as well as students of dentistry and law faculties. He is a reviewer in several international journals, and he has published over 200 articles in refereed journals, chapters in textbooks, and abstracts in scientific meetings. His publications have been cited more than 500 times.

Contents

Preface

Wound healing and its treatment are subjects that have been discussed for centuries in the medical literature. Wounds are everywhere, occurring in the young and elderly and in hospital and at home, and affect patients in every clinical specialty around the world. With an improved understanding of the wound healing process, regenerative treatments have been developed. In the historical process, the pathophysiology of wound healing was better understood, especially with advances in cellular and molecular techniques. The factors affecting wound healing are: size, site, and shape of the wound, injury method, agents used and recurring trauma, foreign objects, hematoma or seroma, heat, amount of oxygen, smoking, infection, nutritional factors, medicines, radiotherapy, and systemic diseases.

In the chapter by Fernando Pereira Beserra et al., the authors review the pathway in the skin healing cascade, relating the major chemical inflammatory mediators, cellular and molecular. Local and systemic factors that interfere with healing and disorders associated with tissue repair deficiency in chronic inflammations, burns, and hypertrophy are also demonstrated. In the third chapter by Christian Agyare et al., biomarkers are discussed relevant to the wound healing process. Non-healing wounds are also identified, where biomarker-guided approaches may be of clinical importance in their management. The fourth chapter by Mohammad Reza Farahpour examines medicinal plants in wound healing and shows wound healing effects by different mechanisms, such as modulation in wound healing, decreasing bacterial count, improving collagen deposition, increasing fibroblasts and fibrocytes, etc.

The fifth chapter by Victor Y. A. Barku deals with plant secondary metabolite antioxidants and briefly reviews antioxidant properties of medicinal plants to highlight the important roles medicinal plants play in wound healing. The sixth chapter by Juin-Hong Cherng discusses the detailed mechanisms and efficacy of natural polysaccharides in accelerating the wound healing process, thereby encouraging the advanced strategies for future wound management. The seventh chapter by Aragona Salvatore Emanuele et al. provides an interesting overview of wound healing: from tissue repair to tissue regeneration. They define wound repair as the incomplete regeneration of the original tissue with hyperproduction of organized collagen, which can lead to the production of new tissue with an 80% similarity to the original tissue.

The eighth chapter by Diego Caicedo and Jesús Devesa focuses on a large amount of experimental and clinical evidence on the action of growth hormones in wound repair and analyzes how the physiological rhythm of growth hormone secretion influences this process. It also looks at one of the most important signaling pathways that mediates the effects of growth hormones on tissue regeneration. The ninth chapter by Peter A. Everts deals with both platelet-rich plasma and mesenchymal stem cell applications. These have the potential to become effective and ideal autologous biological cell-based therapies, which can be applied to chronic wounds to effectively change the wound bed microenvironment to enable and accelerate wound closure.

The tenth chapter by Yan Wang and Wenjing Wu discusses wound healing and the biomechanics of corneal refractive procedures to better understand corneal wound healing from the biomechanical viewpoint. This is mandatory if refractive surgery is ever to achieve more predictable and safer refractive results. The eleventh chapter by Manuel Cadena and Juan José Santivañez provides a comprehensive review of the open abdomen. This is the most challenging of wounds that a surgeon faces because of the metabolic, physiological, and dynamic implications that this condition entails. The twelfth chapter by Girish J. Kotwal et al. discusses facilitation of wound healing with current general wound care, following laparoscopic and conventional surgery with dressings, patches, antibiotics, etc. The last chapter by Raffaele Capoano et al. addresses multidisciplinary approaches to the stimulation of wound healing and use of dermal substitutes in chronic phlebostatic ulcers.

The purpose of presenting this book is to provide an insight into current perspectives on wound healing processes.

Kamil Hakan Dogan
Selcuk University Faculty of Medicine
Department of Forensic Medicine
Konya, Turkey

Chapter 1

Introductory Chapter: An Overview of Wound Healing

Kamil Hakan Dogan

Additional information is available at the end of the chapter

http://dx.doi.org/10.5772/intechopen.84494

1. Introduction

Wound is the deterioration of the normal integrity of the body by the physical damage of any agent. Erosion, ulcer, and fissure expressions are used in wound statement. Erosion is an expression that determines the focal epidermis losses that do not go into the dermis. Fissure is the tissue loss that determines vertical fractures in the form of cracks and it can hold the epidermis and/or dermis. Ulcers are focal wounds with the dermis and tissue loss in the epidermis. Ulcers may become chronic and may cause difficult treatment for clinicians. The wound healing progress depends on many factors ranging from the general condition of the patient to the treatment and the cause of the wound. Wound healing, complications, and scar development include multifactorial and highly complex pathophysiological components.

One of the results of advances in medical technology is increased longevity; associated with this is an increased prevalence of chronic diseases and consequently chronic wounds. There is a need to provide an evidence-based approach to the management of chronic wounds. The amount of knowledge about the processes of wound healing has significantly increased in recent years. It has become more difficult to select the most appropriate therapy for a specific type of wound. Wound healing overlaps into the many disciplines of medicine in general. Dermatologists, surgeons, internists, and geriatricians are becoming increasingly involved in the field of wound care. General practitioners and family physicians are frequently required to treat acute and chronic wounds.

There are two types of wounds: acute and chronic. After trauma or excisional surgery, acute wounds result. If the wound does not heal within 6 weeks, it is chronic. The factors such as involvement of underlying structures, depth of wound, primary wound care, and tissue use are effective in chronic wound formation. The main reason is inadequate circulation in all of the circumstances. Infection; trauma; thermal, chemical, and electrical burns; foreign bodies; postoperative dehiscence; diabetic ulcers; pressure sores; and trophic changes following spinal injury are common etiologies [1]. There are regeneration and tissue repair processes involving a number of molecular and cellular events for the reconstitution of damaged tissue. The exudative, proliferative, and extracellular matrix remodeling phases are sequential events that occur during wound healing. These events involve soluble mediators, blood cells, and parenchymal cells. Tissue edema develops after injury. In the proliferative stage, the area of tissue injury is reduced by fibroplasia and contracting myofibroblasts. Angiogenesis and reepithelialization may still be observed at this stage. Endothelial cells can differentiate into mesenchymal components. A set of signaling proteins are reported to have role in this process [2]. Chronic wounds are a major health problem. There are several local and systemic factors that affect wound healing. Management of a patient with a chronic wound requires close cooperation of physicians and other healthcare workers from related departments. Wound assessment is vital for evaluating the effectiveness of planned treatment in chronic wounds. Accurate and comprehensive wound assessment depends on meticulous and consistent clinical observation and on the use of quantitative measurement methods.

The most important point in the treatment of chronic wounds is to determine the causes of the wound, if possible, to eliminate the causes and to provide a suitable environment for the wound healing mechanisms of the body to work. In order for a wound to heal, there should be no circulatory problems in the area of the wound, and there should be plenty of clean blood flow, elimination or reduction of the discharge of the wound, removal of the wound, and pressure of the wound (if it is pressured, pressed, or pressed by any object such as shoes). Dead tissue and foreign bodies in the wound should be removed. Chronic wounds can be treated by conventional treatment methods. However, this may prolong the treatment period or make it difficult. The modern wound care products used today eliminate the deficiencies in the wound healing process and accelerate the healing by correcting the healing stage where the wound is inserted. A majority of these products are tools and equipment that helps in healing. These products allow the wound to heal in a shorter time and with minimal cosmetic loss. These products provide a moist environment for wound healing, prevent and treat infection, control discharge, and reduce the odor and pain caused by the wound. They reduce the frequency of dressing and provide acceptable esthetic appearance and functionality by the patient in their daily life. Although at first glance the unit costs may seem high, they reduce the total cost of treatment by reducing infection and shortening the wound healing time.

There are many publications about wound healing, but this book intends to give an overview of the current perspectives on wound healing, to be useful to practice care in wound healing and for improving the quality of life. It is considered that this book will be useful for clinicians who are interested with wound care. I gratefully acknowledge the help and support of the authors from five continents and nine countries of the world who contributed to this book.

Author details

Kamil Hakan Dogan

Address all correspondence to: drhakan2000@gmail.com

Selcuk University, Turkey

References

[1] Bhattacharya V, Agarwal NK, Bhattacharya S. Measurement of wound healing and tissue repair. In: Mani R, Romanelli M, Shukla V, editors. Measurements in Wound Healing. London: Springer-Verlag; 2012. pp. 73-92

[2] Gonzalez AC, Costa TG, Andrade ZA, Medrado ARAP. Wound healing—A literature review. Anais Brasileiros de Dermatologia. 2016;**91**(5):614-620

Chapter 2

Regulatory Mechanisms and Chemical Signaling of Mediators Involved in the Inflammatory Phase of Cutaneous Wound Healing

Fernando Pereira Beserra,
Lucas Fernando Sérgio Gushiken,
Maria Fernanda Hussni and
Cláudia Helena Pellizzon

Additional information is available at the end of the chapter

http://dx.doi.org/10.5772/intechopen.81731

Abstract

Wound healing is a highly complex biological process composed of three overlapping phases: inflammatory, proliferative, and remodeling. The acute inflammatory response has being an integral role in tissue healing and fundamental for the homeostasis and reestablishment. This phase depends on the interaction of cytokines, growth factors, chemokines, and chemical mediators from cells to perform regulatory events and complex interactions of the extracellular matrix, extracellular molecules, soluble mediators, various resident cells such as fibroblasts and keratinocytes, and infiltrated leukocyte subtypes that act to restore or replace the integrity of the skin. If this well-orchestrated response becomes deregulated, the wound can become chronic or progressively fibrotic, with both outcomes impairing tissue function, which can ultimately lead to organ failure and death. In this chapter, we will review the pathway in the skin healing cascade, relating the major chemical inflammatory mediators, cellular and molecular, as well as demonstrating the local and systemic factors that interfere in healing and disorders associated with tissue repair deficiency in chronic inflammations, burns and hypertrophy.

Keywords: wound healing, inflammation, cytokines, growth factors, chemokines

IntechOpen

1. Introduction

1.1. Skin wound healing

Skin is the largest organ of all vertebrates, and it is very important to protect the organism against external damage [1]. When the loss of structural integrity of the skin occurs, the organism starts the wound healing process, involving some coordinated, interdependent, and overlapping mechanisms—such as inflammation, cell proliferation, reepithelialization of wounded area, and extracellular matrix remodeling—to restructure the skin homeostasis [2, 3]. The initial mechanism of wound healing is the fibrin clot synthesis to avoid bleeding and to keep the local hemostasis, leading to the platelet retention and activation of local vascular mediators [4, 5]. From now on, there is the dilatation of the local vessels due to the release of histamine and serotonin, as well as the increase of vessel permeability, improving the leukocyte migration to the wounded area and starting the inflammatory process. In the first 5 days after the lesion, neutrophils are attracted to the region, removing pathogenic antigens and dead tissue through phagocytosis and protease secretion. After 3 days, there is the macrophage migration to the wounded area, with the maintenance of inflammatory response [5]. Due to the tissue destruction, the local keratinocytes release interleukin-1β (IL-1β) and tumor necrosis factor-α (TNF-α), essential cytokines in the inflammatory mechanism, through recruitment and activation of leukocytes in the region and with important roles coordinating other wound healing mechanisms. With these facts, keratinocytes, macrophages, platelets, and endothelial cells of wounded area release some mediators such as growth factors (EGF, FGF, PDGF, TGF-β), cytokines (IL-1β, IL-6, IL-8, IL-10, TNF-α, IFN-γ), and chemokines, which will control other subsequent mechanisms in skin wound healing [6, 7].

Therefore, the inflammatory mechanism is an important step to the correct and well-coordinated wound healing, modulating the subsequent mechanisms of healing. Furthermore, the comprehension of inflammatory response can lead to new treatments to wound repair and decrease of healing disorders like hypertrophic scars, keloids, chronic inflammation, skin infections, and unwounded lesions [8].

2. Materials and methods

The search for this chapter was carried out on PubMed, Scopus, and Web of Science until June 2018, using "inflammation", "inflammatory process", "skin wound healing", "cytokines", "chemokines"

Model	Mediator	Target/signaling protein	Biologic effect	References
In vivo BALB/c mice	CD4 cells	IL1β, IL-6, IL-17, IFN-γ, and CXCL-1 IL-4	The absence of CD4 and CD8 lymphocytes changes in cytokine expression and inflammatory cell infiltrate, but does not influence wound breaking strength, collagen content, or angiogenesis	Chen et al. [50]
	CD8 cells	IL1β, IL-6, TNF-α, CXCL-1 and CCL-2, IL-4		

Model	Mediator	Target/signaling protein	Biologic effect	References
In vivo BALB/c mice	Neutrophil	MPO, macrophages, and collagens	Neutrophil depletion exhibited significantly accelerated re-epithelialization, without altering the macrophage infiltration or the collagen content in the wound bed	Dovi et al. [51]
In vivo C57BL/6 mice	Epinephrine	IL-6, IL-1β, TNF-α, IL-1α, and GM-CSF and PMN	Epinephrine altered the neutrophil (PMN)-dependent inflammatory response to a cutaneous wound through an IL-6 mediated mechanism via β2 adrenergic receptor-dependent	Kim et al. [52]
In vivo C57Bl/wild-type mice	IL-1β	Human recombinant IL-1β, occludin, claudin-1, claudin2, claudin-3, and claudin-5	IL -1β induced increased claudin -1 expression in cell culture	Rozlomiy and Markov [53]
In vivo BALB/C mice	IL-12	Recombinant murine IL-12-rMuIL-12/collagen structure and alignment	IL-12 induced a rapid onset and higher metabolic activity in wounded skin at early time	Li et al. [54]
In vivo BALB/C mice	EFG	EGFR/vaccination extracellular domain (ECD)	Not change the wound healing and inflammatory speed	Fuentes et al. [55]
In vivo BALB/C mice and IL-6 KO mice	IL-6	IL-6/ICAM-1 VCAM-1 IL-1α Il-1β MIP-1α	Delayed angiogenesis and collagen deposition, by the reduced expression of angiogenic and fibrogenic growth factors Reduced inflammatory response	Lin et al. [56]
In vitro Keratinocytes	IL-1β and TGF-β1	IL-1β TGF-β1/tissue type plasminogen activator (tPa)	IL-1 β interacts com PA by tPA TGF-β1inibits functional tPA	Lian et al. [57]
In vitro Human and mice fibroblasts	Platelet-derived growth factor (PDGF)	IL-8	Fetal fibroblasts produced less IL-8. Much less IL-8 in stimulated fetal fibroblasts than in adults	Liechty et al. [58]
In vivo C57/Bl6 mice and Mgl2DTR/GFP mice	CD301b macrophage	IL-10, platelet-derived growth factor–β and TGF-β1	CD301b-expressing subpopulation of macrophages is critical for activation of reparative process	Shook et al. [59]
In vivo Levels and role of chemokine CX3CL1 (fractalkine) and its receptor CX3CR1 in mouse model	CX3CL1 and CX3CR1	MPO, Hydroxyproline (collagen accumulation at the wound sites), TGF-1, VEGF	Inflammation, fibrosis, neovascularization, and regeneration of parenchymal cells were affected by the receptor	Ishida et al. [31]

Model	Mediator	Target/signaling protein	Biologic effect	References
In vivo db/db mice as a diabetic skin wound model.	Peptide inhibitor of complement C1 (PIC1)	complement system (CS), Signal transducer, activator of transcription 4 (STAT4), Leukocyte infiltration, C5a, C3, C3a	PIC1 loaded into the derma CELL did reduce the number of inflammatory cells in the wound bed	Cunnion et al. [60]
In vivo kCYC/mice	IL-10	Mast cells migrating, Macrophages, IL-10, IL-6, aFGF, bFGF, TGF-1, PDGF, TNF-α mRNA	kCYC/mice mast cell increased. IL-10: increased, bFGF decreased in kCYC/mice. IL-10 plays an important role in delayed wound healing	Kimura et al. [61]
In vivo C57BL/6J mice	IL-1β	p38, MAPK, ERK	IL-1β stimulates PTGS2 in fibroblast and p38-MAPK in other cells. PGE2 activates INHBA	Arai et al. [62]
In vivo Sprague Dawley Rats	IL-4, IL-12, IL-6, IGF-1 and IFN-α e γ	—	IGF-1, IL-4, IL-6, and IL-3 important in inflammatory phase	Lania et al. [63]
In vivo Mouse model with conditional depletion of macrophages	Inducible diphtheria toxin receptor + diphtheria toxin injections + mice lacking the TGF-b receptor type II (TbRII), Depletion of macrophages	Number of macrophages, neutrophils, and cells positive for activated caspase-3, VEGF-A, or TGF-β1	Inflammatory phase: reduced formation of vascularized granulation tissue, leading to minimized scar formation. Phase of tissue formation: severe hemorrhage in the wound. Wound closure did not occur. No significant impact in tissue maturation phases.	Lucas et al. [64]
In vivo C57Bl/6J mice	Ly6cloMHCIIhi macrophage	IL-17	Ly6cloMHCIIhi macrophages had a non-inflammatory transcriptomic profile and demonstrated that inhibition of IL-17 in mice accelerated normal and delayed healing.	Rodero et al. [65]
In vivo C57BL/6mice	$\gamma\delta$ T Cell	FGF-7, FGF-10, IGF-1, JAML	$\gamma\delta$T Lymphocytes stimulate the gene and protein expression of important mediators in acute healing model	Xu et al. [66]
Mutant mice ICOS −/− ICOSL -?-	IL-6 and IL-4	—	IL6 and ICOS-ICOSL signaling the skin wound healing in mutant mice	Maeda et al. [67]
In vivo C57BL/6 mice and human acute wounds	Macrophage M1 and M2	IRF-8	IRF-8 is an inflammatory mediator. Inhibition of IRF-8 impairs wound healing.	Guo et al. [68]

Model	Mediator	Target/signaling protein	Biologic effect	References
			IRF8 coordinates M1 macrophage population (decrease of M1 mediators IL-1 β, IL-6, TNF-α, iNOS), with no interference in M2 macrophage mediators (arg-1, mrc-1, IL-10)	
In vitro Human skin fibroblasts CCD966-SK and HaCaT keratinocytes In vivo BALB/C mice	Fibroblasts and keratinocytes IL-19	IL-19	IL-19 upregulates KGF expression in fibroblasts and KGF induces IL-19 expression in keratinocytes KGF promotes keratinocyte proliferation. IL-19 induces keratinocyte migration	Sun et al. [69]
In vivo SKH-1 mice	COX-2	COX-1 and COX-2	Selective inhibition of COX-2 and nonselective inhibition of COX-1 and COX-2 did not affect the healing of sutured surgical incisions in mouse skin.	Blomme et al. [70]
In vivo BALB/c mice	IFN-γ and TGF-β1	MPO, TGF-β, Stat1, P-Stat1, Smad2, P-Smad2, Smad3, Smad7, α-Tubulin, VEGF, CD3, IL-12p35, IL-12p40, IL-18, COLIAI	Crosstalk between the IFN-γ/Stat1 and TGF-β1/Smad signaling pathways in the skin wound healing.	Ishida et al. [71]
In vivo Wistar rats	—	EGF, VEGF, IGF and FGF	Growth factors accelerated the healing process promoting greater angiogenic activity and accelerated fibroplasia and the deposition of type I collagen	de Masi et al. [72]
In vivo C3H/Hej TLR4-deficient and wild-type C3H/HeOuj mice In vitro NHEK and THP1 cell line	TLR4	CD3+, T cells, Ki67, NF-κB, p-p38, and p-JNK	TLR4 is activated in early skin wound healing, with a functional mutation of TLR4 results in altered inflammatory cell infiltration, differential cytokine production, and impaired wound closure, besides IL-1β production by injured keratinocytes is induced through the TLR4-p38/JNK pathway	Chen et al. [73]
In vivo C57BL/6 mice	Vγ4 T cells	IL-17A, IGF-1, CCL20, NF-κB p65, p-NF-κB p6, STAT3, p-STAT3, IL-1β, IL-23p19	Mechanistic link between Vγ4 T cell-derived IL-17A, epidermal IL-1β/IL-23, DETC-derived IGF-1, and wound healing responses in the skin	Li et al. [74]

Model	Mediator	Target/signaling protein	Biologic effect	References
In vitro Primary keratinocytes and fibroblasts of IL-6 KO or C57BL/6 mice	IL-6 from keratinocytes and fibroblasts	IL-6, STAT3	IL-6 induces keratinocyte migration indirectly, through the STAT3 activation cascade in fibroblasts, with the synthesis of a fibroblast-derived factor	Gallucci et al. [75]
In vivo Ja18KO (iNKT cell-deficient) mice and C57BL/6 mice	Invariant natural killer T cells (iNKT) and neutrophils	MIP-2, KC, IL-17A, MCP-1, RANTES	MIP-2, KC, IL-17A (neutrophil attractors) were increased in JA18KO mice. MCP-1 and RANTES (macrophage and lymphocyte attractors) were decreased in Ja18KO mice. Decrease of neutrophil apoptosis in Ja18KO mice. iNKT ciNKT cells promote skin wound healing by regulating neutrophil apoptosis	Tanno et al. [76]
In vivo PPAR-γ KO mice and C57BL/6 J male mice	PPAR-γ from macrophages	PPAR-γ, TNF-α, VEGF, collagen 1	Increase of TNF-α in PPAR-γ KO mice and delay in wound healing	Chen et al. [77]
In vivo Human incision model	IL-4 from mast cells	IL-4, MCP-1	Increased MCP-1 chemoattractant activity in mast cell migration. Increase of IL-4 synthesis by mast cells IL-4 stimulates fibroblast activation	Trautmann et al. [78]
In vivo WBB6F1/J-KitW/KitW–v mast cell KO female mice and WBB6F1 female mice	Mast cells	TNF-α, MIP-2, VEGF, FGF-2	Decrease of neutrophil infiltration in KO mice. Increase of FGF-2 in KO mice. Mast cells modulate neutrophil infiltration in wound site, with unlikely influence in proliferative phase of wound healing	Egozi et al. [79]
In vivo miR-31 loss-of-function mice	miR-31	NF-kB, STAT3, RAS/MAPK	Increase of miR-31 in wound edge keratinocytes during inflammation through NF-kB and STAT3 pathways miR-31 regulates keratinocyte migration through RAS/MAPK pathway	Shi et al. [80]
In vitro Primary normal human	IL-6, IL-8, TNF-α	STAT3, p38, JNK, EGFR	STAT3, p38, JNK, and NF-kB activation lead to IL-6, IL-8, and TNF-a increase in	Han et al. [81]

Model	Mediator	Target/signaling protein	Biologic effect	References
keratinocytes In vivo BALB/c female mice			infected wounds. Mixidin2 and mixidin3 modulated inflammatory signaling with anti-inflammatory activity	
In vivo B57BL6/J, B57BL6/NJ, CD301bGFP-DTR, and Il27Ra−/− mice	IL-27 (dendritic cells)	Keratin-6 (keratinocytes)	IL-27 is synthesized by dendritic cells and modulates keratinocyte proliferation, migration, and differentiation after skin injury	Yang et al. [82]

Table 1. Chemical mediators involved in the inflammatory response of skin wound healing.

and "growth factors" as keywords. The articles published in the last 20 years were considered (1998–2018). The results are displayed in **Table 1**.

3. Results and discussion

3.1. Mediators involved in the inflammatory phase of wound healing

Wound healing is an extremely dynamic and interactive biological process involving complex interactions of extracellular matrix, extracellular molecules, soluble mediators, multiple resident cells (fibroblasts and keratinocytes), and subtypes of infiltrating leukocytes that together act to restore integrity of the damaged tissue and replace the lost. This process comprises three sequential and overlapping stages, regardless of the amount of injured tissue: hemostasis/inflammation; cell proliferation and matrix repair; and reepithelialization and remodeling of scar tissue, which involve complex biochemical and cellular mechanisms [9].

The inflammatory phase, hemostasis, leukocyte migration, and the beginning of the tissue repair cascade occur. Initially, in response to inflammatory agents, there is reduction of blood flow by vasoconstriction, and with extravasation of blood from the injured vessel, platelets are activated causing the coagulation process to begin [10]. During this process, there is a progressive increase in vascular permeability to migrant cells and biologically active substances. From this process, essential elements for the physiological continuation of healing appear: a fibrin framework, necessary for the migration of the cells that will reach the lesion site, and pro and anti-inflammatory chemo/cytokines that will aid in cell activation and migration [11].

3.2. Neutrophils and macrophages

Neutrophils are the first immune cells recruited into wounded tissue to play a role in reestablishing tissue homeostasis through pathogen phagocytosis and macrophage recruitment as well as excessive neutrophil activity which can contribute to the development of nonhealing wounds. They play a central role in both killing microbes and promoting wound healing [12]. These cells are extremely important in the inflammatory process, but once recruited into wound sites in such large numbers with exacerbated cytokine secretion, overproduction of reactive oxygen species (ROS), causing extracellular matrix (ECM) and cell membrane damage, and resulting in premature cell senescence [13].

Monocyte-derived macrophages are often considered to be the most important immune cell type in this process. In intact skin, these cells are the most abundant cell types performing sentinel and homeostatic function. The monocytes migrate from vascular circulation to wound. Both infiltrating and resident macrophages on skin are activated by local signals and developed into several subpopulations defined by their different functional phenotypes [14]. Many studies have confirmed that macrophages are critical for proper skin wound healing [15–17]. Upon initial infiltration, proinflammatory macrophages, also called M1, are also responsible for removing cellular debris, damaged matrix, microbes, and neutrophils [17].

3.3. Cytokines

Wound healing is regulated by growth factors and cytokines that are essential not only in the inflammatory process but also in the cell proliferation and maintenance in the repair process by various mechanisms [18].

Cytokines released by neutrophils during apoptosis are chemotactic for monocytes, which start to arrive 5–6 h post injury. IL-1β is a key interleukin of antimicrobial response by inflammatory response amplification; it stimulates leukocyte recruitment, the release of acute phase proteins, and the increase of permeability of blood vessels [19]. Some authors consider this cytokine as part of a proinflammatory positive feedback loop that sustains a persistent proinflammatory wound macrophage phenotype, contributing to impaired healing of diabetic wounds [18].

TNF-α is a second proinflammatory cytokine that contributes to a chronic wound state. It acts on several stages of leukocyte recruitment mechanism, neutrophils and macrophages, inducing molecular adhesion regulation, chemokine production, and metalloproteinase matrix, as well as tissue inhibitors of metalloproteinases [20]. Interleukin IL-6 is a soluble proinflammatory mediator with pleiotropic activities in inflammation, hematopoiesis, and immune responses [21]. Together with TNF-α and IL-1β, IL-6 is present in high concentrations in inflammatory processes. After IL-6 is secreted into the area of injury at the beginning of the inflammatory process, it is directed to the liver through the bloodstream, transmitting the information and inducing the hepatocytes to produce certain inflammatory agents [22]. Another important cytokine in the inflammatory phase is IL-8, which also acts as a chemokine (CXCL8). This cytokine is mainly produced by monocytes and in smaller amounts by fibroblasts, endothelial cells, keratinocytes, melanocytes, hepatocytes, and chondrocytes. It usually receives stimuli from other cytokines, such as IL-1, TNF-α, and IFN-γ [23]. The main action of IL-8 is the migration to cells of the immune system, mainly neutrophils, also determining an increase in the expression of endothelial adhesion molecules cells [13].

Since prolonged presence of proinflammatory cytokines may prevent resolution and both pro and anti-inflammatory cytokines are necessary for wound healing, sequential delivery of pro and anti-inflammatory cytokines could be an interesting strategy for improving chronic wound healing [17]. For example, IL-22, considered a proinflammatory cytokine, helped the wound healing of diabetic mice by inducing keratinocyte proliferator and signal transduction and activation of transcription 3 (STAT3) [24]. In this same context but in other tissues, to improve bone repair, decellularized bone was engineered to sequentially release IL-4 (proinflammatory cytokine) and implanted in mice at the site of injury. The sequential release promoted macrophage polarization to switch from a pro to an anti-inflammatory phenotype, resulting in improved wound healing [25].

IL-10 is a regulatory cytokine, which can be secreted by many kinds of immune cells, including Th1, Th2, Th17, Treg, and CD8+ T cells, B cells, dendritic cells, macrophages, NK cells, eosinophils, neutrophils, basophils, and MCs, as well as nonimmune cells including keratinocytes. This cytokine is considered an anti-inflammatory cytokine because it is capable of inhibiting the production of other proinflammatory cytokines, such as TNF-α, IL-1β, and IL-6 [26]. In addition to its potent anti-inflammatory effects, IL-10 has been shown to regulate fibrogenic cytokines, such as transforming growth factor-β (TGF-β), as a part of its role in the regulation of tissue remodeling [27].

3.4. Chemokines

Chemokines are small molecules that induce chemotaxis and activation of certain subsets of leukocytes. They are classified into four types: CC chemokines, CXC chemokines, C chemokines, and CX3C chemokine. Chemokines play important roles in wound healing and are important for maintaining skin homeostasis, and their disruption can result in skin pathologies [28]. They also play important roles in establishing microenvironment in which migratory immune cells, together with skin-resident cells, cause prolonged inflammation [29].

CX3CL1 is expressed by inflamed endothelial cells and epithelial cells, including macrophage, keratinocytes, and vascular smooth muscle cells, whereas CX3CR1 is mainly expressed by neutrophils, monocytes, mast cells, T cells, and NK cells [30]. In the cutaneous wound healing, CX3CL1 has been shown to be expressed by macrophages and endothelial cells, while CX3CR1 is expressed by macrophages and fibroblasts. Decreased expression of macrophage-related cytokines, such as TGF-β and VEGF, and reduced deposition and α-smooth muscle actin and collagen were shown in the injured skin of CX3CR1−/− mice [31].

3.5. Growth factors

Growth factors are naturally occurring endogenous mediators capable of controlling the control of cell growth, proliferation, migration, and differentiation [32]. Once bound specifically to its receptor, the ligand-receptor interaction is able to activate intracellular signal transduction pathways that regulate different cellular functions [33].

PDGF plays a crucial role in the healing process in both chronic and normal wounds. This growth factor is released from degranulating platelets following an injury into the wound fluid [34]. PDGF stimulates mitogenicity and chemotaxis of cells, such as neutrophils, macrophages, fibroblasts, and smooth muscle cells to the site of the wound, initiating the inflammatory process stage [35]. Its function has already been described during the stage of epithelialization of wound healing by upregulating the production of growth factors, such as insulin-like growth factor (IGF)-1 and thrombospondin-1, in turn IGF-1 increases the motility of keratinocyte cells and thrombospondin-1 inhibits proteolytic and enzymatic degradation of PDGF [36].

Angiogenesis is an extremely important process in normal development and tissue homeostasis and repair, besides contributes directly also to various forms of pathology, such as tumor development and metastasis, psoriasis, rheumatoid arthritis, and wet macular degeneration [37]. One of the most important proangiogenic mediators is vascular endothelial growth factor (VEGF), responsible for stimulating new blood vessels formation, tissue proliferation, migration, differentiation, and survival, which contribute to the angiogenesis process, in addition to influencing the repair and wound closure and granulation tissue formation [38]. The VEGF family has several members, and one of its members such as VEGF-A begins the process of wound healing promoting biological events linked to angiogenesis and migration of endothelial cells [39]. Administration of VEGF-A has been reported to restore impairment of angiogenesis in diabetic ischemic limbs in an animal model as well as to improve the reepithelialization process of diabetic wounds [40].

Epidermal growth factor (EGF) stimulates proliferation and differentiation of various cells, including fibroblasts, endothelial cells, and epithelial cells, and shows mitogenic and migratory activity on the edge keratinocytes of the lesions [41]. EGF participates in this mechanism, which is considered essential in the cutaneous wound healing, which begins a few hours after the injury, but presents a more evident activity in the proliferative phase of wound healing, and continues until the extracellular matrix remodeling phase [42].

Another growth factor that involves healing process activity is the family of fibroblast growth factors (FGF), which have already been reported to play crucial events in the wound healing process [43]. FGFs are secreted by keratinocytes, fibroblasts, endothelial cells, smooth muscle cells, chondrocytes, and mast cells [44]. During an acute cutaneous wound process, it has been reported an increase in the production of FGF-2 and that they are responsible for formation of granulation tissue, reepithelialization, and tissue remodeling [45]. Moreover, functions such as synthesis, deposition of various constituents of the extracellular matrix, and increased motility of keratinocytes are regulated by FGF-2 [46].

Transforming growth factor type-β (TGF-β) activity in the healing process was analyzed by being one of the proteins with the greatest spectrum of activities, with effect on cell proliferation, differentiation and production of extracellular matrix, and immunological modulation [46, 47]. Moreover, TGF-β has many biological activities and is thought to be a particularly important contributor to fibrosis, angiogenesis, and tissue repair. This growth factor can also influence T cells, including Th17 and Treg cells, as well as B cells, dendritic cells, NK cells, neutrophils, and eosinophils [48, 49].

4. Conclusion

Increasing scientific knowledge has contributed to define highly coordinated molecular and cellular events involved in the cutaneous wound healing. Recent findings show that there is a clear correlation between the stage of the wound and its effectiveness in the healing process, and endogenous mediators, such as cytokines, chemokines, and growth factors, indicate important and crucial steps in the normal healing and are useful as prognostic indicators. Although much is known about the cellular and molecular basis of normal skin healing, there are still avenues of research left to unravel that will guide us to better therapies, new therapeutic targets, and strategies for the skin wound treatment, especially chronic wounds.

Conflict of interest

The authors declare no conflict of interests.

Author details

Fernando Pereira Beserra[1], Lucas Fernando Sérgio Gushiken[1], Maria Fernanda Hussni[2] and Cláudia Helena Pellizzon[1]*

*Address all correspondence to: claudia@ibb.unesp.br

1 Department of Morphology, Institute of Biosciences of Botucatu, São Paulo State University (UNESP), São Paulo, Brazil

2 Undergraduate Student School of Veterinary Medicine and Animal Science, São Paulo State University (UNESP), São Paulo, Brazil

References

[1] Fikru A, Makonnen E, Eguale T, Debella A, Mekonnen GA. Evaluation of in vivo wound healing activity of methanol extract of *Achyranthes aspera* L. Journal of Ethnopharmacology. 2012;**143**:469-474. DOI: 10.1016/j.jep.2012.06.049

[2] Martins VL, Caley M, O'Toole EA. Matrix metalloproteinases and epidermal wound repair. Cell and Tissue Research. 2013;**351**:255-268. DOI: 10.1007/s00441-012-1410-z

[3] Agha R, Ogawa R, Pietramaggiori G, Orgill DP. A review of the role of mechanical forces in cutaneous wound healing. The Journal of Surgical Research. 2011;**171**:700-708. DOI: 10.1016/j.jss.2011.07.007

[4] Gurtner GC, Werner S, Barrandon Y, Longaker MT. Wound repair and regeneration. Nature. 2008;**453**:314-321. DOI: 10.1038/nature07039

[5] Tziotzios C, Profyris C, Sterling J. Cutaneous scarring: Pathophysiology, molecular mechanisms, and scar reduction therapeutics. Journal of the American Academy of Dermatology. 2012;**66**:13-24. DOI: 10.1016/j.jaad.2011.08.035

[6] Reinke JM, Sorg H. Wound repair and regeneration. European Surgical Research. 2012;**49**: 35-43. DOI: 10.1159/000339613

[7] Singer AJ, Clark RAF. Cutaneous wound healing. The New England Journal of Medicine. 1999;**341**:738-746. DOI: 10.1056/NEJM199909023411006

[8] Eming SA, Krieg T, Davidson JM. Inflammation in wound repair: Molecular and cellular mechanisms. The Journal of Investigative Dermatology. 2017;**127**:514-525. DOI: 10.1038/sj.jid.5700701

[9] Boateng JS, Matthews KH, Stevens HNE, Eccleston GM. Wound healing dressings and drug delivery systems: A review. Journal of Pharmaceutical Sciences. 2008;**97**:2892-2923. DOI: 10.1002/jps.21210

[10] Martin P, Feng Y. Inflammation: Wound healing in zebrafish. Nature. 2009;**459**:921-923. DOI: 10.1038/459921a

[11] Morin C, Roumegous A, Carpentier G, Barbier-Chassefière V, Garrigue-Antar L, Caredda S, et al. Modulation of inflammation by Cicaderma ointment accelerates skin wound healing. The Journal of Pharmacology and Experimental Therapeutics. 2012;**343**:115-124. DOI: 10.1124/jpet.111.188599

[12] Wilgus TA, Roy S, McDaniel JC. Neutrophils and wound repair: Positive actions and negative reactions. Advances in Wound Care. 2013;**2**:379-388. DOI: 10.1089/wound.2012.0383

[13] Kolaczkowska E, Kubes P. Neutrophil recruitment and function in health and inflammation. Nature Reviews. Immunology. 2013;**13**:159-175. DOI: 10.1038/nri3399

[14] Murray PJ, Wynn TA. Protective and pathogenic functions of macrophage subsets. Nature Reviews. Immunology. 2012;**11**:723-737. DOI: 10.1038/nri3073.Protective

[15] Nagaoka T, Kaburagi Y, Hamaguchi Y, Hasegawa M, Takehara K, Steeber DA, et al. Delayed wound healing in the absence of intercellular adhesion molecule-1 or L-selectin expression. The American Journal of Pathology. 2000;**157**:237-247. DOI: 10.1016/S0002-9440(10) 64534-8

[16] Mori R, Kondo T, Ohshima T, Ishida Y, Mukaida N. Accelerated wound healing in tumor necrosis factor receptor p55-deficient mice with reduced leukocyte infiltration. The FASEB Journal. 2002;**16**:963-974

[17] Larouche J, Sheoran S, Maruyama K, Martino MM. Immune regulation of skin wound healing: Mechanisms and novel therapeutic targets. Advances in Wound Care. 2018;**7**(7): 209-231. DOI: 10.1089/wound.2017.0761

[18] Zhao R, Liang H, Clarke E, Jackson C, Xue M. Inflammation in chronic wounds. International Journal of Molecular Sciences. 2016;**17**:1-14. DOI: 10.3390/ijms17122085

[19] MacLeod AS, Rudolph R, Corriden R, Ye I, Garijo O, Havran WL. Skin-resident T cells sense ultraviolet radiation-induced injury and contribute to DNA repair. Journal of Immunology. 2014;**192**:5695-5702. DOI: 10.4049/jimmunol.1303297

[20] Gragnani A, Müller BR, da Silva IDCG, de Noronha SMR, Ferreira LM. Keratinocyte growth factor, tumor necrosis factor-alpha and interleukin-1 beta gene expression in cultured fibroblasts and keratinocytes from burned patients. Acta Cirurgica Brasileira. 2013;**28**:551-558 papers3://publication/uuid/29D2218B-4653-4A36-AF38-4DAC5ACDC4E0

[21] Tanaka T, Narazaki M, Kishimoto T. IL-6 in inflammation, immunity, and disease. Cold Spring Harbor Perspectives in Biology. 2014;**6**:a016295

[22] Scheller J, Chalaris A, Schmidt-arras D, Rose-john S. The pro- and anti-inflammatory properties of the cytokine interleukin-6. Biochimica et Biophysica Acta. 2011;**1813**:878-888. DOI: 10.1016/j.bbamcr.2011.01.034

[23] Mayadas TN, Cullere X, Lowell CA. The multifaceted functions of neutrophils. Annual Review of Pathology Mechanisms of Disease. 2014;**9**:181-218. DOI: 10.1146/annurev-pathol-020712-164023

[24] Avitabile S, Odorisio T, Madonna S, Eyerich S, Guerra L, Eyerich K, et al. Interleukin-22 promotes wound repair in diabetes by improving keratinocyte pro-healing functions. The Journal of Investigative Dermatology. 2015;**135**:2862-2870. DOI: 10.1038/jid.2015.278

[25] Spiller KL, Nassiri S, Witherel CE, Anfang RR, Ng J, Nakazawa KR, et al. Sequential delivery of immunomodulatory cytokines to facilitate the M1-to-M2 transition of macrophages and enhance vascularization of bone scaffolds. Biomaterials. 2015;**37**:194-207. DOI: 10.1016/j.biomaterials.2014.10.017.Sequential

[26] Saraiva M, O'Garra A. The regulation of IL-10 production by immune cells. Nature Reviews. Immunology. 2010;**10**:170-181. DOI: 10.1038/nri2711

[27] Yamamoto T, Eckes B, Krieg T. Effect of Interleukin-10 on the gene expression of type I collagen, fibronectin, and decorin in human skin fibroblasts: Differential regulation by transforming growth factor-β and monocyte chemoattractant protein-1. Biochemical and Biophysical Research Communications. 2001;**281**:200-205. DOI: 10.1006/bbrc.2001.4321

[28] Nakayama T, Watanabe Y, Oiso N, Higuchi T, Shigeta A, Mizuguchi N, et al. Eotaxin-3/CC chemokine ligand 26 is a functional ligand for CX3CR1. Journal of Immunology. 2010;**185**: 6472-6479. DOI: 10.4049/jimmunol.0904126

[29] Sugaya M. Chemokines and skin diseases. Archivum Immunologiae et Therapiae Experimentalis (Warsz). 2015;**63**:109-115. DOI: 10.1007/s00005-014-0313-y

[30] White GE, Greaves DR. Fractalkine: A survivor's guide chemokines as antiapoptotic mediators. Arteriosclerosis, Thrombosis, and Vascular Biology. 2012;**32**:589-594. DOI: 10.1161/ATVBAHA.111.237412

[31] Ishida Y, Gao J-L, Murphy PM. Chemokine receptor CX3CR1 mediates skin wound healing by promoting macrophage and fibroblast accumulation and function. Journal of Immunology. 2008;**180**:569-579. DOI: 10.4049/jimmunol.180.1.569

[32] Barrientos S, Stojadinovic O, Golinko MS, Brem H, Tomic-Canic M. Growth factors and cytokines in wound healing. Wound Repair and Regeneration. 2008;**16**:585-601. DOI: 10.1111/j.1524-475X.2008.00410.x

[33] Koria P. Delivery of growth factors for tissue regeneration and wound healing. BioDrugs. 2012;**26**:163-175. DOI: 10.2165/11631850-000000000-00000

[34] Uysal AC, Mizuno H, Tobita M, Ogawa R, Hyakusoku H. The effect of adipose-derived stem cells on ischemia-reperfusion injury: Immunohistochemical and ultrastructural evaluation. Plastic and Reconstructive Surgery. 2009;**124**:804-815. DOI: 10.1097/PRS.0b013e3181b17bb4

[35] Mardani M, Asadi-Samani M, Rezapour S, Rezapour P. Evaluation of bred fish and seawater fish in terms of nutritional value, and heavy metals. Journal of Chemical and Pharmaceutical Sciences. 2016;**9**:1277-1283

[36] Mardani M, Mahmoud B, Moradmand JS, Salehi A, Davoodi M, Ghobadi S, et al. Comparison of the descurainia sophia and levostatin effect on the ldl cholesterol reduction, a clinical trial study. Journal of Chemical and Pharmaceutical Sciences. 2016;**9**:1329-1333

[37] Nagy JA, Dvorak AM, Dvorak HF. Vascular hyperpermeability, angiogenesis, and stroma generation. Cold Spring Harbor Perspectives in Medicine. 2012;**2**:a006544. DOI: 10.1101/cshperspect.a006544

[38] Kim HR, Lee JH, Kim KW, Kim BM, Lee SH. The relationship between synovial fluid VEGF and serum leptin with ultrasonographic findings in knee osteoarthritis. International Journal of Rheumatic Diseases. 2016;**19**:233-240. DOI: 10.1111/1756-185X.12486

[39] Huang SP, Hsu CC, Chang SC, Wang CH, Deng SC, Dai NT, et al. Adipose-derived stem cells seeded on acellular dermal matrix grafts enhance wound healing in a murine model of a full-thickness defect. Annals of Plastic Surgery. 2012;**69**:656-662. DOI: 10.1097/SAP.0b013e318273f909

[40] Song SH, Lee MO, Lee JS, Jeong HC, Kim HG, Kim WS, et al. Genetic modification of human adipose-derived stem cells for promoting wound healing. Journal of Dermatological Science. 2012;**66**:98-107. DOI: 10.1016/j.jdermsci.2012.02.010

[41] Singh B, Carpenter G, Coffey RJ. EGF receptor ligands: Recent advances. F1000Research. 2016;**5**:2270. DOI: 10.12688/f1000research.9025.1

[42] Werner S, Grose R. Regulation of wound healing by growth factors and cytokines. Physiological Reviews. 2003;**83**:835-870

[43] Ghafarzadeh M, Eatemadi A. Clinical efficacy of liposome-encapsulated Aloe vera on melasma treatment during pregnancy. Journal of Cosmetic and Laser Therapy. 2017;**19**:181-187. DOI: 10.1080/14764172.2017.1279329

[44] Nie C, Yang D, Xu J, Si Z, Jin X, Zhang J. Locally administered adipose-derived stem cells accelerate wound healing through differentiation and vasculogenesis. Cell Transplantation. 2011;**20**:205-216. DOI: 10.3727/096368910X520065

[45] Jaferian S, Soleymaninejad M, Negahdari B, Eatemadi A. Stem cell, biomaterials and growth factors therapy for hepatocellular carcinoma. Biomedicine and Pharmacotherapy. 2017;**88**:1046-1053. DOI: 10.1016/j.biopha.2017.01.154

[46] Lee SH, Lee JH, Cho KH. Effects of human adipose-derived stem cells on cutaneous wound healing in nude mice. Annals of Dermatology. 2011;**23**:150-155. DOI: 10.5021/ad.2011.23.2.150

[47] Leask A, Abraham DJ. TGF-beta signaling and the fibrotic response. The FASEB Journal. 2004;**18**:816-827. DOI: 10.1096/fj.03-1273rev

[48] Biernacka A, Dobaczewski M, Frangogiannis NG. TGF-b signaling in fibrosis. Growth Factors. 2011;**29**:196-202. DOI: 10.3109/08977194.2011.595714

[49] Sanjabi S, Oh SA, Li MO. Regulation of the immune response by TGF-B: From conception to autoimmunity and infection. Cold Spring Harbor Perspectives in Biology. 2017;**9**: a022236. DOI: 10.1101/cshperspect.a022236

[50] Chen L, Mehta ND, Zhao Y, DiPietro LA. Absence of CD4 or CD8 lymphocytes changes infiltration of inflammatory cells and profiles of cytokine expression in skin wounds, but does not impair healing. Experimental Dermatology. 2014;**23**:189-194. DOI: 10.1021/nn300902w. Release

[51] Dovi JV, He LK, DiPietro L. Accelerated wound closure in neutrophil-depleted mice. Journal of Leukocyte Biology. 2003;**73**:448-455. DOI: 10.1189/jlb.0802406

[52] Kim MH, Gorouhi F, Ramirez S, Granick JL, Byrne BA, Soulika AM, et al. Catecholamine stress alters neutrophils trafficking and impairs wound healing by beta2 adrenergic receptor mediated upregulation of IL-6. The Journal of Investigative Dermatology. 2014;**134**: 809-817. DOI: 10.1038/jid.2013.415.Catecholamine

[53] Rozlomiy VL, Markov AG. Effect of interleukin-1beta on the expression of tight junction proteins in the culture of HaCaT keratinocytes. Bulletin of Experimental Biology and Medicine. 2010;**149**:280-283

[54] Li J, Bower AJ, Vainstein V, Gluzman-Poltorak Z, Chaney EJ, Marjanovic M, et al. Effect of recombinant interleukin-12 on murine skin regeneration and cell dynamics using in vivo multimodal microscopy. Biomedical Optics Express. 2015;**6**:4277. DOI: 10.1364/BOE.6.004277

[55] Fuentes D, Chacón L, Casacó A, Ledón N, Fernández N, Iglesias A, et al. Effects of an epidermal growth factor receptor-based cancer vaccine on wound healing and inflammation processes in murine experimental models. International Wound Journal. 2014;**11**: 98-103. DOI: 10.1111/j.1742-481X.2012.01074.x

[56] Lin ZQ. Essential involvement of IL-6 in the skin wound-healing process as evidenced by delayed wound healing in IL-6-deficient mice. Journal of Leukocyte Biology. 2003;**73**: 713-721. DOI: 10.1189/jlb.0802397

[57] Lian X, Yang L, Gao Q, Yang T. IL-1α is a potent stimulator of keratinocyte tissue plasminogen activator expression and regulated by TGF-β1. Archives of Dermatological Research. 2008;**300**:185-193. DOI: 10.1007/s00403-007-0828-8

[58] Liechty KW, Crombleholme TM, Cass DL, Martin B, Adzick NS. Diminished interleukin-8 (IL-8) production in the fetal wound healing response. The Journal of Surgical Research. 1998;**77**:80-84. DOI: 10.1006/jsre.1998.5345

[59] Shook B, Xiao E, Kumamoto Y, Iwasaki A, Horsley V. CD301b+ macrophages are essential for effective skin wound healing. The Journal of Investigative Dermatology. 2016;**136**: 1885-1891. DOI: 10.1038/ng.3641.Punctuated

[60] Cunnion KM, Krishna NK, Pallera HK, Pineros-Fernandez A, Rivera MG, Hair PS, et al. Complement activation and STAT4 expression are associated with early inflammation in diabetic wounds. PLoS One. 2017;**12**:1-19. DOI: 10.1371/journal.pone.0170500

[61] Kimura T, Sugaya M, Blauvelt A, Okochi H, Sato S. Delayed wound healing due to increased interleukin-10 expression in mice with lymphatic dysfunction. Journal of Leukocyte Biology. 2013;**94**:137-145. DOI: 10.1189/jlb.0812408

[62] Arai KY, Ono M, Kudo C, Fujioka A, Okamura R, Nomura Y, et al. IL-1β stimulates activin βA mRNA expression in human skin fibroblasts through the MAPK pathways, the nuclear factor-κB pathway, and prostaglandin E2. Endocrinology. 2011;**152**:3779-3790. DOI: 10.1210/en.2011-0255

[63] Lania BG, Morari J, De Souza AL, Da Silva MN, De Almeida AR, Veira-Damiani G, et al. Topical use and systemic action of green and roasted coffee oils and ground oils in a cutaneous incision model in rats (Rattus norvegicus albinus). PLoS One. 2017;**12**:1-17. DOI: 10.1371/journal.pone.0188779

[64] Lucas T, Waisman A, Ranjan R, Roes J, Krieg T, Muller W, et al. Differential roles of macrophages in diverse phases of skin repair. Journal of Immunology. 2010;**184**:3964-3977. DOI: 10.4049/jimmunol.0903356

[65] Rodero MP, Hodgson SS, Hollier B, Combadiere C, Khosrotehrani K. Reduced IL-17a expression distinguishes a Ly6c lo MHCIIhimacrophage population promoting wound healing. The Journal of Investigative Dermatology. 2013;**133**:783-792. DOI: 10.1038/jid.2012.368

[66] Xu P, Fu X, Xiao N, Guo Y, Pei Q, Peng Y, et al. Involvements of γδT lymphocytes in acute and chronic skin wound repair. Inflammation. 2017;**40**:1416-1427. DOI: 10.1007/s10753-017-0585-6

[67] Maeda S, Fujimoto M, Matsushita T, Hamaguchi Y, Takehara K, Hasegawa M. Inducible costimulator (ICOS) and ICOS ligand signaling has pivotal roles in skin wound healing via cytokine production. The American Journal of Pathology. 2011;**179**:2360-2369. DOI: 10.1016/j.ajpath.2011.07.048

[68] Guo Y, Yang Z, Wu S, Xu P, Peng Y, Yao M. Inhibition of IRF8 negatively regulates macrophage function and impairs cutaneous wound healing. Inflammation. 2017;**40**: 68-78. DOI: 10.1007/s10753-016-0454-8

[69] Sun D, Yeh C-H, So E, Wang L, Wei T, Chang M, et al. Interleukin (IL)-19 promoted skin wound healing by increasing fibroblast keratinocyte growth factor expression. Cytokine. 2013;**62**:360-368. DOI: 10.1016/j.cyto.2013.03.017

[70] Blomme EAG, Chinn KS, Hardy MM, Casler JJ, Kim SH, Opsahl AC, et al. Selective cyclooxygenase-2 inhibition does not affect the healing of cutaneous full-thickness incisional wounds in SKH-1 mice. The British Journal of Dermatology. 2003;**148**:211-223. DOI: 10.1046/j.1365-2133.2003.05065.x

[71] Ishida Y, Kondo T, Takayasu T, Iwakura Y, Mukaida N. The essential involvement of cross-talk between IFN- and TGF- in the skin wound-healing process. Journal of Immunology. 2004;**172**:1848-1855. DOI: 10.4049/jimmunol.172.3.1848

[72] De Masi ECDJ, Campos ACL, De Masi FDJ, Ratti MAS, Ike IS, De Masi RDJ. A influência de fatores de crescimento na cicatrização de feridas cutâneas de ratas. Brazilian Journal of Otorhinolaryngology. 2016;**82**:512-521. DOI: 10.1016/j.bjorl.2015.09.011

[73] Chen L, Guo S, Ranzer MJ, Dipietro LA. Toll-like receptor 4 plays an essential role in early skin wound healing. Journal of Investigative Dermatology. 2013;**133**:258-267. DOI: 10.1038/jid.2012.267.Toll-like

[74] Li Y, Wang Y, Zhou L, Liu M, Liang G, Yan R, et al. $V\gamma 4$ T cells inhibit the pro-healing functions of dendritic epidermal T cells to delay skin wound closure through IL-17A. Frontiers in Immunology. 2018;**9**:1-19. DOI: 10.3389/fimmu.2018.00240

[75] Gallucci RM, Sloan DK, Heck JM, Murray AR, O'Dell SJ. Interleukin 6 indirectly induces keratinocyte migration. The Journal of Investigative Dermatology. 2004;**122**:764-772. DOI: 10.1111/j.0022-202X.2004.22323.x

[76] Tanno H, Kawakami K, Kanno E, Suzuki A, Takagi N, Yamamoto H, et al. Invariant NKT cells promote skin wound healing by preventing a prolonged neutrophilic inflammatory response. Wound Repair and Regeneration. 2017;**25**:805-815. DOI: 10.1111/wrr.12588

[77] Chen H, Shi R, Luo B, Yang X, Qiu L, Xiong J, et al. Macrophage peroxisome proliferator-activated receptor B deficiency delays skin wound healing through impairing apoptotic cell clearance in mice. Cell Death and Disease. 2015;**6**:1-13. DOI: 10.1038/cddis.2014.544

[78] Trautmann A, Toksoy A, Engelhardt E, Bröcker E-B, Gillitzer R. Mast cell involvement in normal human skin wound healing: Expression of monocyte chemoattractant protein-1 is correlated with recruitment of mast cells which synthesize interleukin-4 in vivo. The Journal of Pathology. 2000;**190**:100-106. DOI: 10.1002/(SICI)1096-9896(200001)190:1<100::AID-PATH496>3.0.CO;2-Q

[79] Egozi EI, Ferreira AM, Burns AL, Gamelli RL, Dipietro LA. Mast cells modulate the inflammatory but not the proliferative response in healing wounds. Wound Repair and Regeneration. 2003;**11**:46-54. DOI: 10.1046/j.1524-475X.2003.11108.x

[80] Shi J, Ma X, Su Y, Song Y, Tian Y, Yuan S, et al. MiR-31 mediates inflammatory signaling to promote re-epithelialization during skin wound healing. The Journal of Investigative Dermatology. 2018;**18**:31857-31858. DOI: 10.1016/j.jid.2018.03.1521

[81] Han HM, Ko S, Cheong MJ, Bang JK, Seo CH, Luchian T, et al. Myxinidin2 and myxinidin3 suppress inflammatory responses through STAT3 and MAPKs to promote wound healing. Oncotarget. 2017;**8**:87582-87597. DOI: 10.18632/oncotarget.20908

[82] Yang B, Suwanpradid J, Sanches-Lagunes R, Choi HW, Hoang P, Wang D, et al. IL-27 facilitates skin wound healing through induction of epidermal proliferation and host defense. The Journal of Investigative Dermatology. 2017;**137**:1166-1175. DOI: 10.1016/j.clinbiochem.2015.06.023.Gut-Liver

Chapter 3

Biomarkers of Wound Healing

Christian Agyare, Newman Osafo and
Yaw Duah Boakye

Additional information is available at the end of the chapter

http://dx.doi.org/10.5772/intechopen.80222

Abstract

The prevalence of conditions that eventually result in poor wound healing abounds as humans advance in age. With the increased possibility of wounds not healing comes a leap in morbidity and mortality with its accompanying socioeconomic impact. It is therefore relevant to understand what accounts for aberrant wound healing and more importantly the molecular markers involved in this pathological state. There are known events associated with the wound healing process, spanning from cellular involvement to the role of specific proteins such as cytokines and growth factors that are significant biomarkers in the wound healing process. This chapter discusses biomarkers relevant to the wound healing process, and these biomarkers go a long way to help identify and stratify nonhealing patients for whom biomarker-guided approaches may be of importance clinically in their management.

Keywords: wound, biomarkers, cytokines, growth factors, proteases

1. Introduction

The concept of biomarkers has existed from the time of the inception of ayurvedic medicine, just around the seventh century when the sweetness of urine was linked to diabetes even though the terminology had not been developed then [1]. The perspective of what constitutes the definition of a biomarker is somewhat diverse. Biomarkers (biological markers) are generally biomolecules whose qualitative and quantitative presence provides an indication of the state of a biological system. A more exhaustive definition as provided by the World Health Organization (WHO) led joint venture on chemical safety that describes a biomarker as any substance, structure, or process that can be measured in the body or its products that can influence or predict the incidence of outcome or disease [2]. The application of biomarkers has attained a vital and grounded position in clinical research, usually as predictors of the clinical outcomes for a varied number of disease conditions and their management [3].

Extensive scientific investigation into the mechanism of wound healing has revealed that the traditional guides in the determination of the wound healing potential, i.e., erythrocyte sedimentation rate (ESR) and C-reactive protein, do not yield enough positive and negative predictive values [4]. In lieu of the scientific evidence available, the focus has shifted to cytokines, chemokines, and proteases which hold the greatest potential as biomarkers [4].

2. Cytokines

Cytokines are proteins of relatively low molecular weight that are secreted to influence or modulate the behavior of immune cells and also other cells [5]. Crucial among them include interleukins, lymphokines, and other signaling molecules such as interferons and tissue necrosis factor (TNF-α). It has been long considered and corroborated by scientific evidence that pro-inflammatory cytokines such as interleukins 1α (IL-1α), 1β (IL-1β), and 6 (IL-6) and TNF-α play essential roles in wound healing process such as the stimulation of keratinocyte and fibroblast proliferation, modulation of immune response, synthesis and breakdown of extracellular matrix proteins, and the chemotaxis of fibroblast to the wound site [6].

Grellner et al. [7, 8] in their work to quantitatively analyze pro-inflammatory cytokines in human skin wounds realized an upregulation of the expression of IL-1α, IL-1β, IL-6, and TNF-α in the inflammatory phase of the wound healing process. The levels of these pro-inflammatory cytokines (TNF-α, IL-1, and IL-6) were higher in nonhealing wounds than healing wounds owing to the fact that nonhealing wounds stay in the inflammatory phase of wound healing process [4]. Bilder et al. [9] also report an increase in the levels of IL-8 in chronic nonhealing wounds as opposed to those with a healing potential. Ligi et al. [10] upon the assessment of several studies which evaluated the level expression of cytokines and chemokines in the microenvironment of a chronic ulcer alluded to a heightened pro-inflammatory condition in a nonhealing wound, thus corroborating other studies. It was however noted that the level of cytokines detectable does not necessarily correlate to its bioactivity due to anti-inflammatory cytokines whose presence counteracts the activity of these pro-inflammatory cytokines [10]. There are also specific cytokine inhibitors and proteolytic enzymes that also act on these cytokines to mask their bioavailability [10]. Patel et al. [4] also report the inconsistency in wound and serum levels of cytokines which poses a challenge in its use as reliable biomarkers of nonhealing wounds.

2.1. Interleukin 1 (IL-1)

The IL-1 family of cytokines is made up of two pro-inflammatory cytokines, namely, IL-α and IL-β. Interleukin 1 is primarily sourced from macrophages in the event of injury, infection, and antigenic challenge although the epidermal, epithelial, lymphoid, and vascular tissues also serve as reservoirs for the polypeptide [11]. The actions of IL-1 span from systemic changes in the neurological, hematologic, endocrinologic, and metabolic systems to some local effects that are particularly relevant in wound healing [12]. By influencing both destructive and repair processes, it contributes the mesenchymal tissue remodeling, and it does so by influencing quite a number of cells. First of all, it stimulates capillary endothelial cells to produce chemokines such as MCP-1 and also cause an upregulation of the synthesis of vascular adhesion molecules such as ICAM-1, VCAM-1, and E-selectin [13, 14]. The combined effect of these two actions is to cause the infiltration of the injury site with mononuclear cells, thus setting the stage for inflammatory response. The expression of matrix metalloproteases (MMPs) from resident fibroblasts is also under the control of IL-1. The call of MMPs to play results in the degradation of the extracellular matrix to allow for enhanced monocyte migration. It also leads to a down-modulation of the inflammatory response as MMPs degrade IL-1. Inhibiting the IL-1 pathway through the use of recombinant antibodies and macrophages from IL-1 receptor knockout mice appeared to turn the tables around as far as the wound microenvironment is concerned by inducing a switch from pro-inflammatory to healing-associated macrophage phenotypes and growth factors [14]. Therefore, there is a negative implication for wound healing in the absence of high expression of IL-1.

2.2. Interleukin 6 (IL-6)

Interleukin 6 is described as the chief contributor to the stimulation of a majority of the acute-phase proteins during inflammation. IL-6-deficient transgenic mice (IL-6 KO) therefore showed a substantial delayed cutaneous wound healing relative to the wild-type control animals by about threefold, the time required for healing [15].

Based on similar animal model studies on IL-6 knockout mice and the administration of recombinant murine IL-6 protein, IL-6 was found to be essential in stimulating the mitogenic activity of keratinocytes, an action that has been linked to scar formation as well as exerting a chemo-attractive action on neutrophils [6]. These effects seek to kick-start the wound healing process. However, a study conducted to determine the indicators of inflammation in the pathogenesis of diabetic foot ulcers identified a positive correlation between high serum IL-6 levels in diabetic patients with foot ulcers and low serum IL-6 levels in those without foot ulcers. This implicates its effect on poor wound healing [16].

This is not surprising as IL-6 has a reputation for dictating the transition from acute to chronic inflammation systemically by its stimulatory effects on T and B cells.

2.3. Tumor necrosis factor-α (TNF-α)

Tumor necrosis factor alpha (TNF-α) is a key pro-inflammatory cytokine involved in the early phase of most inflammatory events in the body. Employing mouse models, the expression of TNF-α at detectable levels was discovered to happen just after wound creation and sees an increase in the first several hours until it reaches a peak within 24 hours after which it returns to the basal level [17]. Vascular endothelial cells, keratinocytes, and fibroblasts are the major sources of TNF-α which cause an initiation of the inflammatory phase of the wound healing by promoting the recruitment of inflammatory leukocytes. TNF-α is also involved in the regulation of the activity of fibroblasts, keratinocytes, and vascular endothelial cells as well as in modulating synthesis of extracellular matrix proteins and matrix metalloproteinase [17, 18]. Based on diabetic models, an increase in TNF-α level coupled with decrease in IL-10 that has anti-inflammatory properties results in sustained expression of chemokines CXCL2 and CCL2 and leads to continuous infiltration of leucocytes to the injury site. This ultimately prolongs the inflammation and reduces the wound healing potential [19].

2.4. Transforming growth factor (TGF)

Transforming growth factor describes the superfamily for pluripotent cytokines which have very important functions to perform during disease, homeostasis, development, and repair. These sets of proteins are structurally related, but functionally distinguishable and relevant among them for wound healing are the isoforms TGF-β 1–3 [20]. The roles of these isoforms in the wound healing process can be both distinct and overlapping. However, the overall nature of their contribution to the wound healing has generated some controversy and thus is among the most studied molecules involved in the process [6]. Transforming growth factor β1 (TNF-β1) however has the widest spectrum of actions, affecting all manners of cell types that are involved in all stages of wound healing. These effects have been reported to be both positive and negative [21]. Historically, the synthesis of TNF-β1 from keratinocytes, platelets, and macrophages is upregulated right after injury, and this is crucial for initiating inflammation and granulation tissue formation. In addition, TNF-β1 contributes to the chemotactic migration of cells during wound repair. Some proteases such as MMP-1, MMP-2, MMP-3, and MMP-9 are also under the control of TNF-β1 [6, 22]. Based on human studies, TNF-β1 was found to stimulate the production of extracellular matrix molecules, including collagens and fibronectin, which strengthen the repaired wound. In spite of this knowledge, available evidence goes to raise questions about the true effects of TNF-β1 levels on wound healing [23]. Wound healing in Smad knockout mice, which have the signaling pathway of TNF-β1 blocked, was rather accelerated to the surprise of the investigators. In similar fashion, TNF-β1 knockout mice showed demonstrated reepithelialization during incisional wound repair, in comparison with wild-type mice. The consensus in the face of current evidence is that the selective inhibition of TNF-β1 in some cells may prove beneficial [24].

3. Growth factors

The growth factors are essentially responsible for the initiation of the proliferation stage of the wound healing process. The platelet-derived growth factor (PDGF), transforming growth factors (TGF-α, TGF-β), insulin growth factor (IGF-1), fibroblast growth factor (FGF), and granulocyte-macrophage colony-stimulating factors (GM-CSF) are examples of growth factors whose roles in wound healing as well as their possible use as biomarkers have been studied extensively based on their expressed levels [25]. In spite of the fact that insight about ideal levels and the spatiotemporal distribution of growth factors is far from complete, available data points to no local growth factor deficiency in chronic leg ulcers with the possible exception of TGF [6]. Trengove et al. [26] after studying wound fluids from both healing and nonhealing wounds arrive at similar conclusion that poor wound healing may be due to inflammatory mediators rather than a deficiency of growth factors.

3.1. Platelet-derived growth factors (PDGF)

Platelet-derived growth factors (PDGFs) are made up of a family of homodimeric or heterodimeric growth factors, including PDGF-AA, PDGF-AB, PDGF-BB, PDGF-CC, and PDGF-DD [27]. PDGF has been established to have chemotactic role for cells that migrate to the healing wound site such as fibroblasts, neutrophils, and monocytes. It was actually the very first growth factor shown to have this function [28]. It additionally stimulates the proliferation of fibroblast and the deposition of extracellular matrix. In vitro studies have also revealed that it stimulates insulin growth factor (IGF) release in fibroblasts which is vital to the initiation of the repair process [28]. Lastly, it stimulates fibroblasts to contract collagen matrices and induces the myofibroblast phenotype in the implicated cells. It has thus been established to be a major player in the wound healing and has formed the basis for studies into its clinical application in the treatment of wound healing disorders.

Owing to the close proximity of the expression sites of the PDGF, which is predominantly in the epidermis, and its receptors which are also in the dermis and granulating tissue, a paracrine mechanism has been suggested for its action [6, 29]. However, unlike other growth factors like fibroblast growth factor (FGF) and vascular epithelial growth factor (VEGF) that see an overexpression in the microenvironment or at the site of a healing wound or one in a granulation phase, the increase in the expression of PDGF-BB is without this spatial limitation as its levels in plasma also increases. It does make it potentially useful as the biomarker in wound healing [10].

4. Proteases

The action of proteases and their inhibitors goes a long way to influence the equilibrium between extracellular matrix (ECM) degradation and deposition which is responsible for the coordinated and timely healing of wounds [30]. There is an overwhelming wealth of evidence to suggest that nonhealing wounds are characterized by an increase in the levels of proteases and an imbalance in the protease/protease inhibitor levels [30, 31]. This manifests as a persistence of proteolysis and degradation of the extracellular matrix causing wound healing to delay. Significant among these proteases are the matrix metalloproteases (MMPs) [32]. MMPs are part of a family of zinc endopeptidase which essentially help in the degradation of provisional extracellular matrix, facilitate the migration of inflammatory cells to the wound site, remodel the granulation tissue, and modulate angiogenesis [28]. MMP activity as measured using Azocoll assay was found to be significantly elevated in chronic wounds as compared to acute wounds, thus implicating it poor wound healing [26].

Proteases as biomarkers for wound healing hold the key to transform clinical approach to the management of wounds. For example, the appropriateness of using protease-modulating dressing and tissue-engineered products, scaffolds, and skin grafts for the treatment can be made by the determination of the levels of proteases [33].

5. Matrix metalloproteinase

Matrix metalloproteinases (MMPs) are a group of endopeptidase that are zinc and calcium dependent and are usually divided into six groups depending on the substrate they act on. These MMPs consist of collagenases (MMP-1, MMP-3, MMP-8); gelatinases (MMP-2, MMP-9); stromelysins (MMP-3, MMP-10); matrilysins (MMP-7, MMP-26); membrane-type MMPs (MT-MMP) like MMP-14, MMP-15, MMP-16, and MMP-24; and other MMPs (MMP-11, MMP-12, MMP-19, MMP-20, MMP-22, MMP-23, MMP-28) [34].

Various MMPs are relevant to the wound healing process at varied points, and the tight control of their proteolytic activity is also essential to conduct the different events of wound healing [36]. MMPs are however generally involved in the inflammatory, proliferative, and remodeling phases of the wound healing process by modulating cytokine/chemokine activity by activating them enzymatically or influencing their availability by cleaving them from cell surface. Additionally, the actions of MMPs involve the breakdown of proteins part of the cell-cell and cell-extracellular matrix interaction [35, 36].

In terms of the predictive roles of MMPs' level for the wound healing process, some studies have focused on the MMP-1 to tissue inhibitor of metalloproteinase (TIMP-1) ratio. In one study, for instance, a significant correlation was found between a high ratio of MMP-1/TIMP-1 and good healing ($r = 0.65$, $p = 0.008$) with receiver operator curve (ROC) analysis showing an MMP-1/TIMP-1 ratio of 0.39 being the best predictive value for wound healing. High levels of MMP-8 and MMP-9 also appear to have negative predictive value for the process of wound healing [32].

6. Conclusion

With the growing research into the therapeutic benefits of biomarkers comes the challenge of identifying biomarkers that satisfy the required characteristics for use clinically. It is prudent to validate new biomarkers affecting the wound healing process by employing innovative, simple, and cost-effective molecular approaches to determine the type, level, and activity of all potential biomarkers. With the advent of trendsetting technical knowhow in defining diseases and other biological processes, it has become increasingly possible to identify and characterize novel biomarkers of the wound healing process. Continuing the research into identification of new biomarkers affecting the wound healing process is imperative since it will eventually have weighty health benefits on patients and offer a relevant guide to wound management. This will significantly lower the risks of microbial colonization and invasion of wounds and loss of structural function as a result of chronic wounds.

Author details

Christian Agyare[1]*, Newman Osafo[2] and Yaw Duah Boakye[1]

*Address all correspondence to: cagyare.pharm@knust.edu.gh

1 Faculty of Pharmacy and Pharmaceutical Sciences, Department of Pharmaceutics, Kwame Nkrumah University of Science and Technology, Kumasi, Ghana

2 Faculty of Pharmacy and Pharmaceutical Sciences, Department of Pharmacology, Kwame Nkrumah University of Science and Technology, Kumasi, Ghana

References

[1] Karley D, Gupta D, Tiwari A. Biomarkers: The future of medical science to detect cancer. Journal of Molecular Biomarkers Diagnosis. 2011;**2**:118

[2] WHO International Programme on Chemical Safety Biomarkers in Risk Assessment: Validity and Validation. 2001. Retrieved from: http://www.inchem.org/documents/ehc/ehc/ehc222.htm

[3] WHO International Programme on Chemical Safety Biomarkers and Risk Assessment: Concepts and Principles. 1993. Retrieved from: http://www.inchem.org/documents/ehc/ehc/ehc155.htm

[4] Patel S, Maheshwari A, Chandra A. Biomarkers for wound healing and their evaluation. Journal of Wound Care. 2016;**25**(1):46-55

[5] Cytokine. In: Stedman's Medical Dictionary. 28th ed. Wolters Kluwer Health, Lippincott: USA: Williams & Wilkins, Philadelphia; 2006

[6] Werner S, Grose R. Regulation of wound healing by growth factors and cytokines. Physiological Reviews. 2003;**83**(3):835-870

[7] Grellner W, Georg T, Wilske J. Quantitative analysis of proinflammatory cytokines (IL-1beta, IL-6, TNF-alpha) in human skin wounds. Forensic Science International. 2000;**113**:251-264

[8] Grellner W, Vieler S, Madea B. Transforming growth factors (TGF-alpha and TGF-beta1) in the determination of vitality and wound age: Immunohistochemical study on human skin wounds. Forensic Science International. 2005;**153**:174-180

[9] Bilder D, Schober M, Perrimon N. Integrated activity of PDZ protein complexes regulates epithelial polarity. Nature Cell Biology. 2003;**5**:53-58

[10] Ligi D, Mosti G, Croce L, Raffetto JD, Mannello F. Chronic venous disease—Part I: Inflammatory biomarkers in wound healing. Biochimica et Biophysica Acta. 2016;**1862**(10):1964-1974

[11] Chamberlain SC, Leiferman ME, Frisch EK, et al. Interleukin expression after injury and the effects of interleukin-1 receptor antagonist. PLoS One. 2013;**8**(8):e71631

[12] Doersch KM, DelloStritto DJ, Newell-Rogers MK. The contribution of interleukin-2 to effective wound healing. Experimental Biology and Medicine. 2017;**242**(4):384-396

[13] Cook-Mills JM, Marchese ME, Abdala-Valencia H. Vascular cell adhesion molecule-1 expression and signaling during disease: Regulation by reactive oxygen species and antioxidants. Antioxidants and Redox Signaling. 2011;**15**(6):1607-1638

[14] Lobmann R, Zemlin C, Motzkau M, Reschke K, Lehnert H. Expression of matrix metalloproteinases and growth factors in diabetic foot wounds treated with a protease absorbent dressing. Journal of Diabetes and its Complications. 2006;**20**(5):329-335

[15] Gallucci RM, Simeonova PP, Matheson JM, Kommineni C, Guriel JL, Sugawara T, Luster MI. Impaired cutaneous wound healing in interleukin-6–deficient and immunosuppressed mice. FASEB Journal. 2000;**14**(15):2525-2531

[16] Sallam AWA, El-Sharawy MHA. Role of interleukin-6 (IL-6) and indicators of inflammation in the pathogenesis of diabetic foot ulcers. Australian Journal of Basic and Applied Sciences. 2012;**6**(6):430-435

[17] Ritsu M, Kawakami K, Kanno E, Tanno H, Ishii K. Critical role of tumor necrosis factor- a in the early process of wound healing in skin. Journal of Dermatology and Dermatologic Surgery. 2017;**21**(1):14-19

[18] Mast BA, Schultz GS. Interactions of cytokines, growth factors, and proteases in acute and chronic wounds. Wound Repair and Regeneration. 1996;**4**:411-420

[19] Sen CK. Wound healing essentials: Let there be oxygen. Wound Repair and Regeneration. 2009;**17**:1-18

[20] Huang T, Schor LS, Hinck PA. Biological activity differences between TGF-β1 and TGF-β3 correlate with differences in the rigidity and arrangement of their component monomers. Biochemistry. 2014;**53**(36):5737-5749

[21] Wang XJ, Han G, Owens P, Siddiqui Y, Li AG. Role of TGF beta-mediated inflammation in cutaneous wound healing. The Journal of Investigative Dermatology. Symposium Proceedings. 2006;**11**(1):112-117

[22] Manicone AM, McGuire JK. Matrix metalloproteinases as modulators of inflammation. Seminars in Cell and Developmental Biology. 2008;**19**(1):34-41

[23] Goncalves MBB, Rabeh SAN, Tercariol CAS. The contribution of distance learning to the knowledge of nursing lecturers regarding assessment of chronic wounds. Revista Latino-Americana de Enfermagem. 2015;**23**(1):122-129

[24] Tejiram S, Kavalukas SL, Shupp JW, Barbul A. Wound healing. Wound Healing Biomaterials. 2016:3-39

[25] Olczyk P, Mencner Ł, Komosinska-Vassev K. The role of the extracellular matrix components in cutaneous wound healing. BioMed Research International. 2014;**2014**:747584, 8 pages

[26] Trengove NJ, Stacey MC, Macauley S, et al. Analysis of the acute and chronic wound environments: The role of proteases and their inhibitors. Wound Repair and Regeneration. 1999;**7**(6):442-452

[27] Rönnstrand L. Signaling by the platelet-derived growth facto receptor family. In: Bradshaw RA, Dennis EA, editors. Handbook of Cell Signaling. Cambridge, Massachusetts, USA: Academic Press. p. 427

[28] Diagn JMB, Gupta A. Wound healing: Assessment by various markers. Journal of Molecular Biomarkers. 2016;**8**(2):8-10

[29] Pastar I, Stojadinovic O, Yin NC, et al. Epithelialization in wound healing: A comprehensive review. Advances in Wound Care. 2014;**3**(7):445-464

[30] McCarty SM, Percival SL. Proteases and delayed wound healing. Advances in Wound Care. 2013;**2**(8):438-447

[31] Demidova-Rice TN, Hamblin MR, Herman IM. Acute and impaired wound healing: Pathophysiology and current methods for drug delivery, part 1: Normal and chronic wounds: Biology, causes, and approaches to care. Advances in Skin & Wound Care. 2012;**25**(7):304-314

[32] Iuonut AM, Dindelegan GC, Ciuce C. Proteases as biomarkers in wound healing. Temporomandibular Journal. 2011;**61**(1-2):65-73

[33] International Consensus. The Role of Proteases in Wound Healing Diagnostics. An Expert Working Group Review. London: Wounds International; 2011. p. 10

[34] Ligi D, Mosti G, Croce L, Raffetto JD, Mannello F. Chronic venous disease—Part II: Proteolytic biomarkers in wound healing. Biochimica et Biophysica Acta. 2016;**1862**(10): 1900-1908

[35] Caley MP, Martins VLC, O'Toole EA. Metalloproteinases and wound healing. Advances in Wound Care. 2015;**4**(4):225-234

[36] Jablonska-Trypuc A, Matejczyk M, Rosochacki S. Matrix metalloproteinases (MMPs), the main extracellular matrix (ECM) enzymes in collagen degradation, as a target for anticancer drugs. Journal of Enzyme Inhibition and Medicinal Chemistry. 2016;**31**(1):177-183

Chapter 4

Medicinal Plants in Wound Healing

Mohammad Reza Farahpour

Additional information is available at the end of the chapter

http://dx.doi.org/10.5772/intechopen.80215

Abstract

Wound healing process is known as interdependent cellular and biochemical stages which are in trying to improve the wound. Wound healing can be defined as stages which is done by body and delayed in wound healing increases chance of microbial infection. Improved wound healing process can be performed by shortening the time needed for healing or lowering the inappropriate happens. The drugs were locally or systemically administrated in order to help wound healing. Antibiotics, antiseptics, desloughing agents, extracts, etc. have been used in order to wound healing. Some synthetic drugs are faced with limitations because of their side effects. Plants or combinations derived from plants are needed to investigate identify and formulate for treatment and management of wound healing. There is increasing interest to use the medicinal plants in wound healing because of lower side effects and management of wounds over the years. Studies have shown that medicinal plants improve wound healing in diabetic, infected and opened wounds. The different mechanisms have been reported to improve the wound healing by medicinal plants. In this chapter, some medicinal plants and the reported mechanisms will be discussed.

Keywords: antibacterial, animal studies, inflammatory phase, medicinal plants, wound healing

1. Introduction

Wound healing is defined as a collection of complex process which comprises different compounds including soluble mediators, blood cells, extracellular matrix, and parenchymal cells [1, 2]. Wound healing is divided into stages including inflammation process, tissue formation, and tissue remodeling. The inflammatory phase involves different stages such as platelet accumulation, coagulation, and leukocyte migration. Re-epithelialization, angiogenesis, fibroplasia, and wound contraction are stages for tissue formation. Remodeling phase may be lasted for 1 month, and the dermis may respond to injury with the production of collagen and matrix proteins and then returns to its pre-injury phenotype [3, 4].

The different treatments are used in order to treat the wound healing. The different treatments have locally and systemically been used in order to help wound healing. The different agents are used in order to wound healing including antibiotics and antiseptics, desloughing agents (chemical debridement, e.g., hydrogen peroxide, eusol and collagenase ointment, wound healing promoters, some substances such as tissue extracts, vitamins, and minerals and a number of plant products [5]. Medicinal plants heal wound healing process by promoting blood clotting, fighting against infection and accelerating wound healing. It can be stated plants and chemical agents obtained from plants improve treatment and manage wound healing [5]. Medicinal plants show wound healing effects by the different mechanisms, such as modulation in wound healing, decreasing bacterial count, improving collagen deposition, increasing fibroblasts and fibrocytes, etc. In this chapter, we will describe different mechanisms in medicinal plants.

2. Medicinal plants

2.1. Cinnamon

Cinnamomum verum, cinnamon, belongs to the *Lauraceae* family. Cinnamon has been traditionally used in traditional systems of medicine. Cinnamon bark is used as spice, condiment and flavoring agent. It has some properties such as antioxidant, antiulcer, antimicrobial, antidiabetic, hypoglycemic, hypolipidemic and anti-inflammatory activity [6], which can be beneficial in types of wound such as diabetic and infected wounds. In addition to mentioned properties, cinnamon is known to have significant levels of polyphenols that may enhance glucose uptake in animals [7]. It increases glucose transporters-1 (GLUT-1) mRNA levels in mice adipocytes [8]. Studies have shown that cinnamon alcoholic and aqueous extracts accelerating the wound healing by their antioxidant properties [9, 10]. In this association, other studies have shown that faulted antioxidant system causes to increase oxidative stress which damages proteins, nucleotides, lipid levels and delays wound healing [11, 12]. On the other hand, anti-inflammatory effects of cinnamon components including cinnamaldehyde [13], 2-hydroxycinnamaldehyde [14] and quercetin [15] can help to accelerating wound healing.

2.2. *Aloe vera*

Aloe vera is a native plant in Africa and is so called lily of the desert or the plant of immortality. The *Aloe vera* extract has some beneficial properties which can decrease inflammation; enhance mature granulation tissue and resulting in help to accelerate wound healing [16]. It also decreases the blood glucose which can be beneficial in diabetic wounds [17]. Topical administration of *Aloe vera* gel is beneficial tool in healing minor burns and application of the *Aloe vera* gel is harmless as hypersensitive reactions to it are rare. However, *Aloe vera* gel may have harmful effects on severe burns and may actually prevent healing [18]. Gels have been traditionally found which contain 96% of water and essential oil, amino acids, minerals, vitamins, enzymes and glycoproteins. In addition, *Aloe vera* extract promotes the wound healing process because of its anti-inflammatory property. Because *Aloe vera* extract contains tannic acid and a type of polysaccharide [19] that help wound healing process. *Aloe vera* extract shows beneficial effects on wound healing by decreasing the inflammatory phase and supplying more mature granulation tissue which finally promotes healing and may be caused to produce a sound well-remodeled scar [16]. The *Aloe vera* leaf gel has beneficial effects on wound healing by antioxidant properties which can be attributed to some compounds including indoles, and alkaloids [20]. The spectrophotometric analyses show that *Aloe vera* contains non-flavonoid polyphenols compounds phytosterols, and indoles that may encourage the symptoms related with diabetes [20]. These compounds also shows antibacterial properties which may help to alleviate the wound healing in infected wounds. Chitra et al. [21] have reported the different mechanisms for wound healing of *Aloe vera* which mainly attributed to enhancing collages turnover rate and level of lysyl oxidase.

2.3. *Anethum graveolens*

Anethum graveolens L. (dill) (Apiaceae) is known as one of the most popular medicinal plants in all over world. *Anethum graveolens* is known to have some properties such as antimicrobial, antidiabetic and anti-inflammatory that can improve wound healing [22]. Some compounds including cis-carvone, limonene, α-phellandrene, and anethofuran are major compounds in dill essential oil [23]. Alpha-phellandrene is other major compounds in dill essential oil which may decrease bacterial growth and colonization and is to be beneficial in infected wounds [24, 25].

2.4. Eucalyptus

Eucalyptus is also known as Dinkum oil and is belonging to family *Myrtaceae*. Eucalyptus contains some compounds such as cineole which is also known as eucalyptol. It not only contains cineole but contains other compounds such as pinene, camphene, and phellandrene, citronellal, geranyl acetate. It is traditionally used for skin care including burns, blisters, herpes, cuts, wounds, skin infections and insect bites [26].

2.5. *Securigera securidaca*

Securigera securidaca, a native plant of Iran, has traditionally been used in the southern part of Iran in order to treatment the diabetes. It is commonly used in order to treat the wound healing. Flavonoids and coumarins are broadly used as major constituents in aerial parts, of *Securigera securidaca* that act as strong antioxidants [27]. It is also known to have antibacterial properties that improve wound healing in infected wounds [28].

2.6. Trigonella foenum

Trigonella foenum-graecum, is so called fenugreek, is extensively used in preparations the Ayurveda and also known to have effects antiulcer action and hypocholesterolaemic effects. Fenugreek (*Trigonella foenum-graecum*) has commonly been used as a condiment and in food preparations. Fenugreek is known to have hypoglycemic effects [29]. Fenugreek seeds have some polysaccharides such as diosgenin, yamogenin, gitogenin, tigogenin, and neotigogens. Saponins can produce steroidal effects which can decrease inflammation in the body. Other bioactive constituents of fenugreek are including mucilage, volatile oils, flavonoids and amino acid, alkaloids. The other active ingredient found in fenugreek is 4-hydroxyisoleucine [30]. It has been reported that fenugreek releases anti-inflammatory substance into wound region and decreases inflammation [31]. In addition, antimicrobial properties of fenugreek may increase its anti-inflammatory responses. A study has shown that flavonoids and triterpenoids may promote the wound healing process because of its antimicrobial properties [32]. Fenugreek is known to have antioxidant properties which can accelerate wound healing [33]. The kinetics of wound contraction and epithelialization were improved in a significant level from topical administration of the fenugreek seed [34].

2.7. Nelumbo nucifera

Nelumbo nucifera is belonging to family Nymphaeaceae which is so called Kamal in Hindi and Lotus in English. It has mud with large flower and is extensively used as natural and traditional healers. Its leaves are known to have wound healer effects [35]. It is reported that methanolic extract of *Nelumbo nucifera* rhizomes in the formulation of ointment could improve types of wound model in rats. This effect was studied in excision wound model, incision wound model and dead space wound model in the different concentrations of 5 and 10% w/w ointment. The both concentrations could significantly improve wound models. The both concentrations could improve contracting activity, wound close time, tensile strength, regeneration of tissue at the wound site and lysyl oxidase activity. The observed effects were similar to standard drugs [36].

2.8. Neem

Neem leaf extracts and essential oil from seeds are known to have antimicrobial effect which may be beneficial in the infected wounds. In addition, it can be stated that neem maintains wound and lesion free from secondary infections through reducing bacterial population. Clinical studies have shown that neem extract prevents inflammation and subsequently increases wound healing [5]. Neem leaf extracts and oil from seeds show antimicrobial effect which is mainly attributed to its compounds including margosic acid, glycerides of fatty acids, butyric acid and trace valeric acid [35].

2.9. Chamomile

Chamomilla recutita is so called as chamomile and is belonging to the *Asteraceae* family. It contains some substances such as chamazulene, alpha bisabolol, bisabolol oxides, spiroethers, and flavonoids which induce therapeutic effects [37]. It is also known to have anti-inflammatory which decreases inflammation during infected wounds [37]. Gholami Dogoury et al. [38] have shown that topical administration of *Chamomilla recutita* could decrease inflammatory phase and increase the proliferative stage. They have also advised to consider *Chamomilla recutita* as safe alternative chemicals for nitrofurazone ointment in wound healing process.

2.10. Bael

Bael which is so called *Aegle marmelos* which is belonging to family *Rutaceae*. It contains carbohydrates, protein, volatile oil, tanines, vitamin C and vitamin A. two alkaloids Omethylhalfordional and isopentylhalfordinol. It is traditionally used to treat wound healing properties [39].

2.11. Linumu sitatissimum

Flaxseed (*Linumu sitatissimum*) is one of oldest cultivated plant and is often cultivated for its fiber and oil. Flaxseed and its derivatives are known as rich sources of the essential fatty acid and alpha-linolenic acid, which are biological precursor for omega-3 and fatty acids such as eicosapentaenoic which may improve wound healing. Dogoury et al. [38] reported that topical administration of *Chamomilla recutita* and *Linumu sitatissimum* could decrease inflammatory phase and enhance the proliferative stage. They have also advised to consider *Chamomilla recutita* and *Linumu sitatissimum* as alternative agents for nitrofurazone ointment in wound healing process.

2.12. Moltkia coerulea

Moltkia coerulea is considered as one of most important plants in *Boraginaceae* that is belonging to *Lithospermeae* subfamily [40]. It is known to have some properties such as antioxidant and antibacterial effects, because of large amounts of flavonoids and phenols [41] which may accelerate wound healing. Farahpour et al. [42] have shown that topical administration of *Moltkia coerulea* improved well-formed clot in wound area, down-regulated the inflammation by exerting antioxidant properties, increased vascularization, promoted the collagen synthesis by up-regulating the fibroblasts and fibrocytes cells proliferation.

2.13. Ribwort plantain

Ribwort plantain (Plantaginaceae) is a perennial plant species with a worldwide distribution and large ecological amplitude. It is also known to have antibacterial properties [43, 44]. Studies have shown that *Ribwort plantain* accelerates epithelialization and wound contraction [45, 46]. Farahpour and Heydari [47] have shown that antioxidant properties reduce inflammation and increase wound contraction in rabbits.

2.14. Rosemary officinalis

Rosemary is belonging to the mint family which is known to have antioxidant properties because of its compounds including carnosic acid, carnosol, rosmarinic acid, diterpene, triterpenoid, phenolic acid and flavonoids [48]. It is also known to have anti-inflammatory [49] and anti-microbial properties [50] which may promote wound healing. In addition, its essential oil contains major levels of terpenoids, limonene, 1, 8-cineol, carnosic acid, rosemarinic acid and α-pinene, that can reduce inflammatory phase and can accelerate the healing process by promoting the proliferation stage [51]. Abu-Al-Basal [52] reported that rosmarinus aqueous extract accelerates wound healing by closure of the wound area and full-thickness epidermal regeneration and organization in diabetic BALB/c mice. Nejati et al. [53] have reported that topical application of rosemary ointment significantly decreased inflammatory cells, increased fibroblast migration and also increased wound contraction in wound healing in infected rat model.

2.15. *Allium sativum*

Allium sativum L. (Amaryllidaceae) is a member of the lily family which contains high levels of alliin, allyl cysteine, allyl disulfide, and allicin and has powerful antioxidant agents [54].

Farahpour et al. [55] have shown that topical administration of *Allium sativum* accelerated wound healing because of its preliminary impact on mast-cell distribution and increased collagen synthesis and up-regulated angiogenesis, and improved the healing process by increasing the intra-cytoplasmic carbohydrate ratio.

2.16. *Vitis vinifera*

Grape *Vitis vinifera* is belonging to *Vitaceae* family and contains vitamin E, linoleic acid, oligomer pro-anthocyanidins compounds and phenolic compounds such as flavonoids, phenolic acids and antioxidants [56] stilbenes and anthocyanins [57]. Active compounds present have beneficial effects including anti-inflammatory and wound healing [58], antimicrobial and diabetes properties [59]. Nejati and Farahpour [60] have shown that *Vitis vinifera* accelerated wound healing process by increasing neovascularization, fibroblast migration and epithelialization and can stimulate the enclosure of burn wounds.

2.17. *Calendula officinalis*

Calendula officinalis L. is so called pot marigold and is one of the medicinal plants in the *Asteraceae* family. Phytochemical evaluations of *Calendula officinalis* showed the presence of the flavonoids, flavonol glycosides, coumarins, saponins, triterpenes, alcohol triterpenes, fatty acid esters, carotenoids, essential oils, hydrocarbons, and fatty acids [61, 62]. Some studies have reported biological activities in *Calendula officinalis* including wound healing and anti-inflammatory effects [61, 62]. Farahpour [63] showed that *Calendula officinalis* aerial part hydroalcoholic extracts, have antinociceptive and anti-inflammatory activities in chemical pain and anti-inflammatory tests.

2.18. *Curcuma longa*

Turmeric (*Curcuma longa L.*) is known as turmeric and is belonging to *Zingiberaceae* family [64]. Turmeric extract contain major amounts of mineral dyes, curcumin, curcuminoids, phenolic compounds and volatile oils including turmerone, atlantone and zingiberene [65]. Farahpour et al. [66] showed that topical application of differential levels of hydroethanolic extract of turmeric rhizome remarkably accelerated wound healing activity by increasing in the rate of wound contraction and re-epithelialization, tensile strength value and collagen deposition in rat as an *in vivo* experimental wound models, and suggested to use various types of wounds in animal and human beings.

2.19. *Pistacia atlantica*

The *Pistacia atlantica* is belonging to *Anacardiaceae* family and is known to have anti-inflammatory, antibacterial, antimicrobial properties [67, 68]. Haghdoost et al. [69] have shown that *Pistacia atlantica* has beneficial effect on burn wound healing. Farahpour et al. [70] shown that the different levels of *Pistacia atlantica* decreased the healing time, improved the wound contraction, up-regulated hydroxyproline content and increased the neovascularization. They have also reported that *Pistacia atlantica* increased collagen deposition simultaneously by up-regulating the mast cells and fibroblast distribution. Finally, obtaining better results from high dose administration of *Pistacia atlantica* suggests that dosing higher concentration contains more constituents that plays major role in shortening healing time. In other study, Farahpour and Fathollahpour [71] have shown that ointment prepared from flaxseed and pistachio oil decreased polymorphonuclear and mononuclear cell distribution, improved new vessel formation and fibroblast distribution in injured rabbits.

2.20. Astragalus membranaceus

Astragalus is known as Huang Qi in China and contains polysaccharides, saponins, flavonoids, amino acids and trace elements. *Astragalus* had high potential in wound healing and its mechanism was by preventing inflammation, accelerating cell cycle and promoting the secretion of repair factors in wound healing model [72].

2.21. *Morinda citrifolia* Linn

Morinda citrifolia Linn (Rubiaceae) is so called noni or Indian mulberry. A significant enhance in the wound-healing activity has reported in the animals treated with the *Morinda citrifolia* extract in comparison to animals receiving the placebo control treatments. *Morinda citrifolia* extract improves wound healing by decreasing wound size and time to epithelialization [14].

2.22. Lucidone

Lucidone is a natural compound in *Lindera erythrocarpa* Makino which is known to have some properties such as antioxidant, anti-inflammatory, neuroprotective and anti-vital efficacies [73]. It has reported that Lucidone prevents free radical-induced oxidative stress and inflammation in human skin HaCaT cells [74]. Lucidone maintains human skin keratinocytes against UVA-induced DNA damage and mitochondrial dysfunction. Lucidone promoted wound healing by cooperation of keratinocyte/fibroblast/endothelial cell growth and migration and macrophage inflammation by PI3K/AKT, Wnt/β-catenin and NF-κB signaling cascade activation [75].

2.23. Genistein

Genistein is one of the most important isoflavones in legumes and has estrogen-like effects [76] antioxidative effects by regulating antioxidant enzyme activities such as super oxide dismutase, heme oxygenase-1 and glutathione peroxidase [77]. Studies have reported that dietary supplementation of genistein improved the regular wound healing process by regulating the antioxidant defense system and pro-inflammatory cytokines [78]. Treatment with genistein improved NLRP3 inflammasome in the basal level and alleviated inflammation and antioxidant defense system at early stage of wound healing in diabetic mice [79]. Eo et al. [79] have also reported that genistein improved wound healing by modulating in inflammation and oxidative stress during inflammatory stage.

2.24. Asiaticoside

Asiaticoside is a glycoside compound which is commonly used in order to wound healing. A study has shown that topical application of 0.4% solution of asiaticoside on the wound of streptozotocin-induced diabetic rats could improve the tensile strength, hydroxyproline content, protein content and epithelialization and accelerate facilitating the wound healing [80]. Another study has shown that 0.2% solution of asiaticoside increased hydroxyproline, tensile strength and quick healing. It also promoted angiogenesis collagen formation, remodeling of the collagen matrix and stimulated of glycosaminoglycan synthesis in a rat wound chamber model [81]. Antioxidants have major important role in the wound healing process that may improve wound healing by antioxidant property.

2.25. Curcumin

Curcumin is a phenolic compound which is isolated from *Curcuma longa Linn* [82] and used for its various biological and therapeutic properties. It also has antioxidant, anti-inflammatory, antimutagenic, anticarcinogenic, anti-infective and anticoagulant effects [82]. Curcumin can improve wound healing by its anti-inflammatory, anti-oxidant and anti-infectious properties and also because of the prevention of STAT, TNF-α, cyclin D1, COX-2, NF-κB, IL (1β, 6, 8) expressions, and down-regulation of MMP- 8 expression [83]. Curcumin also increases collagen deposition, tissue remodeling, fibroblast proliferation, granulation tissue formation and vascular density [82]. It also prevented the growth of dangerous pathogens like methicillin-resistant *Staphylococcus aureus* (MRSA) [84], P. *gingivalis, P. intermedia, F. nucleatum,* and *T. denticola* [85].

3. Conclusion

In this chapter, the possible mechanisms were described. We only mentioned some medicinal plants. The most medicinal plants act through antioxidant and antibacterial properties. However, some medicinal herbs and especially active compounds act by gene expression. It cannot certainly be stated efficiency medicinal plants in improving wound healing, but they have major potential for improving wound healing. The use of active compounds is a new strategy to improve the wound healing. Medicinal plants and active compounds help to decrease the inflammation. Future studies will be needed to determine the more mechanisms.

Conflict of interest

None.

Author details

Mohammad Reza Farahpour

Address all correspondence to: mrf78s@gmail.com

Department of Clinical Sciences, Faculty of Veterinary Medicine, Urmia Branch, Islamic Azad University, Urmia, Iran

References

[1] Bullers S, Berry H, Ingham E, Southgate J. The resolution of inflammation during the regeneration of biological scaffolds by human tissue. Journal of Tissue Engineering and Regenerative Medicine. 2012;**6**:218-218

[2] Pesce M, Patruno A, Speranza L, Reale M. Extremely low frequency electromagnetic field and wound healing: Implication of cytokines as biological mediators. European Cytokine Network. 2013;**24**:1-10. DOI: 10.1684/ecn.2013. 0332

[3] Castillo-Briceno P, Bihan D, Nilges M, Hamaia S, Meseguer J, Garcia-Ayala A, et al. Arole for specific collagen motifs during wound healing and inflammatory response of fibroblasts in the teleost fishgil the adseabream. Molecular Immunology. 2011;**48**:826-834. DOI: 10.1016/j.molimm 2010:12-24

[4] Bainbridge P. Wound healing and the role of fibroblasts. Journal of Wound Care. 2013; **22**:407-412

[5] Raina R, Prawez S, Verma PK, Pankaj NK. Medicinal plants and their role in wound healing. Vet Scan. 2008;**3**(1):1-24

[6] Vaibhavi J, Rakesh R, Pankaj K. Cinnamon: A pharmacological review. Journal of Advanced Science and Engineering Research. 2010;**1**:19-23

[7] Qin B, Nagasaki M, Ren M, Bajotto G, Oshida Y, Sato Y. Cinnamon extract prevents the insulin resistance induced by a high-fructose diet. Hormone and Metabolic Research. 2004;**36**:119-125

[8] Cao H, Gravesc DJ, Anderson RA. Cinnamon extract regulates glucose transporter and insulin-signaling gene expression in mouse adipocytes. Phytomedicine. 2010; **17**:1027-1032

[9] Kamath JV, Rana AC, Chowdhury AR. Pro-healing effect of Cinnamomum zeylanicum bark. Phytotherapy Research. 2003;**17**:970-972

[10] Farahpour MR, Habibi M. Evaluation of the wound healing activity of an ethanolic extract of Ceylon cinnamon in mice. Veterinary Medicine. 2012;**57**:53-57

[11] Rahman K. Studies on free radicals, antioxidants, and co-factors. Clinical Interventions in Aging. 2007;**2**:219-225

[12] Sharma P, Jha AB, Dubey RS, Pessarakli M. Reactive oxygen species, oxidative damage, and antioxidative defense mechanism in plants under stressful conditions. Journal of Botany. 2012;**24**:1-26

[13] Yang D, Liang XC, Shi Y, Sun Q, Liu D, Liu W, Zhang H. Anti-oxidative and anti-inflammatory effects of cinnamaldehyde on protecting high glucose-induced damage in cultured dorsal root ganglion neurons of rats. Chinese Journal of Integrative Medicine. 2015;**17**:1-9

[14] Lee SH, Lee SY, Son DJ, Lee H, Yoo HS, Song S, Oh KW, Han DC, Kwon BM, Hong JT. Inhibitory effect of 2′-hydroxycinnamaldehyde on nitric oxide production through

inhibition of NF-κB activation in RAW 264.7 cells. Biochemical Pharmacology. 2005; **69**:791-799

[15] Caddeo C, Díez-Sales O, Pons R, Fernàndez-Busquets X, Fadda AM, Manconi M. Topical anti-inflammatory potential of quercetin in lipid-based nanosystems: In vivo and in vitro evaluation. Pharmacological Research. 2014;**1**:959-968

[16] Abdel Hamid AAM, Solaiman MFM. Effect of topical aloe vera on the process of healing of full-thickness skin burn: A histological and immunohistochemical study. Journal of Histology & Histopathology. 2015;**2**:1-9. DOI: 10.7243/2055-091X-2-3

[17] Daburkar M, Lohar V, Rathore AS, Bhutada P, Tangadpaliwar S. An in vivo and in vitro investigation of the effect of Aloe vera gel ethanolic extract using animal model with diabetic foot ulcer. Journal of Pharmacy and Bioallied Sciences. 2014;**6**(3):205-212

[18] Schmidt JM, Greenspoon JS. *Aloe vera* dermal wound gel is associated with a delay in wound healing. Obstetrics and Gynecology. 1991;**78**:115-117

[19] Schäfer M, Werner S. Oxidative stress in normal and impaired wound repair. Pharmacological Research. 2008;**58**:165-171

[20] Nejatzadeh-Barandozi F. Antibacterial activities and antioxidant capacity of Aloe vera. Organic and Medicinal Chemistry Letters. 2013;**3**:5 http://www.orgmedchemlett.com/content/3/1/5

[21] Chitra P, Sajithlal GB, Chandrakasan G. Influence of Aloe vera on collagen turnover in healing of dermal wounds in rats. Indian Journal of Experimental Biology. 1998; **36**:896-901

[22] Heamalatha S, Swarnalatha S, Divya M, Gandhi-Lakshmi R, Ganga-Devi A, Gomathi E. Pharmacognostical, pharmacological, investigation on Anethum graveolens Linn: A review. Research Journal of Pharmaceutical, Biological and Chemical Sciences. 2011;**2**:564-574

[23] Radulescu V, Popescu ML, Ilies DC. Chemical composition of the volatile oil from different plant parts of *Anethum graveolens L.*(Umbelliferae) cultivated in Romania. Farmácia. 2010;**58**:594-600

[24] Singh G, Maurya S, Lampasona MP, Catalan C. Chemical constituents, antimicrobial investigations, and antioxidative potentials of *Anethum graveolens L.* essential oil and acetone extract. Journal of Food Science. 2005;**70**:208-215

[25] Zhang JH, Sun HL, Chen SY, Zeng L, Wang TT. Anti-fungal activity, mechanism studies on α-Phellandrene and nonanal against Penicillium cyclopium. Botanlcal Study. 2017;**58**:13-21

[26] Hukkeri VT, Karadi RV, Akki KS, Savadi RV, Jaiprakash B, Kuppast J, Patil MB. Wound healing property of Eucalyptus globulus leaf extract. Indian Drugs. 2002;**39**:481-483

[27] Tofighi Z, Asgharian P, Goodarzi S, Hadjiakhoondi A, Ostad SN, Yassa N. Potent cytotoxic flavonoids from Iranian Securigera securidaca. Medicinal Chemistry Research. 2014;**23**:1718-1724

[28] Amin GH. Popular Medicinal Plants of Iran. 2nd ed. Tehran: Tehran University of Medical Sciences Publications; 2005. p. 240

[29] Hasan M, Rahman M. Effect of fenugreek on Type 2 diabetic patients. International Journal of Environmental Research and Public Health. 2016;**10**:251-255

[30] Acharya SN, Srichamoren A, Basu S, Ooraikul B, Basu T. Improvement in the nutraceutical properties of fenugreek (Trigonella foenum-graecum L.) Songklanakarin J. Science and Technology. 2006;**28**(1):1-9

[31] Muhammed DO, Salih NA. Effect of application of fenugreek (Trigonella foenum-graecum) on skin wound healing in rabbits. AL-Qadisiyah Journal of Veterinary Medicine Sciences. 2012;**2**:86-93

[32] Badri PN, Renu S. Role of medicinal plants in wound healing. Research Journal of Medicinal Plants. 2011;**5**:392-405

[33] Kaur C, Kapoor HC. Anti-oxidant activity and total phenolic content of some Asian vegetables. International Journal of Food Science and Technology. 2002;**37**:153-161

[34] Sumitra M, Manikandan P, Suguna L, Hittar GCE. Study of dermal wound healing activity of Trigonella foenum graceum seeds in rats. Journal of Clinical Biochemistry and Nutrition. 2008;**200**:59-67

[35] Sabale P, Bhimani B, Prajapati C, Sabale V. An overview of medicinal plants as wound healers. Journal of Applied Pharmaceutical Science. 2012;**2**(11):143-150

[36] Mukherjee PK, Mukherjee K, Pal M, Saha BP. Wound healing potential of Nelumba nucifera (Nymphaceae) rhizome extract. Phytomedicine. 2000;**7**:66-73

[37] Mann C, Staba EJ. The chemistry, pharmacology, and commercial formulations of chamomile. In: Craker LE, Simon JE, editors. Herbs, Spices, and Medicinal Plants: Recent Advances in Botany, Horticulture and Pharmacology. Vol. 1. Phoenix, AZ: Oryx Press; 1986. pp. 235-280

[38] Gholami Dogoury H, Farahpour MR, Amniattalab A. Comparison effect of chamomile (*Chamomilla Recutita*) hydroethanolic extract and flaxseed oil (*Linum Ustatissum*) alone and simultaneous administration with nitrofurazone in wound healing process. Indian Journal of Fundamental and Applied Life Sciences. 2015;**10**:2231-6345

[39] Jaswanth A, Loganathan V, Manimaran S, Rukmani S. Wound healing activity of Aegle marmelos. Indian Journal of Pharmaceutical Sciences. 2001;**63**:41-44

[40] Azimova SS, Glushenkova AI. Lipids, lipophilic components and essential oils from plant sources. New York: Springer Science Business Medical LLC; 2012. p. 163

[41] Koncic MZ, Kremer D, Gruz J, et al. Antioxidant and antimicrobial properties of Moltkia petraea (Tratt.) Griseb. Flower, leaf and stem infusions. Food and Chemical Toxicology. 2010;**48**:1537-1542

[42] Farahpour MR, Dilmaghanian A, Faridy M, Karashi E. Topical Moltkia coerulea hydroethanolic extract accelerates the repair of excision wound in a rat model. Chinese Journal of Traumatology. 2016;**19**:97-103

[43] Kumar VP, Chauhan NS, Padh H, Rajani M. Search for antibacterial and antifungal agents from selected Indian medicinal plants. Journal of Ethnopharmacology. 2006;**107**:182-188

[44] Braga FG, Bouzada MLM, Fabri RL, de O Matos M, Moreira FO, Scio E, Coimbra ES. Antileishmanial and antifungal activity of plants used in traditional medicine in Brazil. Journal of Ethnopharmacology. 2007;**111**:396-402

[45] Scortichini M, Rossi MP. Preliminary in vitro evaluation of the antimicrobial activity of terpenes and terpenoids towards Erwinia amylovora (Burrill) Winslow et al. Journal of Applied Microbiology. 1991;**71**:109-112

[46] Sasidharan S, Nilawatyi R, Xavier R, Latha LY, Amala R. Wound healing potential of Elaeis guineensis Jacq leaves in an infected albino rat model. Molecules. 2010;**15**:3186-3199

[47] Farahpour MR, Heydari A. Wound healing effect of hydroethanolic extract of *Ribwort plantain* leaves in rabbits. Research Opinions in Animal and Veterinary Sciences. 2014;**5** (3):143-147

[48] Erkan N, Ayranci G, Ayranci E. Antioxidant activities of rosemary (Rosmarinus Officinalis L.) extract, black seed (Nigella sativa L.) essential oil, carnosic acid, rosmarinic acid and sesamol. Food Chemistry. 2008;**110**(1):76-82

[49] Mengoni ES, Vichera G, Rigano LA, Rodriguez-Puebla ML, Galliano SR, Cafferata EE, Pivetta OH, Moreno S, Vojnov AA. Suppression of COX-2, IL-1β and TNF-α expression and leukocyte infiltration in inflamed skin by bioactive compounds from Rosmarinus officinalis L. Fitoterapia. 2011;**82**(3):414-421

[50] Moreno S, Scheyer T, Romano CS, Vojnov AA. Antioxidant and antimicrobial activities of rosemary extracts linked to their polyphenol composition. Free Radical Research. 2006;**40**(2):223-231

[51] Jiang Y, Wu N, Fu YJ, Wang W, Luo M, Zhao CJ, Zu YG, Liu XL. Chemical composition and antimicrobial activity of the essential oil of rosemary. Environmental Toxicology and Pharmacology. 2011;**32**(1):63-68

[52] Abu-Al-Basal MA. Healing potential of Rosmarinus officinalis L. on full-thickness excision cutaneous wounds in alloxan-induceddiabetic BALB/c mice. Journal of Ethnopharmacology. 2010;**131**:443-450

[53] Nejati H, Farahpour MR, Neyriz NM. Topical rosemary officinalis essential oil improves wound healing against disseminated Candida albicans infection in rat model. Comparative Clinical Pathology. 2015. DOI: 10.1007/s00580-015-2086-z

[54] Chung LY. The antioxidant properties of garlic compounds: Allyl cysteine, alliin, allicin, and allyl disulfide. Journal of Medicinal Food. 2006;**9**:205-213

[55] Farahpour MR, Hesaraki S, Faraji D, Zeinalpour R, Aghaei M. Hydroethanolic *Allium sativum* extract accelerates excision wound healing: Evidence for roles of mast-cell infiltration and intracytoplasmic carbohydrate ratio. Brazilian Journal of Pharmaceutical Sciences. 2017. http://dx.doi.org/10.1590/s2175-97902017000115079

[56] Mureşan A, Alb C, Suciu S, Clichici S, Filip A, Login C. Studies on antioxidant effects of the red grapes seed extract from Vitis Vinifera, Burgund Mare, Recaş in pregnant rats. Acta Physiologica Hungarica. 2010;**97**(2):240-246

[57] Maier T, Schieber A, Kammerer DR, Carle R. Residues of grape (Vitis vinifera L.) seed oil production as a valuable source of phenolic antioxidants. Food Chemistry. 2009; **112**(3):551-559

[58] Hemmati AA, Aghel N, Rashidi I, Gholampur-Aghdami A. Topical grape (Vitis vinifera) seed extract promotes repair of full thickness wound in rabbit. International Wound Journal. 2011;**8**(5):514-520

[59] Xia E-Q, Deng G-F, Guo Y-J, Li H-B. Biological activities of polyphenols from grapes. International Journal of Molecular Sciences. 2010;**11**(2):622-646

[60] Nejati H, Farahpour MR. Effect of topical red grape seed hydroethanol extract on burn wound healing in rats. Indian Journal of Chemical Technology. 2014;**6**:2340-2346 2014

[61] Parente LML, Júnior L, de Souza R, Tresvenzol LMF, Vinaud MC, de Paula JR, et al. Wound healing and anti-inflammatory effect in animal models of pot marigold growing in Brazil. Evidence-Based Complementary and Alternative Medicine. 2012;**2012**

[62] Preethi KC, Kuttan R. Wound healing activity of flower extract of calendula Officinalis. Journal of Basic and Clinical Physiology and Pharmacology. 2009;**20**(1):73-80

[63] Farahpour MR. Antioxidant activity, Antinociceptive and anti-inflammatory effects of pot marigold hydroalcoholic extract on experimental animals. International Journal of PharmTech Research. 2014;**6**(5):1640-1646

[64] Chan EWC, Lim YY, Wong SK, Lim KK, Tan SP, Lianto FS, Yong MY. Effects of different drying methods on the antioxidant properties of leaves and tea of ginger species. Journal of Food Chemistry. 2009;**113**:166-172

[65] Li S, Yuan W, Deng G, Wang P, Yang P, Aggarwal BB. Chemical composition and product quality control of turmeric (Curcuma longa L.). Journal of Pharmaceutical Crops. 2011;**2**:28-54

[66] Farahpour MR, Emami P, Jangkhahe GS. In vitro antioxidant properties and wound healing activity of hydroethanolic turmeric rhizome extract (Zingiberaceae). International Journal of Pharmacy and Pharmaceutical Sciences. 2014;**8**:474-478

[67] Ali-Shtayeh M, Abu Ghdeib SI. Antifungal activity of plant extracts against dermatophytes. Mycoses. 1999;**42**:665-672

[68] Magiatis P, Melliou E, Skaltsounis AL, Chinou IB, Mitaku S. Chemical composition and antimicrobial activity of the essential oils of Pistacia lentiscus var. chia. Planta Medicine. 1999;**65**:749-752

[69] Haghdoost F, Baradaran Mahdavi MM, Zandifar A, Sanei MH, Zolfaghari B, Javanmard SH. *Pistacia atlantica* resin has a dose-dependent effect on angiogenesis and skin burn wound healing in rat, Evidence-Based Complementary and Alternative Medicine; 2013. 8 p. http://dx.doi.org/10.1155/2013/893425. Article ID 893425

[70] Farahpour MR, Mirzakhani N, Doostmohammadi J, Ebrahimzadeh M. Hydroethanolic Pistacia atlantica hulls extract improved wound healing process; evidence for mast cells infiltration, angiogenesis and RNA stability. International Journal of Surgery. 2015; **17**:88-98

[71] Farahpour MR, Fathollahpour S. Topical co-administration of flaxseed and pistachio ointment promoted wound healing; evidence for histopathological features. Comparative Clinical Pathology. 2015. DOI: 10.1007/s00580-015-2097-9

[72] Zhao B, Zhang X, Han W, Cheng J, Qin Y. Wound healing effect of an *Astragalus membranaceus* polysaccharide and its mechanism. Molecular Medicine Reports. 2017;**15**:4077-4083

[73] Chen W, Wang S, Chiu C, Tseng C, Lin C, Wang H, Lee J. Lucidone suppresses hepatitis C virus replication by Nrf2-mediated heme oxygenase-1 induction. Antimicrobial Agents and Chemotherapy. 2013;**57**:1180-1191

[74] Kumar KS, Yang H, Tsai Y, Hung P, Chang S, Lo H, Shen P, Chen S, Wang H, Wang S. Lucidone protects human skin keratinocytes against free radical-induced oxidative damage and inflammation through the up-regulation of HO-1/Nrf2 antioxidant genes and down-regulation of NF-κB signaling pathway. Food and Chemical Toxicology. 2013;**59**:55-66

[75] Yang H, Tsai Y, Korivi M, Chang C, Hseu Y. Lucidone promotes the cutaneouswound healing process via activation of the PI3K/AKT, Wnt/β-catenin and NF-κB signaling pathways. Biochimica et Biophysica Acta. 1864;**2017**:151-168

[76] Wang TT, Sathyamoorthy N, Phang JM. Molecular effects of genistein on estrogen receptor mediated pathways. Carcinogenesis. 1996;**17**:271-275

[77] Mezei O, Banz WJ, Steger RW, Peluso MR, Winters TA, Shay N. Soy isoflavones exert antidiabetic and hypolipidemic effects through the PPAR pathways in obese Zucker rats and murine RAW 264.7 cells. The Journal of Nutrition. 2003;**133**:1238-1243

[78] Park E, Lee SM, Jung IK, Lim Y, Kim J. Effects of genistein on early-stage cutaneous wound healing. Biochemical and Biophysical Research Communications. 2011;**410**:514-519

[79] Eo H, Lee H-J, Lim Y. Ameliorative effect of dietary genistein on diabetes induced hyper-inflammation and oxidative stress during early stage of wound healing in alloxan induced diabetic mice. Biochemical and Biophysical Research Communications. 2016;**478**:1021-1027

[80] Maquart FX, Chastang F, Simeon A, Birembaut P, Gillery P, et al. Triterpenes from Centella asiatica stimulate extracellular matrix accumulation in rat experimental wounds. European Journal of Dermatology. 1999;**9**(4):289-296

[81] Rosen H, Blumenthal A, McCallum J. Effect of asiaticoside on wound healing in the rat. Proceedings of the Society for Experimental Biology and Medicine. 1967;**125**(1):279-280

[82] Mahmood K, Zia KM, Zuber M, Salman M, Anjum MN. Recent developments in curcumin and curcumin based polymeric materials for biomedical applications: A review. International Journal of Biological Macromolecules. 2015;**81**:877-890

[83] Ghosh S, Banerjee S, Sil PC. The beneficial role of curcumin on inflammation, diabetes and neurodegenerative disease: A recent update. Food and Chemical Toxicology. 2015;**83**:111-124

[84] Mun SH, Joung DK, Kim YS, Kang OH, Kim SB, et al. Synergistic antibacterial effect of curcumin against methicillin resistant Staphylococcus aureus. Phytomedicine. 2013; **20**(8-9):714-718

[85] Izui S, Sekine S, Maeda K, Kuboniwa M, Takada A. Antibacterial activity of curcumin against periodontopathic bacteria. Journal of Periodontology. 2016;**87**(1):83-90

Chapter 5

Wound Healing: Contributions from Plant Secondary Metabolite Antioxidants

Victor Y.A. Barku

Additional information is available at the end of the chapter

http://dx.doi.org/10.5772/intechopen.81208

Abstract

Plants by their genetic makeup possess an innate ability to synthesize a wide variety of phytochemicals that help them to perform their normal physiological functions and/or to protect themselves from microbial pathogens and animal herbivores. The synthesis of these phytochemicals presents the plants their natural tendency to respond to environmental stress conditions. These phytochemicals are classified either as primary or secondary metabolites. The secondary metabolites have been identified in plants as alkaloids, terpenoids, phenolics, anthraquinones, and triterpenes. These plant-based compounds are believed to have diverse medicinal properties including antioxidant properties. Plants have therefore been a potential source of antioxidants which have received a great deal of attention since increased oxidative stress has been identified as a major causative factor in the development and progression of several life-threatening diseases, including neurodegenerative and cardiovascular diseases and wound infection. Consequently, many medicinal plants have been cited and known to effect wound healing and antioxidant properties. This chapter briefly reviews antioxidant properties of medicinal plants to highlight the important roles medicinal plants play in wound healing.

Keywords: wound healing, antioxidants, phytochemicals, reactive oxygen species, plants

1. Introduction

Plant-derived drugs have been part of the human race in the healthcare for thousands of years [1]. Throughout the world, a huge percentage of population depends upon the use of plant-based medicine because of their easy availability and also due to the lack of better healthcare alternatives. Plant-based medicines or herbal medicines have been effective and safe traditional methods practiced in many countries including China, India, and most African countries for the treatment of various diseases [2]. A large number of plant extracts, concoctions, poultices, decoctions, or pastes are equally used in many countries for treatment of diseases, cuts, wounds, and burns. Thus, since antiquity, several medicinal plants and plant-based strategies are widely known for their significant role in wound healing and skin regeneration as well as their therapeutic applications [2].

Wound is an injury that damages the dermal layer of the skin. Several factors contribute to wound generation, e.g., accidental traumas or surgery, and in certain cases, this dermal injury may have a devastating outcome [2, 3]. Wound healing is the natural process which leads to restore the structural and functional integrities of injured tissues. It involves several biochemical and cellular pathways, in order to repair the lesions and to restore the physiological conditions. Fortunately, the human body has the inbuilt capacity to promote this repairing process. However, there can be impairment of this sophisticated repairing process leading to chronic or non-healing wounds, which may result in severe clinical complications or even patient death. Deficiencies in nutritional factors which are essential in cellular differentiation, immune functioning, and collagen formation may result to the failure of wound healing process [4]. Additionally, oxygen- and nitrogen-centered reactive species are known to play crucial roles in regulating healing [2, 5]. Hence, high concentrations of these reactive species are present in wound sites. Unfortunately, these substances can induce harmful effects on cells and tissues and even promote oxidative stress that generates lipid peroxidation, damage of deoxyribonucleic acid (DNA), and enzyme inactivation, including free radical scavenger enzymes [6]. This necessitates the involvement or use of antioxidants which may represent potential therapeutic tools to enhance and accelerate wound healing process.

Several phytoconstituents such as triterpenes, alkaloids, and polyphenols show antioxidant and antimicrobial effects and are able to promote one or more mechanisms of the reparative process [7]. Accordingly, numerous plant extracts have been employed to promote wound healing with a high degree of success [8]. Many wound healing medicinal plants have been investigated to possess antioxidant properties. In other dimensions, numerous studies conducted over the years showed the great potential of plants in promoting wound healing, by virtue of their high contents in antioxidant properties. This document therefore intends to throw more light on the existing literature on wound healing potentials of medicinal plants and their antioxidant properties.

2. Wound

A physical, chemical, thermal, microbial, or immunological action on the living tissue may result in disruption of a cellular, anatomical, and functional continuity of the living tissue [9]. This phenomenon results in an injury to the skin or the underlying tissue or organ termed a wound. A wound is therefore damage or disruption to the normal anatomical structure and function [10, 11]. This can range from a simple break in the epithelial integrity of the skin or it can be deeper, extending into subcutaneous tissue with damage to other structures such as tendons, muscles, vessels, nerves, parenchymal organs, and bones [12, 13].

Wound can result through accident or intentional etiology or as a result of a disease process. Wounding, irrespective of the cause and whatever the form, damages the tissue and disrupts the local environment within it [14].

2.1. Types of wounds

Based on the underlying cause of wound creation, wounds may be classified into two main groups: open and closed wounds. In open wounds, the skin is broken, and the underlying tissue is exposed to the outside environment allowing blood to leave the body. These are wounds in which there is loss of superficial surface covering the tissue such as loss of skin. Such wounds are opened to invasion by microorganisms [15]. Open wounds consist of abrasion or glazes, laceration, incision, puncture, avulsion, cuts, blisters, penetration, and gunshot wounds. In closed wounds, the skin is intact, and the underlying tissue is not directly exposed to the outside world. The superficial surface covering the wound is not lost. The wound occurs under the surface of the skin without affecting the skin and hence does not involve any external bleeding. Infection of these wounds is rare, and it may resolve without any treatment if it is not extensive. Examples of closed wounds are contusion (bruises), hematomas, and crush injuries.

Wound can also be classified as either internal or external based on the wound origin. Internal wounds result from impaired immune and nervous system functions and/or decreased supply of blood, oxygen, or nutrients to that area, such as in cases of chronic medical illness (diabetes, atherosclerosis, and deep vein thrombosis). External wounds are usually caused by penetrating objects or non-penetrating trauma. Penetrating wounds result from trauma that breaks through the full thickness of the skin, reaching down to the underlying tissue and organs, and include stab wounds (trauma from sharp objects, such as knives), skin cuts, surgical wounds (intentional cuts in the skin to perform surgical procedures), and gunshot wounds (wounds resulting from firearms).

Non-penetrating wounds are usually the result of blunt trauma or friction with other surfaces; the wound does not break through the skin and may include abrasions (scraping of the outer skin layer), lacerations (a tear-like wound), contusions (swollen bruises due to accumulation of blood and dead cells under the skin), and concussions (damage to the underlying organs and tissue on the head with no significant external wound).

Depending on the healing time, wound can further be classified as either acute or chronic wounds [14]. Acute wounds heal uneventfully (with no complications) in the predicted amount of time, while chronic wounds take a longer time to heal and might have some complications.

The presence of foreign material and bacteria leads to another way to classify wounds. A wound that has dirt, fragments of the causative agent, bacteria, or other foreign materials is determined to be contaminated or infected. A wound with no foreign materials or debris inside is determined to be clean [15].

3. Wound healing

Wound healing is a complex and dynamic process of replacing devitalized and missing cellular structures and tissue layers. The wound healing process can be divided into three or four distinct basic phases. Inflammatory, fibroblastic or proliferation, and maturation or remodeling constitutes the three-phase division [16, 17]. In the four-phase concept, there are the hemostasis phase, the inflammatory phase, the proliferation phase, and the remodeling phase. In the three-phase approach, the hemostasis phase is contained within the inflammatory phase [18]. The normal physiology of wound healing depends on low levels of reactive oxygen species (ROS) and oxidative stress [19, 20]. An overexposure to oxidative stress leads to impaired wound healing. Free radicals are highly unstable molecules, and ROS are a form of free radicals that include the oxygen atom as well as reactive molecules such as superoxides and peroxides. Although normally formed as a by-product of metabolism and are reactive to invading organisms, overproduction leads to an increased load of free radicals and ROS known as oxidative stress. Free radicals attack and remove electrons from all types of molecules in the cell, including nucleic acids in DNA, proteins, and polyunsaturated fatty acids in cell membranes or organelle membranes. When free radicals attack proteins, they break peptide bonds in the protein backbone, changing the protein structure and altering its functionality [21]. All of these processes are detrimental to the proliferation of new cells in the healing process of epithelial wounds. ROS are likely needed at some basal level for wound healing. The importance of ROS to wound healing is illustrated by studies demonstrating that total suppression of oxidant production results in impaired healing, just as excessive amounts of oxidants do. ROS have also been implicated as important mediators of cell signaling and inflammation in wound repair. Although ROS production is physiologic, excessive production can be harmful.

3.1. Reactive oxygen species (ROS)

Oxidation is a basic part of the aerobic life and our metabolism. The body uses oxygen (O_2) to produce energy by oxidizing glucose. In the biochemical process involving oxygen, i.e., during oxidation, many highly unstable reactive molecules called free radicals are produced. The free radicals are atoms or molecules having odd number of electrons. Atoms of oxygen or nitrogen having central unpaired electron are called reactive oxygen or nitrogen species [22, 23]. These species are natural by-products produced by the normal metabolism of oxygen in living organisms. These reactive oxygen species (ROS) are various forms of activated oxygen which causes oxidative damage. They include free radicals such as superoxide anion radicals $(O_2)^-$, hydroxyl radicals ($OH^\cdot$), and non-free radical species such as peroxyl radicals $(O_2)^{-2}$ and singlet oxygen ($^1O_2$) which are various forms of activated oxygen generated in the body [24].

In small amounts, these ROS can be beneficial as signal transducers and growth regulators. However, during oxidative stress, large or excessive amounts of these ROS can be produced and may be dangerous and harmful to the body. The free radicals have the potential to damage biological tissues by disrupting cell membranes. This then affects the ability of the cell to transport substances across the membranes. The immune system is vulnerable to oxidative stress. Oxidative stress refers to an imbalance between the production of free radicals and the antioxidant defense system. It is the accumulated damage due to free radical activity in the human body. Excessive amounts of ROS may be a primary cause of biomolecular oxidation. The ROS have the ability to attack numerous molecules in the membrane that contain carbon–carbon double bonds (C=C). For instance, polyunsaturated fatty acids are particularly sensitive to free radicals. The free radicals are destructive to these molecules including proteins and lipids through oxidation [25]. As a result, ROS have the potential of causing peroxidation of membrane lipids, aggression of tissue membranes and proteins, or damage to DNA and enzyme and generally by oxidizing low-density lipoproteins (LDL). This may result in significant damage to cell structure, contributing to various diseases, such as cancer, stroke, diabetes, arthritis, hemorrhagic shock, coronary artery diseases, cataract, cancer, and acquired immune deficiency syndrome (AIDS) as well as age-related degenerative brain diseases [26]. Under normal circumstances, the cell can reduce the impact of these free radicals and ROS by an endogenous system, i.e., by the body's natural antioxidant defense mechanisms. Physiologic antioxidant defenses include the ROS-detoxifying enzymes superoxide dismutase (SOD), catalase, glutathione peroxidases, and peroxiredoxins [27]. However, the following factors or conditions may contribute to the overproduction of ROS and antioxidant depletion: the mitochondrial electron transport chain; excessive stimulation of nicotinamide adenine dinucleotide phosphate (NADPH); exposure to environmental pollutants such as cigarette smoke, ultraviolet (UV) rays, radiation and toxic chemicals which weaken the body's defense system; and exposure to explosion-generated shock waves [28, 29]. It becomes evidently clear that the devastating impact of ROS can only be reduced successfully through exogenous systems. There is therefore the need to provide the body with a constant supply of antioxidants through dietary supplementation. Antioxidants are postulated to help control wound oxidative stress and thereby accelerate wound healing. They are important mediators in regulating the damage that is potentially incurred by biological molecules such as DNA, protein, lipids, and body tissue in the presence of reactive species.

3.2. Antioxidants

Antioxidants are substances that prevent oxidation to occur. They are compounds that detoxify ROS to prevent their damaging effects through multi-mechanisms. Antioxidants may offer resistance against the oxidative stress by scavenging free radicals, inhibiting lipid peroxidation and thus preventing disease. Antioxidants have the ability to prevent, delay, or ameliorate many of the effects of free radicals. During certain diseased state, as well as during aging, there is a need to boost the antioxidant abilities, thereby potentiating the immune mechanism [30]. The antioxidants preserve and stimulate the function of immune cells against homeostatic disturbances [31].

Synthetic antioxidants such as butylated hydroxyanisole (BHA), butylated hydroxytoluene (BHT), and tertiary butylhydroquinone (TBHQ) are commonly employed as preservatives or additives by pharmaceutical, cosmetic, and food companies [32]. The free radicals are known to be scavenged by these synthetic antioxidants. However, reports on the involvement of synthetic antioxidants in chronic diseases and their adverse side effects leading to carcinogenicity have restricted their use in foods. Therefore, attention has been focused on natural antioxidants mainly from plant sources [33, 34].

3.3. Plants as important sources of natural antioxidants in wound healing

There is great interest in the use of natural products, which include compounds derived from fruits, plants, and herbs. Plants have an innate ability to synthesize a wide variety of phytochemicals. Plants do not only provide the carbohydrates, proteins, and fats necessary in the diet of man and other animals but also produce a vast range of organic materials to perform their normal physiological functions and to protect themselves from microbial pathogens and animal herbivores and to respond to environmental stress conditions. Hence plants accumulate a range of low- and high-molecular weight secondary metabolites that play important roles in ROS metabolism and avoidance of uncontrolled oxidation of essential biomolecules.

Consequently, plants have efficient complex enzymatic and non-enzymatic antioxidant defense systems to avoid the toxic effects of free radicals. Enzymatic systems include SOD, catalase (CAT), glutathione peroxidase (GPx), and glutathione reductase (GR), while non-enzymatic systems consist of low-molecular weight antioxidants (ascorbic acid, glutathione, proline, carotenoids, phenolic acids, flavonoids, etc.) and high-molecular weight secondary metabolites such as tannins [35, 36]. **Figure 1** gives a summary of the different classifications of antioxidants.

Among all secondary metabolites, phenolic compounds have been mentioned to be largely the contributory compound to antioxidant activity of plants since they have shown promising antioxidant activity in many in vivo and in vitro studies. Phenolic compounds exhibit a considerable free radical scavenging (antioxidant) activity, which is determined by their reactivity as hydrogen or electron-donating agents, the stability of the resulting antioxidant-derived radical, their reactivity with other antioxidants, and finally their metal-chelating properties [37, 38]. Similarly, polyphenols derived from plants are of great importance because of their potential antioxidant and antimicrobial properties [39]. Plant phenolics are mainly classified into five major groups as phenolic acids, flavonoids, lignans, stilbenes, and tannins. These classes of phytochemicals are found to have excellent antioxidant activity and are widely available for the treatment of a multitude of cutaneous ailments. Many studies have presented plants to possess great potential for wound healing because they are versatile as antioxidant and antimicrobial sources. Medicinal plants and their active compounds have been used in medicine since ancient times and are well known for their abilities to promote wound healing and prevent infection without grave side effects [40].

Flavonoids are a group of polyphenolic compounds with known properties which include free radical scavenging, inhibition of hydrolytic and oxidative enzymes, and anti-inflammatory action [41]. The best-described property of almost every group of flavonoids is their capacity to act as antioxidants. The flavones and catechins seem to be the most powerful flavonoids for protecting the body against reactive oxygen species. Flavonoids may have an additive effect to the endogenous scavenging compounds. Many in vitro studies have demonstrated the potent peroxyl radical scavenging abilities of flavonoids, which contribute to inhibiting lipid peroxidation and oxidation of LDL [42].

Flavonoids are known to possess protective effects in biological systems due to their capacity to transfer free radical electrons, chelate metal catalysts, activate antioxidant enzymes, reduce alpha-tocopherol radicals, and inhibit oxidases [43]. Flavonoids have lower redox potentials hence are able to reduce highly oxidizing free radicals by forming less reactive flavonoid radicals. As a result, they are able to prevent lipid peroxidation which is one of the most important actions of free radicals that leads to cellular membrane damage and, ultimately, to cell death [44]. Flavonoids are also able to scavenge nitric oxide which forms in combination with superoxide free radicals the highly damaging peroxynitrite and also to inhibit xanthine oxidase, an important biological source of superoxide radicals that can react with hydrogen peroxide to produce a more toxic hydroxyl radical [44].

Other flavonoids such as quercetin, kaempferol, myristin, apigenin, and luteolin also have anti-oxidative activity in many in vitro studies [45]. It has been observed that anthocyanins, which were one of the main antioxidant components in red wine, were the most effective, both in scavenging ROS and in inhibiting lipoprotein oxidation [46]. Quercetin is also known to have inhibited iron-catalyzed Fenton reaction (reaction between superoxide radicals with hydrogen peroxide).

The exogenous (dietary) antioxidants are mainly derived from food and medicinal plants, such as fruits, vegetables, cereals, mushrooms, beverages, flowers, spices, and traditional medicinal herbs [47]. A large number of plant species and their phytochemicals have diverse medicinal properties, and almost majority of these plants have been found to possess excellent antioxidant activity within in vitro assays.

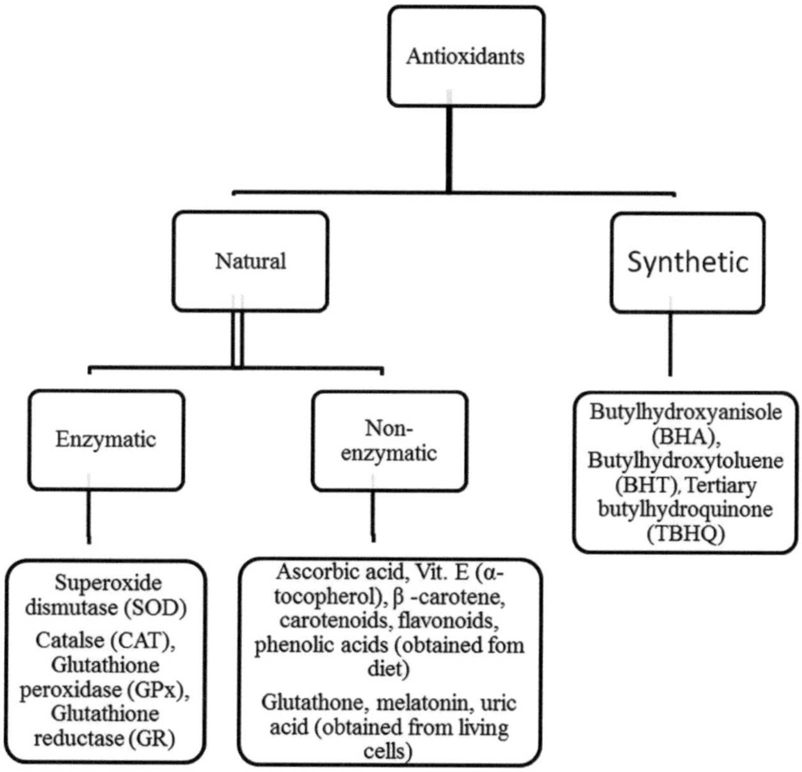

Figure 1. Flow chart showing the different classifications of antioxidants.

The natural function of vitamin E which is present in vegetable oils, nuts, and other fatty plant-based foods is to prevent oxidation. Vitamin E therefore acts as antioxidant when consumed. It helps to prevent degradation of cell membranes in regions containing C=C bonds. Some other antioxidants operate by different mechanisms, reacting with oxygen molecules (O_2) to prevent the production of free radicals. Additionally, there are numerous dietary antioxidants that can be consumed which contribute to an enhanced cellular protection. Ascorbic acid, for example, effectively scavenges ROS and resynthesizes α-tocopherol [48].

Similarly, a number of plants and plant isolates have been reported to protect free radical-induced damage in various experimental models. In recent times, focus on plant research has increased all over the world, and a large body of evidences has been collected to show the immense potential of medicinal plants used in various traditional systems. Green tea, for example, contains catechin components that are known to stimulate antioxidant activity by scavenging free radicals, inhibiting pro-oxidant enzymes and stimulating antioxidant enzymes [49]. Majority of these plants are endowed with free radical scavenging molecules, such as vitamins, terpenoids, phenolic acids, lignins, stilbenes, tannins, flavonoids, quinones, coumarins, alkaloids, amines, betalains, and other metabolites, which are rich in antioxidant activities [50].

Various plant products have been used in the treatment of wounds over the years. Wound healing phytochemical compounds fight infection, promote blood clotting, and accelerate the healing process. Numerous phytochemical compounds have been identified and synthesized from medicinal plants that have unique properties associated with the mechanism of wound healing. Interestingly, many of these wound healing plants investigated displayed antioxidant potential as their major unique properties. A plethora of examples of medicinal plants appears in literature to have shown both wound healing and antioxidant properties.

Clausena anisata (Willd) Hook. (Rutaceae) is a shrub widely used in many parts of West Africa including Ghana as therapeutic alternatives for the management of wounds and treatment of other bacterial and fungal infections. In a study conducted on the ethanol leaf, extract of *C. anisata* was found to exhibit antioxidant property with the half maximal inhibitory concentration (IC50) of 32.9 μg/mL. The extract enhanced the rate of wound closure and also exhibited high influence on proliferation of fibroblasts and levels of fibrous connective tissues in the wound bed [51].

Croton bonplandianum has been credited with potential to cure liver diseases, swelling of the body, cure against ring worms, and skin diseases. An investigation on the ethanolic and aqueous extracts of the dried leaves of *C. bonplandianum* on experimental excision wounds inflicted on Wistar Albino rats of either sex showed a definite, positive effect on wound healing, with significant increase in wound contraction. Antioxidant property of the extracts was also confirmed by 2,2-diphenyl-1-picryl-hydrazyl (DPPH) and nitric oxide scavenging activity [52].

Leucas lanata Wall. ex Benth. (Lamiaceae) is a medicinal plant whose juice has been traditionally used by local peoples to treat stomachache, headache, whooping cough, and as an antidote for reptile poison. Fresh leaves are applied externally for wound healing and for absorbing pus when placed on the affected area. A study designed to evaluate wound healing potential of *L. lanata* through the excision wound model and functional changes in biochemical indicators of antioxidant parameters using 10% (w/w) ointment of 50% ethanol extract showed a remarkable wound healing activity. In the study of uninfected wounds, epithelization period was reduced from 24.66 ± 0.97 for the control group treated with blank ointment to 12.16 ± 0.36 for the group treatment. Similarly, in the case of infected wounds with *Staphylococcus epidermidis*, the percentage of wound contraction was significantly enhanced. Also, the extract significantly increased superoxide dismutase and catalase and reduced glutathione when compared with the control group of infected and uninfected wounds [11].

Limonia acidissima Linn. is used traditionally in India for the treatment of tumors, asthma, wounds, cardiac debility, and hepatitis. Wound healing investigations using the excision, incision, and dead space wound models were carried out on the 200 and 400 mg/kg methanol extract doses. The wound contracted progressively when treated with the extracts. In the wounding healing, results for the incision and dead space models, breaking strength, hydroxyproline, and granulation tissue weight, as well as SOD and catalase all increased significantly ($p < 0.05$), following treatment with the extract and standard drug, when compared with the control group. Thus, the extract not only promoted wound healing but also exerted antioxidant activity [53].

Marrubium vulgare L. (Lamiaceae) is a gray-leaved herbaceous perennial medicinal plant well known for several pharmaceutical activities. It is traditionally employed against respiratory infections such as bronchitis, coughs, and asthma. An experiment carried out on the hydroalcoholic leaf extract showed a good activity, with the half maximal effective concentration (EC50) of 38.56 ± 0.10 µg/mL (DPPH assay). A preliminary MTT [3-(4,5-dimethylthiazol-2-yl)-2,5-diphenyltetrazolium bromide-tetrazolium dye] test with 5 µg/mL concentration was noncytotoxic and able to improve fibroblast growth. This capability was subsequently confirmed by the results of in vitro wound healing test that led to the conclusion that *M. vulgare* might be effective against skin injuries [2].

Morinda citrifolia (Noni) has been traditionally used to treat broken bones, deep cuts, bruises, sores, and wounds. It is also reported to have a broad range of nutritional and therapeutic values for cancer, infection, arthritis, diabetes, asthma, hypertension, and pain. Investigating the effect of *M. citrifolia* leaves on experimental wounds and lipid peroxide levels in rats resulted in ample evidences confirming that *M. citrifolia* enhances wound healing by acting on various phases of the wound healing process. There was a significant increase in wound contraction rate, skin breaking strength that reflected increased collagen levels. The findings from the investigation also showed a decrease in lipid peroxide level in the *M. citrifolia*-treated group [54].

Musa paradisiaca (plantain) is a crop in the genus *Musa* that is indigenous to tropical and subtropical countries. To validate the ethnotherapeutic claims of the plant in skin diseases, wound healing activity was studied, besides antioxidant activity to understand the mechanism of wound healing activity. Methanol and hexane extracts of *M. paradisiaca* peel were used to evaluate the biological activity (antioxidant and wound healing) on the regenerative process of the epithelial tissue. The two extracts showed a good inhibition of DPPH radical; the hexane has an activity of 94.25% and methanol 87.33% at a concentration of 125 µg/mL compared with BHT 43.22% as a control. Wound closure was significantly more advanced in the treated groups (methanol 94.62%, hexane 88.39%) compared with control groups 81.75% at

15 days. The results suggested that extracts obtained with methanol has potential to stimulate the healing process in a close relation to antioxidant properties more that hexane extracts [55].

Phaleria macrocarpa is a traditional medicinal plant from New Guinea, Papua Island, and Indonesia. It is used to treat cancer, diabetes, ulcers, and hypercholesterolemia. Topical application of *P. macrocarpa* fruit extracts on skin excision wounds in rats resulted in an improved wound contraction rate and considerable reduction in healing time. The extract showed significant healing effect on excision wounds and demonstrated an important role in the inflammation process by increasing antioxidant enzyme activities, thereby accelerating the wound healing process and reducing tissue injury [56].

Polygonatum odoratum is an important herbal medicine used in folk medicine for the treatment of various elements. Its leaf extract is known to have possessed strong antioxidant, antibacterial, and anti-breast cancer activity. Topical application of ethanol leaf extract of this plant on the rate of wound healing closure using male Sprague Dawley rats in an excision wound healing model significantly accelerated the rate of wound healing with less inflammatory cells and more collagen with angiogenesis [57].

Sphaeranthus amaranthoides is a medicinal plant used in folklore medicine in India for the treatment of skin diseases. The evaluation of antioxidant activity of the methanol extract and its flavonoid fraction by using DPPH free radical scavenging activity, total antioxidant capacity, and total phenolic content showed variable degrees of antioxidant activity. When wound healing activity was studied in excision wound model in rats, both the methanol extract and the flavonoid fraction exhibited better wound healing activity than the standard drug (silver sulfadiazine). The methanolic extract and flavonoid fraction significantly enhanced the rate of wound contraction and the period of epithelialization comparable to silver sulfadiazine [58].

In my study of wound healing medicinal plants, 26 wound healing plants used among the people of Kpando Traditional Area for effective wound healing have been identified. In vitro investigations on four of these plants, namely, *Anogeissus leiocarpus*, *Amaranthus spinosus*, *Corchorus olitorius*, and *Combretum dolichopetalum*, exhibited wound healing efficacies and antioxidant properties.

The enhanced wound healing potency of various herbal extracts, therefore, may be partly attributed to free radical scavenging action of the phytoconstituents present in plant extracts.

4. Conclusions

Many plants used traditionally in treatment of wound possess antioxidant activity. It is evidently clear that wound healing and repair are accelerated by applying plant extracts that are rich in antioxidant phytochemicals. The assertion made that wound healing and antioxidant activity coexist, to some extent, can be confirmed. Researchers are encouraged to intensify their search for plants for the treatment of wounds with novel antioxidant activity that could be beneficial in therapeutic practice.

Acknowledgements

I am grateful to the University of Cape Coast for their support.

Conflict of interest

Author declared no conflict of interest.

Author details

Victor Y.A. Barku

Address all correspondence to: vbarku@ucc.edu.gh

Department of Chemistry, School of Physical Sciences, University of Cape Coast, Ghana

References

[1] Balachandar R, Saran Prakash L, Ashok Kumar K, Ragavi A, Gurumoorthy P. Antioxidant activity and wound healing potential of selected medicinal plants. Journal of Chemical and Pharmaceutical Sciences. 2014;**2**:100-103

[2] Amri B, Martino EID, Vitulo EID, Corana F, Ben-Kaâb LB, Rui M, et al. *Marrubium vulgare* L. leave extract: Phytochemical composition, antioxidant and wound healing properties. Molecules. 2017;**22**:1851. DOI: 10.3390/molecules22111851T

[3] Frykber RG, Banks J. Challenges in the treatment of chronic wounds. Advances in Wound Care. 2015;**4**:560-582

[4] Mackay D, Miller AL. Nutritional support for wound healing. Alternative Medicine Review. 2003;**8**:359-377

[5] Schwentker A, Vodovotz Y, Weller R, Billiar TR. Nitric oxide and wound repair: Role of cytokines? Nitric Oxide. 2002;**7**:1-10

[6] Edwards J, Howley P, Cohen IK. In vitro inhibition of human neutrophil elastase by oleic acid albumin formulations from derivatized cotton wound dressings. International Journal of Pharmaceutics. 2004;**284**:1-12

[7] Somashekar Shetty B. Wound healing and indigenous drugs: Role as antioxidants: A review. Research and Reviews: Journal of Medical and Health Sciences. 2013;**2**(2):5-15

[8] Fikru A, Makonnen E, Eguale T, Debella A, Mekonnen GA. Evaluation of in vivo wound healing activity of methanol extract of *Achyranthes aspera* L. Journal of Ethnopharmacology. 2012;**143**:469-474

[9] Ammar I, Bardaa S, Mzid M, Sahnoun Z, Rebaii T, Attia H, et al. Antioxidant, antibacterial land in vivo dermal wound healing effects of Opuntia flower extracts. International Journal of Biological Macromolecules. 2015;**81**:483-490

[10] Paarakh PM, Chansouria JPN, Khosa RL. Wound healing activity of *Annona muricata* extract. Journal of Pharmacy Research. 2009;**2**:404-406

[11] Dixit V, Verma P, Agnihotri P, Paliwal AK, Rao CV, Husain T. Antimicrobial, antioxidant and wound healing properties of *Leucas lanata* Wall. ex Benth. The Journal of Phytopharmacology. 2015;**4**(1):9-16

[12] Kayode OA. Epidemiological study on wound distribution pattern in horses presented at two veterinary clinics in south west, Nigeria between 2007-2010. Journal of Dairy, Veterinary & Animal Research. 2017;**5**(4):00148. DOI: 10.15406/jdvar.2017.05.00148

[13] Alonso JE, Lee J, Burgess AR, Browner BD. The management of complex orthopaedic injuries. The Surgical Clinics of North America. 1996;**76**(4):879-903

[14] Velnar T, Bailey T, Smrkolj V. The wound healing process: An overview of the cellular and molecular mechanisms. The Journal of International Medical Research. 2009; **37**:1528-1542

[15] Open Wound Basics. https://www.woundcarecenters.org/article/wound-basics/open-wound-basics

[16] Gilmore MA. Phases of wound healing. Dimensions in Oncology Nursing. 1991;**5**(3):32-34

[17] Mercandetti M. Wound Healing and Repair, 2017. Available from: https://emedicine.medscape.com/article/1298129-overview

[18] Maxson S, Lopez EA, Yoo D, Danilkovitch-Miagkova A, Leroux MA. Concise review: Role of mesenchymal stem cells in wound repair. Stem Cells Translational Medicine. 2012;**1**(2):142-149

[19] Dunnill C, Patton T, Brennan J, Barrett J, Dryden M, Cooke J, et al. Reactive oxygen species (ROS) and wound healing: The functional role of ROS and emerging ROS-modulating technologies for augmentation of the healing process. International Wound Journal. 2017;**14**:89-96. DOI: 10.1111/iwj.12557

[20] Nita M, Grzybowski A. The role of the reactive oxygen species and oxidative stress in the pathomechanism of the age-related ocular diseases and other pathologies of the anterior and posterior eye segments in adults. Oxidative Medicine and Cellular Longevity. 2016;**2016**:3164734. DOI: 10.1155/2016/3164734

[21] Underdown MJ. Antioxidants and wound healing [thesis]. East Tennessee: East Tennessee University; 2013

[22] Finkel T, Holbrook NJ. Oxidants, oxidative stress and the biology of ageing. Nature. 2000;**408**(6809):239-247

[23] Sathya M, Kkilavani R. Phytochemical screening and in vitro antioxidant activity of *Saccharum spontaneum Linn*. International Journal of Pharmaceutical Sciences Review and Research. 2013;**18**(11):75-79

[24] Visioli F, Keaney JF, Halliwell B. Antioxidants and cardiovascular disease; pancrease or tonics for tired sheep. Cardiovascular Research. 2000;**47**(3):409

[25] Tosun M, Ercisli S, Sengul M, Oezr H, Polat T, Ozturk E. Antioxidant properties and phenolic content of eight salvia species from Turkey. Biological Research. 2009;**42**:175-181

[26] Parr A, Bolwell GP. PhEnols in the plant and in man: The potential for possible nutritional enhancement of the diet by modifying the phenols content or profile. Journal of the Science of Food and Agriculture. 2000;**80**:985-1015

[27] Arouma OI. Nutrition and health aspect of free radical and antioxidants. Food and Chemical Toxicology. 1994;**32**:671-683

[28] Elsayed NM, Gorbunov NV. Interplay between high energy impulse noise (blast) and antioxidants in the lung. Toxicology. 2003;**189**:63-67

[29] Valkov M, Leibfritz D, Moncol J, Cronin MTD, Mazur M, Telser J. Free radicals and antioxidants in normal physiological functions and human disease. The International Journal of Biochemistry & Cell Biology. 2006;**7**(1):45-78

[30] Devasagayam TPA, Sainis KB. Immune system and antioxidants, especially those derived from Indian medicinal plants. Indian Journal of Experimental Biology. 2002;**40**:639-655

[31] De la Fuente M, Victor M. Antioxidants as modulators of immune function. Immunology and Cell Biology. 2000;**78**(1):n49-n54

[32] Nguyen Q, Eun J. Antioxidant activity of solvent extracts from Vietnamese medicinal plants. Journal of Medicinal Plant Research. 2011;**5**(13):2798-2811

[33] Dehghan G, Shafiee A, Ghahremani M, Ardestani S, Abdollahi M. Antioxidant potential of various extracts from Ferulaszovitsiana in relation to their phenolic contents. Pharmaceutical Biology. 2007;**45**(9):1-9

[34] Kai-Wei L, Chiung-Hui L, Huang-Yao T, Horng-Huey K, Bai-Luh W. Antioxidant prenylflavonoids from *Artocarpus communis* and *Artocarpus elasticus*. Food Chemistry. 2009; **115**:558-562

[35] Lobo V, Patil A, Phatak A, Chandra N. Free radicals, antioxidants and functional foods: Impact on human health. Pharmacognosy Reviews. 2010;**4**(8):118-126. DOI: 10.4103/0973-7847.70902

[36] Kasote DM, Katyare SS, Hegde MV, Bae H. Significance of antioxidant potential of plants and its relevance to therapeutic applications. International Journal of Biological Sciences. 2015;**11**(8):982-991. DOI: 10.7150/ijbs.12096

[37] Tuadhar ET, Rao A. Plasma protein oxidation and total antioxidant power in premenstrual syndrome. Asian Pacific Journal of Tropical Medicine. 2010;**3**(3):237-240

[38] Wojdylo A, Oszmianski J, Czmerys R. Antioxidant phenolic compounds in 32 selected herbs. Food Chemistry. 2007;**105**:940-949

[39] Kumbhare MR, Guleha V, Sivakumar T. Estimation of total phenolic content, cytotoxicity and in vitro antioxidant activity of stem bark of Moringa oleifera. Asian Pacific Journal of Tropical Disease. 2012; **2**(2):144-150

[40] Budovsky A, Yarmolinsky L, Ben-Shabat S. Effect of medicinal plants on wound healing. Wound Repair and Regeneration. 2015;**23**:171-183

[41] Frankel EN, Waterhouse AL, Kinsella JE. Inhibition of human LDL oxidation by resveratrol. Lancet. 1995;**341**:454-457

[42] Castelluccio C, Paganga G, Melikian N, Bolwell GP, Pridham J, Sampson J, et al. Antioxidant potential of intermediates in phenylpropanoid metabolism in higher plants. FEBS Letters. 1995;**368**:188-192

[43] Hirano R, Sasamoto W, Matsumoto A, Itakura H, Igarashi O, Kondo K. Antioxidant ability of various flavonoids against DPPH radicals and LDL oxidation. Journal of Nutritional Science and Vitaminology (Tokyo). 2001;**47**:357-362

[44] Cuyckens F, Claeys M. Mass spectrometry in structural analysis of flavonoids. Journal of Mass Spectrometry. 2004;**39**:1-15

[45] Frankel EN, Kanner J, German JB, Parks E, Kinsella JE. Inhibition of oxidation of human low-density lipoprotein by phenolic substances in red wine. Lancet. 1993;**341**:454-457

[46] Ghiselli A, Nardini M, Baldi A, Scaccini C. Antioxidant activity of different phenolic fractions separated from an Italian red wine. Journal of Agricultural and Food Chemistry. 1998;**46**:361-367

[47] Dong-Pi X, Li Y, Meng X, Zhou T, Zhou Y, Zheng J, et al. Natural antioxidants in foods and medicinal plants: Extraction, assessment and resources. International Journal of Molecular Sciences. 2017;**18**:96. DOI: 10.3390/ijms18010096

[48] Williamson J, Hughes CM, Davison GW. Exogenous plant-based nutraceutical supplementation and peripheral cell mononuclear DNA damage following high intensity exercise. Antioxidants. 2018;**7**:70. DOI: 10.3390/antiox7050070

[49] Modi AJ, Khadabadi SS, Deokate UA, Farooqui IA, Deore SL, Gangwani MR. *Argyreia speciosa* Linn. F: Phytochemistry, pharmacognosy and pharmacological studies. Journal of Pharmacognosy and Phytotherapy. 2010;**293**:34-42

[50] Amutha Iswarya Devi J, Kottai Muthu A. Phytochemical screening, antioxidant activities and total phenolic content of ethanolic extract from whole plant of *Saccharum spontaneum* (Linn.). International Journal of Chemical and Pharmaceutical Sciences. 2014;**5**(2):112-118

[51] Agyepong N, Agyare C, Ossei PPS, Duah Boakye Y. Antioxidant and in vivo wound healing activities of *Clausena anisata*. European Journal of Medicinal Plants. 2015;**10**(2):1-8

[52] Divya S, Naveen Krishna K, Ramachandran S, Dhanaraju MD. Wound healing and in vitro antioxidant activities of *Croton bonplandianum* leaf extract in rats. Global Journal of Pharmacology. 2011;**5**(3):159-163

[53] Ilango K, Chitra V. Wound healing and anti-oxidant activities of the fruit pulp of *Limonia Acidissima* Linn (Rutaceae) in rats. Tropical Journal of Pharmaceutical Research. 2010;**9**(3):223-230

[54] Pandurang Rasal VP, Sinnathambi A, Ashok P, Yeshmaina S. Wound healing and antioxidant activities of *Morinda citrifolia* leaf extract in rats. Iranian Journal of Pharmacology and Therapeutics. 2008;**7**:49-52

[55] Canales-Aguirre A, Carvallo-Aceves A, Manzano-Chávez L, Padilla-Camberos E, Lugo-Cervantes E. Wound healing and antioxidant activities of extracts from *Musa paradisiaca* L. peel. Planta Medica. 2008;**74**:PD9. DOI: 10.1055/s-0028-1084684

[56] Abood WN, Al-Henhena NA, Abood AN, Al-Obaidi MMJ, Ismail S, Abdulla MA, et al. Wound-healing potential of the fruit extract of Phaleria macrocarpa. Bosnian Journal of Basic Medical Sciences. 2015;**15**(2):25-30

[57] Mughrabi FF, Hashim H, Mahmood AA, Suzy SM, Salmah I, Zahra AA, et al. Acceleration of wound healing activity by *Polygonatum odoratum* leaf extract in rats. Journal of Medicinal Plant Research. 2014;**8**(13):523-528. DOI: 10.5897/JMPR10.451

[58] Geethalakshmi R, Sakravarthi C, Kritika T, Arul Kirubakaran M, Sarada DVL. Evaluation of antioxidant and wound healing potentials of *Sphaeranthus amaranthoides* Burm.f. Bio Med Research International. 2013;**2013**:7. DOI: 10.1155/2013/607109

Chapter 6

The Strategies of Natural Polysaccharide in Wound Healing

Juin-Hong Cherng

Additional information is available at the end of the chapter

http://dx.doi.org/10.5772/intechopen.80812

Abstract

Severe or chronic wounds related to diseases or serious incidents have received big attention from not only a scientific standpoint but also a business perspective. Therefore, an effective treatment to abridge the long-term hospitalization of severe wound becomes indispensable. Glycosaminoglycan (GAG), one of the extracellular matrix molecules produced by fibroblasts, participates in cell-cell and cell-matrix interactions, in cell proliferation and migration, and in cytokine and growth factor signaling associated with all phases of wound recovery. Natural polysaccharide, for example, calcium alginate, which consists of mainly differing ratios of D-mannuronic and L-guluronic acid and rich of calcium ions, has been demonstrated to functionalize the glycosaminoglycan activity during wound healing. Once the trigger of the underlying wound healing mechanisms was understood, it should be possible to find ways to enhance and resolve the wound healing process in the patient with conditions and may lead to the potential for treatment alternatives in the future clinical field.

Keywords: glycosaminoglycan (GAG), extracellular matrix (ECM) molecules, cytokines, natural polysaccharide, wound healing

1. Introduction

Wound injuries are the most common health problem people faced in decades and continuously demand advanced wound management strategies to obtain optimal healing. Wound injuries can range from small wounds caused by daily activities to chronic or severe wounds caused by diseases or serious incidents. Besides the type of wound being treated, the effectiveness of wound management also involves a better understanding of different factors such as the healing process and the physical-chemical properties of the available dressings [1]. Mostly in small wounds, tissue injuries will heal completely with normal healing phases within weeks [2]. On the other hand, severe or chronic wounds are hard to heal within months or a year and often reoccur with persistent inflammation [3], which represent major challenges to patients medically and financially. Therefore, proper wound dressings that have the ability to accelerate the wound healing phases and reduce the healing time simultaneously are required to overcome this problem.

Glycosaminoglycans (GAG) are extracellular matrix molecules that have significant roles in the control of the all wound healing phases, either an acute wound or severe wound, such as an effective mediator of angiogenesis and inflammation [4, 5] and promote the wound recovery by leading to rapid granulation, vascularization, and reepithelialization [6]. As a GAG-rich content, the use of natural polysaccharide as wound dressing-based material is proposed to enhance the healing phases, especially to abridge the long-term healing mechanism in severe wound injury, determined by several studies and clinical trials. This chapter will further discuss the detail mechanisms and efficacy of natural polysaccharide in accelerating the wound healing process, thereby intended to encourage the advanced strategies for future wound management.

2. The involvement of glycosaminoglycan during wound healing

Generally, wound healing has been represented with the complexity and overlapping of its phases. These processes integrate a dynamic interaction between cells and extracellular matrix (ECM) that trigger tissue or organ regeneration. The significant roles of ECM and its components during each stage of the healing process are represented by structural matrix provision and function of signal transduction compliance in the dynamic of biological reactions during each stage of the healing process [7, 8–11].

ECM provides structural and functional integrity to connective tissues and organs [12]; yet its synthesis and deposition mainly occur in response to growth factors, cytokines, and mechanical signals mediated via cell surface receptors [13]. In the case of wound healing, ECM consists of at least four major classes [8]: (1) structural proteins such as the collagens and elastin; (2) multidomain adhesive glycoproteins such as fibronectin, vitronectin, and laminin; (3) glycosaminoglycan (GAG) such as hyaluronic acid (HA), proteoglycans (PGs) including versican, syndecans, glypicans, aggrecan, and perlecan (chondroitin sulfate (CS)/dermatan sulfate (DS), and heparin sulfate (HS))—and keratin sulfate (KS), often in large amounts; and (4) matricellular proteins such as secreted protein acidic and rich in cysteine (SPARC, also known as osteonectin and BM-40), thrombospondins 1 and 2, tenascin C and X, and osteopontin.

GAG is the important constituent of the extracellular matrix found on cell surfaces [14] and widely distributed in connective tissues. GAG is composed of characteristic repeating disaccharides, with specific monosaccharides sulfated at each of C_2, C_3, C_4, and C_6 [15]. These compounds are highly anionic polymers, which interact with many cationic species (such as ions and proteins) due to the presence of the carboxylic acid and sulfate functional groups [16]. The negative ion charge of GAG molecules carries was considered substantial in many biological processes.

Among the various molecules secreted by ECM, the GAG has partners that have significant roles in the control of the all wound healing phases, either acute wound or severe wound. Those molecules participate in cell-cell and cell-matrix interactions, in cell proliferation and migration, and in cytokine and growth factor signaling, thus locally modulating their biologic activities. In an acute wound, the healing progresses through the normal phases of wound healing (hemostasis, inflammation, proliferation, and remodeling) within weeks, while in a severe wound, those phases do not progress normally, mostly within months or years, thus needing an appropriate supplementary treatment to enhance the healing process. Therefore, GAG or GAG-containing material treatment is expected to become a key to turning and accelerating not only acute wound but also especially severe or chronic wound healing problems.

2.1. Role of glycosaminoglycan in acute wound healing

2.1.1. Hemostasis phase of wound healing

Hemostasis is the beginning of the wound healing process and may be defined as the interaction between platelets and vessel of vascular injury. The vital mediators of hemostasis are fibrin, platelets, and blood vessels. In the first 1 or 2 hours after injury, wound repair starts with the formation of a fibrin matrix through the proteolytic cleavage of fibrinogen by thrombin, and fibrin directly binds to platelets to produce a clot [17–21]. The α granules of platelets release numerous growth factors, such as PDGF, TGF-α, TGF-β, bFGF, IGF-1, and VEGF [22, 23]. Further, PDGF and IGF-1 call up and activate the fibroblasts as well as synthesize GAG and collagen to lead the migration and proliferation of the cells into the wound site [24, 25].

The enzymes of the fibrinolytic resist the clot formation. On the other hand, serpins ensure that excessive fibrinolytic activity does not occur. The ECM contains a network of scaffold proteins that are linked by GAG. GAG, especially HS, plays a key role as anticoagulants that have important acts to manage the regulations of many of the serpins [15]. HS represents 50–90% of the total GAG content [25] and is only in contact with blood when an injury occurs [26, 27]. HS has been identified binding with more than 100 proteins involved in hemostasis, many growth factors, proteins involved in lipid metabolism, and proteins of the ECM [28]. In addition, HS maintains hemostasis as an effective mediator of angiogenesis at the surface of endothelial cells [4].

Summarily, the hemostasis phase begins the healing process, generates blood clot formation which maintains the structure of vessels, and provides a temporary matrix, secreting cytokines and other growth factors, in order to prepare the wound bed for the next phase of the healing process.

2.1.2. Inflammatory phase of wound healing

The inflammatory response is elicited by infection or tissue injury involved in the distribution of blood components (plasma and leukocytes) to the damage site [29, 30]. This phase occurs in the next 24–48 hours after injury on average accompanied by inflammation symptoms, such as redness, body heat, swelling, and pain around the wounded place [31]. Once the bleeding is controlled, the key cells of the inflammatory response such as neutrophils, macrophages, and lymphocytes assemble into the wound site, simultaneously release a large number of active mediators (cytokines and growth factors), and thus stimulate the inflammatory phase [32–34].

HA, a non-sulfated GAG of the ECM, is involved in a significant process of the inflammatory phase. During this phase, HA assembles in the wound bed and regulates early inflammation to modulate inflammatory cell and fibroblast cell migration, pro-inflammatory cytokine synthesis, and the phagocytosis of invading microbes [5]. Moreover, HA may bind and improve the efficiency of chemokines to neutrophils. Butler et al. revealed that HA appeared able to present stimuli to neutrophils [35]. HA on the endothelial surface was increased as well as the efficiency of recruitment of neutrophils. In the inflammatory phase, neutrophils collagenase and elastase eliminate damaged tissue from the temporary matrix of the wound site, while monocytes transform into macrophages and phagocytose fragments of denatured ECM debriding the wound site and inactivating any source of microbial infection through the activity of secreted proteases.

At sites of inflammation, the low-molecular-weight HA fragments (accumulated from degradation of high-molecular-weight HA) can initiate Toll-like receptor 2 and Toll-like receptor 4 induction of pro-inflammatory cytokines IL-6, TNF-α, and IL-1β [36]. Furthermore, the growth factors and cytokines released by the inflammatory cells induce the migration and proliferation of fibroblast and keratinocyte, which synthesize the levels of HA. All along the reepithelialization process, where epithelial cells migrate across the new tissue to form a barrier between the wound and the environment, the level of HA was found significantly elevated [37]. The secretion of cytokines such as TGF-β, PDGF, FGF-2, IL-1, and TNF-α modulate collagen deposition by fibroblasts and penetration of new blood vessels into the wound site.

2.1.3. Proliferation phase of wound healing

During the proliferation phase of wound healing, over the next 2 or 3 days and lasts for about 2 weeks thereafter, the layer of a new matrix by fibroblasts restores the tissue at the wound site. The other mesenchymal cells also enter the inflammatory site of the wound in response to growth factors that are necessary for the stimulation of cell proliferation [38]. Moreover, fibroblasts, endothelial cells, and keratinocytes produce IGF-I, FGF-2, TGF-β, PDGF, and VEGF, promoting cell migration and proliferation, matrix synthesis, and angiogenesis.

The fibroblasts synthesize collagen and PGs. Both of them act to form an unstructured connective tissue medium that provides new cells to migrate. A number of PGs were presented in the wound site, and their GAG side chains were involved in the stabilization and activation of growth factors [15]. Sulfated PGs with CS and DS contribute in collagen polymerization [39], and HS PGs on cells can create anchors to the surrounding matrix [40]. The PGs provide a matrix for cellular attachment, and some PGs (hyalectans) form ternary complexes with HA hydrating the tissue promoting cell survival and migration above the granulation tissue to cover the wound site.

2.1.4. Remodeling phase of wound healing

Remodeling is the final phase of wound healing which is achieved over longer periods of up to a year after the initial wound injury [41]. This phase is characterized by wound surface contraction [42]. During this phase, new epithelium forms along with the transition of granulation tissue to a mature scar. This process is accompanied by high mechanic strength of the formed tissue, reduction of capillary amounts by combining into bigger blood vessels, lowering cell density and metabolic activity of the tissue, and lowering the content of GAG [43, 44]. The mechanic strength of the formed tissue equals 25% related to the dermis and equals 80% related to the unchanged tissue after many months of reconstruction [43, 45, 46]. Considering that GAG activities are able to reduce the inflammatory responses and ECM deposition in the early phases of wound healing, a proper wound handling in the beginning of injury with a GAG-rich-containing material is expected to heal the wound more closely to normal skin and reduce the period of this phase.

2.2. Role of glycosaminoglycan in severe or chronic wound healing

Severe or chronic wounds, hard-to-heal wounds related to diseases or serious incidents, were also commonly encountered instead of acute wounds. Mostly, this issue has been associated with the aging of the population. Unlike acute wounds, the treatment and management of severe wounds represent major challenges to patients medically and financially, resulting in a long-term recovery.

Severe wounds are frequently characterized by persistent injury and prolonged inflammation, high incidence of bacterial biofilms, and excessive proteolysis [3]. Impairment of macrophage function and angiogenic response is also suggested, which are mostly related to severe wounds healing process [47, 48]. Due to the prolonged inflammation, an excessive recruitment of inflammatory cells to the wound bed will be incurred and produced by the large numbers of neutrophils. It is known that neutrophils can eliminate damaged tissue from the temporary matrix of the wound site and prevent microbial infection. On the other hand, however, the unmanageable neutrophils' potential to kill pathogens also can lead to excessive protease production that initiates significant tissue damage to the host which is harmful to wound healing as they cause degradation of the ECM and growth factors [16]. Furthermore, the inefficient cell proliferation due to ECM molecule degradation within the wound leads to impaired angiogenesis that indicates further wound bed defacement and impaired healing. Hence, in order to conquer this issue, the prevention of prolonged inflammation is a goal strategy in severe wound therapy.

GAG has been found to bind to neutrophils, macrophages, and lymphocytes which are the key cells of the inflammatory response. The effect of excessive protease production caused by too many activated neutrophils in the wound site can be inhibited by electrostatic binding with certain anionic polymers such as GAG or functionalized dextrans [16]. The highly anionic nature of GAG that was expected would be ion pairing with the cationic neutrophils to interfere the activity of these cationic proteins via charge interactions. Therefore, it may be possible that by this mechanism the excessive neutrophil recruitment is reduced and the wound can pass from the inflammatory stage to the next stage of healing.

However, after serious tissue injury, the glycanases and proteases can destroy GAG [49]. The lack of GAG in severe wounds can be fixed with the addition of GAG-containing material, such as a natural polysaccharide, directly into the wound site as a wound dressing. With the rich source of GAG at the wound environment and a better understanding of GAG roles in healing processes, it has been possible to formulate therapeutic strategies which are expected to accelerate severe wound healing.

3. Natural polysaccharide in wound healing

3.1. The properties of natural polysaccharide

Glycosaminoglycan (GAG) has been shown to perform significant roles in cell signaling and development, angiogenesis, anticoagulation, and co-receptors for growth factors, which belong to the control of the all wound healing phases, both of acute wound and severe wound. GAG is an enormous complex of carbohydrate molecules that interact with several proteins involved in physiological and pathological processes [50, 51]. GAG, with a molecular weight roughly around 10–100 kDa, is a linear negatively charged polysaccharide. This electrostatic characteristic is useful for managing the excessive protease production through ion pairing with the cationic neutrophils and interfering the activity of these cationic proteins via charge interactions [16]. Once the excessive neutrophil recruitment is reduced as well as the excessive protease production, the wound can pass efficiently from the inflammatory stage to the next stage of healing, especially for severe wound injury.

Polysaccharides, especially natural polysaccharide, have been extensively used in wound-dressing development due to their properties such as being biocompatible, nonimmunogenic, and antimicrobial [52–54]. They appeared as abundant sources in many different forms of plants and production in the body. Based on their availability, a natural polysaccharide with different chemical structures and physical properties represents a large source of materials for progressive applications in the future, especially in the domain of biomaterials for the medical field [55, 56].

Containing a beta-1,3-D-glucan linker, natural polysaccharides contribute to the wound healing process because of their ability to stimulate immune system activation by activating macrophages that clean up the wound site after injury [57]. The macrophage is one of the major inflammatory cells in wounds. It has many substantial functions during wound healing, such as host defense, the promotion and resolution of inflammation, the removal of apoptotic cells, and the support of cell proliferation and tissue restoration following injury [58]. In several studies, natural polysaccharides have been shown to enhance macrophage cytotoxic activity against tumor cells and microorganisms and activate phagocytic activity by escalated reactive oxygen species (ROS) and nitric oxide (NO) production [59–61]. These abilities are useful for enhancing the quality of the wound healing process.

3.2. The effect of natural polysaccharide structure in wound healing: animal studies

Alginate, chitosan, and hyaluronic acid are mainly natural polysaccharides that are considered as good candidates for the management of wounds in decades. Alginate, as a prominent example of a natural polysaccharide with the abundance of GAG, has been utilized to become platforms used for fabricating wound dressing materials. Spun as calcium alginate wound dressing, a severe wound injury in swine model treated with this material exhibited a rapid reepithelialization and less scar formation, which appeared with a smooth wound, compared to commonly used wound dressing [62]. The ability of natural polysaccharide reduces scar formation in severe wound injury due to its rich content of GAG which was known to promote wound healing and leads to rapid granulation, vascularization, and reepithelialization, thus yielding a minimum scar formation certainly [6]. As well, once the dressing is attached with the wound, an ion exchange reaction occurs between the calcium in the alginate and the sodium in the exudate, producing a soluble gel which in turn helps maintain a moist wound environment [63]. A moist wound environment will prevent the scab's formation and facilitate the growth and migration of cells to optimize the formation of new tissues.

Regarding immune system activation, the release of pro-inflammatory cytokines, such as IL-1β, IL-6, IL-8, IFN-γ, and TNF-α, after wound injury also takes an important part during the wound healing process. Various crucial processes at the wound site, such as stimulation of keratinocyte and fibroblast proliferation, synthesis and breakdown of ECM proteins, and regulation of immune response, were handled with these cytokines [64]. Their expressions were shown to be intensely upregulated during the inflammatory phase of healing and strongly reduced after wound healing was impaired [65].

Natural polysaccharide, by its oligosaccharides (β-glucan, xyloglucan, chitin, pectin, D-mannuronic, and L-guluronic), can stimulate human cells to produce cytokines [66, 67]. Particularly, the mechanism of β-glucan is mediated by several receptors including dectin-1 receptor, Toll-like receptors (2, 4, 6), complement receptor 3, scavenger receptor, and lactosylceramide [68]. Once binding to the dectin-1, as the most important receptor, β-glucan stimulates the production of many cytokines or activates other immune and nonimmune reaction mechanisms [69]. Martins et al. demonstrated that a polysaccharide-rich fraction of *Agaricus brasiliensis* is able to regulate the host response by activating both pro- and anti-inflammatory mechanisms, thus increasing the production of TNF-α and IL-1β by human monocytes through modulation of Toll-like receptor 4 and Toll-like receptor 2 expression [70]. In addition, even after TLR blockade, these polysaccharides still activated the monocytes to produce considerable levels of IFN-γ, IL-1β, and IL-10. TNF-α and IFN-γ were recognized as the important agents of the anti-mycobacterial cytokine cascade, and IL-10 was considered as an inhibitory cytokine which is important to the adequate balance between inflammatory and immunopathological responses [71]. On the other hand, IL-1β is known as a critical mediator of inflammation which is involved in neutrophil mobilization, cellular adhesion to the endothelium, and white blood cell infiltration [72, 73]. Zhao et al. determined the wound healing effect of an *Astragalus membranaceus* polysaccharide treatment and its mechanism through in vitro and in vivo studies. The results showed that this polysaccharide was able to promote human skin fibroblast propagation and accelerate cell cycle progression, as well as the reepithelialization, revascularization, and cytokine secretion of TGF-β1, bFGF, and EGF which significantly confirmed the accelerated wound closure in mouse wound model [74]. TGF-β1 is an important promoter in the fibroblast proliferation and the secretion of ECM and inhibits its degradation, while EGF and bFGF are important stimulators in the formation of reepithelialization and keratinocyte migration in wound healing [75]. Moreover, the pain and the mechanism of pain signals including peripheral and central processing are also related to the modulation of TGF-β, which is implicated in the pathogenesis of keloids and hypertrophic scarring [76]. The use of calcium alginate dressing for severe wound injury treatment in the animal model demonstrated high levels of TGF-β1, TGF-β2, and TGF-β3, suggesting that it might contribute to reduced pain perception [62].

3.3. The application of natural polysaccharide in clinical trials

There are also several clinical trials of natural polysaccharide for wound repair. A natural polysaccharide that contains rich GAG has been widely used in the medical field as electrospun regenerative materials in the act of matrices that mimic tissues which are being replaced during wound healing. HA-based dressings have been used for chronic wound ulcer treatment of various etiologies, burns, and epithelial surgical wounds. The results revealed that HA significantly upgraded the healing process of wounds compared to traditional standards of care [77]. In line with this result, chitosan and alginate, fabricated as gelling fiber dressing, have been examined to accelerate the healing of patients with chronic non-healing wounds [78, 79]. This dressing has the ability to gel when in contact with wound fluid, less painful to remove, suitable for moderate to high exudate, reduced bioburden, and maintain hemostasis. Taken together, all of these benefits nominate natural polysaccharide as an advisable material in accelerating the wound healing process.

4. Limitation to using natural polysaccharide in wound healing

Generally, natural polysaccharide has demonstrated considerable merit as a treatment for chronic wounds for their anti-inflammatory and moist wound environment preservation abilities. Despite, especially for atopy people (the people with genetic tendency to develop allergic diseases), a natural polysaccharide may induce the immune system to overreact and cause irritation due to its heterogeneous complex structure. Hence, the control of the molecular weight of natural polysaccharide is expected to overcome this limitation. Through the selection of desirable molecular weight, we could simplify or remove the excessive part of natural polysaccharide that may cause the hypersensitivity reaction. Additionally, in the dry wound, these properties may also lead to the inefficiency of the wound healing process. They may cause dehydration to the dry wound, thus reducing blood flow and the epithelial cells' migration ability around the wound site which interrupts the creation of new tissue. As evidence, reepithelialization of the wound site is more rapid under moist conditions than under dry ones with natural polysaccharide wound dressing treatment [80–82]. With controllable molecular weight, it is probable that the potential of natural polysaccharide in accelerating the wound healing process can be utilized as well into several types of wound injury and patient background.

A natural polysaccharide is the element of human dermal ECM [83–86]. As naturally occurring compounds, they have been demonstrated as a great potential for medical, pharmaceutical, and biomedical applications, including wound dressings, biomaterials, and tissue regeneration, due to their economical, less toxic, and favorable compatibility profile. However, possessing a lack of protein structure, natural polysaccharide exhibits a very poor bio-stability and difficulty to assemble a "matrix" to bridge the damaged tissue during wound healing process, therefore facilitating wound contraction and leading to scar formation [87–89]. To address this limitation, natural polysaccharide has been combined with the other natural polymers or synthetic polymers to yield the desired bioactive material.

http://dx.doi.org/10.5772/intechopen.80812

5. Conclusion and future perspective

Wound dressings have a significant function in the management of wound recovery and have been continuously developed upon to improve the quality of the healing process. In this respect, a natural polysaccharide, with GAG-rich content, has been shown as a potential candidate to enhance the healing process of the wound, especially a severe wound, due to its outstanding properties. The detailed mechanism of natural polysaccharide involvement in wound healing was presented in this chapter, and it is expected to raise further wound management strategies. For example, recently, 3D bioprinting was expanded in tissue engineering for personalized regenerative medicine; hence, natural polysaccharide can be considerably utilized as the bio-ink for the printing of various types of structures as scaffolds as the desired function. The combined therapeutic potential of natural polysaccharide and proper development technique would be a promising potential not only in the wound management field but also the other medical applications.

Acknowledgements

The author would like to thank Dr. Chih-Hsin Wang (Department of Plastic and Reconstructive Surgery), Dr. Cheng-Che Liu (Department and Graduate Institute of Physiology and Biophysics), and Dr. Yi-Wen Wang (Department and Graduate Institute of Biology and Anatomy) at the Tri-Service General Hospital, National Defense Medical Center, Taipei, Taiwan (ROC) for their helpful discussion during this chapter writing, as well as thanks to Dewi Sartika MS for her help in documentation.

Conflict of interest

The author declared no potential conflicts of interest with respect to the research, authorship, and/or publication of this article.

Author details

Juin-Hong Cherng[1,2,3]

Address all correspondence to: i72bbb@gmail.com

1 Department and Graduate Institute of Biology and Anatomy, National Defense Medical Center, Taipei, Taiwan, R.O.C.

2 General Clinical Research Center for New Drug Trial, Tri-Service General Hospital, National Defense Medical Center, Taipei, Taiwan, R.O.C.

3 Department of Gerontological Health Care, National Taipei University of Nursing and Health Sciences, Taipei, Taiwan, R.O.C.

References

[1] Morgan DA. Wounds—What should a dressing formulary include? Hospital Pharmacist. 2002;**9**:261-266

[2] Percival JN. Classification of wounds and their management. Surgery. 2002;**20**(5):114-117. DOI: 10.1383/surg.20.5.114.14626

[3] Demidova-Rice TN, Hamblin MR, Herman IM. Acute and impaired wound healing: Pathophysiology and current methods for drug delivery, part 1: Normal and chronic wounds: Biology, causes, and approaches to care. Advances in Skin & Wound Care. 2012;**25**(7):304-314. DOI: 10.1097/01.ASW.0000416006.55218.d0

[4] Shriver Z, Liu D, Sasisekharan R. Emerging views of heparin sulfate glycosaminoglycan structure/activity relationships modulating dynamic biological functions. Trends in Cardiovascular Medicine. 2002;**12**:71-77. DOI: 10.1016/S1050-1738(01)00150-5

[5] Chen WYJ, Abatangelo G. Functions of hyaluronan in wound repair. Wound Repair and Regeneration. 1999;**7**(2):79-89. DOI: 10.1046/j.1524-475X.1999.00079.x

[6] Kirker KR, Luo Y, Nielson JH, Shelby J, Prestwich GD. Glycosaminoglycan hydrogel films as bio-interactive dressings for wound healing. Biomaterials. 2002;**23**:3661-3671. DOI: 10.1016/S0142-9612(02)00100-X

[7] Raghow R. The role of extracellular matrix in postinflammatory wound healing and fibrosis. The FASEB Journal. 1994;**8**(11):823-831. DOI: 10.1096/fasebj.8.11.8070631

[8] Schultz GS, Wysocki A. Interactions between extracellular matrix and growth factors in wound healing. Wound Repair and Regeneration. 2009;**17**(2):153-162. DOI: 10.1111/j.1524-475X.2009.00466.x

[9] Hodde JP, Johnson CE. Extracellular matrix as a strategy for treating chronic wounds. American Journal of Clinical Dermatology. 2007;**8**(2):61-66. DOI: 10.2165/00128071-200708020-00001

[10] Tran KT, Griffith L, Wells A. Extracellular matrix signaling through growth factor receptors during wound healing. Wound Repair and Regeneration. 2004;**12**(3):262-268. DOI: 10.1111/j.1067-1927.2004.012302.x

[11] Frenkel JS. The role of hyaluronan in wound healing. International Wound Journal. 2014;**11**:159-163. DOI: 10.1111/j.1742-481X.2012.01057.x

[12] Carey DJ. Control of growth and differentiation of vascular cells by extracellular matrix proteins. Annual Review of Physiology. 1991;**53**:161-177. DOI: 10.1146/annurev.ph.53.030191.001113

[13] Boudreau NJ, Jones PL. Extracellular matrix and integrin signalling: The shape of things to come. The Biochemical Journal. 1999;**339**(3):481-488. DOI: 10.1042/bj3390481

[14] D'Ardenne AJ. Ground substance. In: McGee JOD, Isaacson PG, Wright NA, editors. Oxford Textbook of Pathology: Principles of Pathology. 1st ed. London: Oxford University Press; 1992

[15] Melrose J. Glycosaminoglycans in wound healing. Bone and Tissue Regeneration Insights. 2016;**7**:29-50. DOI: 10.4137/BTRI.S38670

[16] Peplow PV. Glycosaminoglycan: A candidate to stimulate the repair of chronic wounds. Thrombosis and Haemostasis. 2005;**94**:4-16. DOI: 10.1160/TH04-12-0812

[17] Mosesson MW, Siebenlist KR, Meh DA. The structure and biological features of fibrinogen and fibrin. Annals of the New York Academy of Sciences. 2001;**936**:11-30. DOI: 10.1111/j.1749-6632.2001.tb03491.x

[18] Ofosu FA, Nyarko KA. Human platelet thrombin receptors: Roles in platelet activation. Hematology/Oncology Clinics of North America. 2000;**14**:1185-1198. DOI: 10.1016/S0889-8588(05)70178-7

[19] Scheraga HA, Laskowski M. The fibrinogen-fibrin conversion. Advances in Protein Chemistry. 1957;**12**:1-19. DOI: 10.1016/S0065-3233(08)60115-1

[20] Blomback B. Studies on the action of thrombotic enzymes on bovine fibrinogen as measured by N-terminal analysis. Arkiv för Kemi. 1958;**12**:321-335

[21] Blomback B, Hessel B, Hogg D, Therkildsen L. A two-step fibrinogen-fibrin transition in blood coagulation. Nature. 1978;**275**:501-505. DOI: 10.1038/275501a0

[22] Reinke JM, Sorg H. Wound repair and regeneration. European Surgical Research. 2012;**49**:35-43. DOI: 10.1159/000339613

[23] Shah JMY, Omar E, Pai DR, Sood S. Cellular events and biomarkers of wound healing. Indian Journal of Plastic Surgery. 2012;**45**(2):220-228. DOI: 10.4103/0970-0358.101282

[24] Olczyk P, Ramos P, Biernas M, Komosinska-Vassev K, Stojko J, Pilawa B. Microwave saturation of complex EPR spectra and free radicals of burnt skin treated with apitherapeutic agent. Evidence-Based Complementary and Alternative Medicine. 2013;**2013**:545201. DOI: 10.1155/2013/545201

[25] Reitsma S, Slaaf DW, Vink H, van Zandvoort MA, oude Egbrink MG. The endothelial glycocalyx: Composition, functions, and visualization. Pflügers Archiv. 2007;**454**:345-359. DOI: 10.1007/s00424-007-0212-8

[26] Shworak NW, Kobayashi T, de Agostini A, Smits NC. Anticoagulant heparin sulfate to not clot—or not? Progress in Molecular Biology and Translational Science. 2010;**93**:153-178. DOI: 10.1016/S1877-1173(10)93008-1

[27] Mertens G, Cassiman JJ, Van den Berghe H, Vermylen J, David G. Cell surface heparan sulfate proteoglycans from human vascular endothelial cells. Core protein characterization and antithrombin III binding properties. The Journal of Biological Chemistry. 1992;**267**:20435-20443

[28] Conrad HE. Heparin-binding Proteins. San Diego, CA: Academic Press; 1998

[29] Majno G, Joris I. Cells, Tissues, and Disease. London: Oxford University Press; 2004

[30] Vinay K, Cotran RS, Robbins SL. Robbins Basic Pathology. Philadelphia, PA: Saunders; 2003

[31] Busti AJ, Hooper JS, Amaya CJ, Kazi S. Effects of perioperative antiinflammatory and immunomodulating therapy on surgical wound healing. Pharmacotherapy. 2005;**25**(11): 1566-1591. DOI: 10.1592/phco.2005.25.11.1566

[32] Broughton G II, Janis JE, Attinger CE. The basic science of wound healing. Plastic and Reconstructive Surgery. 2006;**117**(7):12S-34S. DOI: 10.1097/01.prs.0000225430.42531.c2

[33] Campos ACL, Groth AK, Branco AB. Assessment and nutritional aspects of wound healing. Current Opinion in Clinical Nutrition and Metabolic Care. 2008;**11**(3):281-288. DOI: 10.1097/MCO.0b013e3282fbd35a

[34] Gosain A, DiPietro LA. Aging and wound healing. World Journal of Surgery. 2004;**28**: 321-326. DOI: 10.1007/s00268-003-7397-6

[35] Butler LM, Rainger GE, Nash GB. A role for the endothelial glycosaminoglycan hyaluronan in neutrophil recruitment by endothelial cells cultured for prolonged periods. Experimental Cell Research. 2009;**315**:3433-3441. DOI: 10.1016/j.yexcr.2009.08.012

[36] Campo GM, Avenoso A, Campo S, D'Ascola A, Nastasi G, Calatroni A. Molecular size hyaluronan differently modulates toll-like receptor-4 in LPS-induced inflammation in mouse chondrocytes. Biochimie. 2010;**92**(2):204-215. DOI: 10.1016/j.biochi.2009.10.006

[37] Clark RAF. Overview and general considerations of wound repair. In: Clark RAF, Henson PM, editors. The Molecular and Cellular Biology of Wound Repair. Boston, MA: Springer; 1998

[38] Martin P. Wound healing—Aiming for perfect skin regeneration. Science. 1997;**276**(5309): 75-81. DOI: 10.1126/science.276.5309.75

[39] Hascall VC. Proteoglycans: Structure and Function. New York, USA: Plenum Press; 1981

[40] Lark MW, Culp LA. Cell-Matrix Interaction: Biochemistry of Close and Tight-Focal Adhesive Contacts of Fibroblasts to Extracellular Matrices. New York, USA: Mercel Decker; 1987

[41] MacKay D, Miller AL. Nutritional support for wound healing. Alternative Medicine Review. 2003;**8**(4):359-377

[42] Sethi KK, Yannas IV, Mudera V, Eastwood M, McFarland C, Brown RA. Evidence for sequential utilization of fibronectin, vitronectin, and collagen during fibroblast mediated collagen contraction. Wound Repair and Regeneration. 2002;**10**(6):397-408. DOI: 10.1046/j.1524-475X.2002.10609.x

[43] Diegelmann RF, Evans MC. Wound healing: An overview of acute, fibrotic and delayed healing. Frontiers in Bioscience. 2004;**9**:283-289

[44] Hoffman M, Harger A, Lenkowski A, Hedner U, Roberts HR, Monroe DM. Cutaneous wound healing is impaired in hemophilia B. Blood. 2006;**108**(9):3053-3060. DOI: 10.1182/blood-2006-05-020495

[45] Gurtner GC, Werner S, Barrandon Y, Longaker MT. Wound repair and regeneration. Nature. 2008;**453**(7193):314-321. DOI: 10.1038/nature07039

[46] Vedrenne N, Coulomb B, Danigo A, Bont'e F, Desmouli'ere A. The complex dialogue between (myo)fibroblasts and the extracellular matrix during skin repair processes and ageing. Pathologie Biologie. 2012;**60**(1):20-27. DOI: 10.1016/j.patbio.2011.10.002

[47] Maruyama K, Asai J, Ii M, Thorne T, Losordo DW, D'Amore PA. Decreased macrophage number and activation lead to reduced lymphatic vessel formation and contribute to impaired diabetic wound healing. The American Journal of Pathology. 2007;**170**: 1178-1191. DOI: 10.2353/ajpath.2007.060018

[48] Galiano RD, Tepper OM, Pelo CR, et al. Topical vascular endothelial growth factor accelerates diabetic wound healing through increased angiogenesis and by mobilizing and recruiting bone marrow-derived cells. The American Journal of Pathology. 2004;**164**:1935-1947. DOI: 10.1016/S0002-9440(10)63754-6

[49] Eming SA, Krieg T, Davidson JM. Inflammation in wound repair: Molecular and cellular mechanisms. The Journal of Investigative Dermatology. 2007;**127**:514-525. DOI: 10.1038/sj.jid.5700701

[50] Jackson RL, Busch SJ, Cardin AD. Glycosaminoglycans: Molecular properties, protein interactions, and role in physiological processes. Physiological Reviews. 1991;**71**: 481-539. DOI: 10.1152/physrev.1991.71.2.481

[51] Casu B, Lindahl U. Structure and biological interactions of heparin and heparan sulfate. Advances in Carbohydrate Chemistry and Biochemistry. 2001;**57**:159-206. DOI: 10.1016/S0065-2318(01)57017-1

[52] Chen JP, Chang GY, Chen JK. Electrospun collagen/chitosan nanofibrous membrane as wound dressing. Colloids and Surfaces A: Physicochemical and Engineering Aspects. 2008;**313**:183-188. DOI: 10.1016/j.colsurfa.2007.04.129

[53] Noh HK, Lee SW, Kim JM, Oh JE, Kim KH, Chung CP, et al. Electrospinning of chitin nanofibers: Degradation behavior and cellular response to normal human keratinocytes and fibroblasts. Biomaterials. 2006;**27**:3934-3944. DOI: 10.1016/j.biomaterials.2006.03.016

[54] Cai Z, Mo X, Zhang K, Fan L, Yin A, He C, et al. Fabrication of chitosan/silk fibroin composite nanofibers for wound-dressing applications. International Journal of Molecular Sciences. 2010;**11**:3529-3539. DOI: 10.3390/ijms11093529

[55] Dumitriu S. Polysaccharides as biomaterials. In: S. Dumitriu, editor. Polymeric Biomaterials. New York: Marcel Dekker; 2002. pp. 1-61

[56] Rinaudo M. Characterization and properties of some polysaccharides used as biomaterials. Macromolecular Symposia. 2006;**245-246**:549. DOI: 10.1002/masy.200651379

[57] Su CH, Sun CS, Juan SW, Hu CH, Ke WT, Sheu MT. Fungal mycelia as the source of chitin and polysaccharides and their applications as skin substitutes. Biomaterials. 1997;**18**:1169-1174. DOI: 10.1016/S0142-9612(97)00048-3

[58] Koh TJ, DiPietro LA. Inflammation and wound healing: The role of the macrophage. Expert Reviews in Molecular Medicine. 2011;**13**(23). DOI: 10.1017/S1462399411001943

[59] Park HR, Hwang D, Suh HJ, Yu KW, Kim TY, Shin KS. Anti-tumor and anti-metastatic activities of rhamnogalacturonan-II-type polysaccharide isolated from mature leaves of green tea via activation of macrophages and natural killer cells. International Journal of Biological Macromolecules. 2017;**99**:179-186. DOI: 10.1016/j.ijbiomac.2017.02.043

[60] Wagener J, MacCallum DM, Brown GD, Gown NAR. *Candida albicans* chitin increases arginase-1 activity in human macrophages, with an impact on macrophage antimicrobial functions. mBio. 2016:e01820. DOI: 10.1128/mBio.01820-16

[61] Lundahl MLE, Scanlan EM, Lavelle EC. Therapeutic potential of carbohydrates as regulators of macrophage activation. Biochemical Pharmacology. 2017;**146**:23-41. DOI: 10.1016/j.bcp.2017.09.003

[62] Wang CH, Chang SJ, Tzeng YS, Shih YJ, Adrienne C, Chen SG, et al. Enhanced wound-healing performance of a phyto-polysaccharide-enriched dressing-a preclinical small and large animal study. International Wound Journal. 2017;**14**:1359-1369. DOI: 10.1111/iwj.12813

[63] Kannon GA, Garrett AB. Moist wound healing with occlusive dressings. A clinical review. Dermatologic Surgery. 1995;**21**:583-590. DOI: 10.1111/j.1524-4725.1995.tb00511.x

[64] Werner S, Grose R. Regulation of wound healing by growth factors and cytokines. Physiological Reviews. 2003;**83**:835-870. DOI: 10.1152/physrev.00031.2002

[65] Hubner G, Brauchle M, Smola H, Madlener M, Fassler R, Werner S. Differential regulation of pro-inflammatory cytokines during wound healing in normal and glucocorticoid-treated mice. Cytokine. 1996;**8**(7):548-556. DOI: 10.1006/cyto.1996.0074

[66] Iwamoto M, Kurachi M, Nakashima T, Kim D, Yamaguchi K, Oda T, et al. Structure–activity relationship of alginate oligosaccharides in the induction of cytokine production from RAW264.7 cells. FEBS Letters. 2005;**579**:4423-4429. DOI: 10.1016/j.febslet.2005.07.007

[67] Ryan CA, Farmer EE. Oligosaccharide signals in plants: A current assessment. Annual Review of Plant Physiology and Plant Molecular Biology. 1991;**42**:651-674. DOI: 10.1146/annurev.pp.42.060191.003251

[68] Bloebaum RM, Grant JA, Sur S. Immunomodulation: The future of allergy and asthma treatment. Current Opinion in Allergy and Clinical Immunology. 2004;**4**:63-67. DOI: 10.1097/01.all.0000113681.18759.5e

[69] Sun L, Zhao Y. The biological role of dectin-1 in immune response. International Reviews of Immunology. 2007;**26**:349-364. DOI: 10.1080/08830180701690793

[70] Martins PR, Soares AMV, Domeneghini AVSP, Golim MA, Kaneno R. Agaricus brasiliensis polysaccharides stimulate human monocytes to capture *Candida albicans*, express toll-like receptors 2 and 4, and produce pro-inflammatory cytokines. Journal of Venomous Animals and Toxins including Tropical Diseases. 2017;**23**:17. DOI: 10.1186/s40409-017-0102-2

[71] Cavalcanti YVN, Brelaz MCA, Neves JKAL, Ferraz JC, Pereira VRA. Role of TNF-alpha, IFN-gamma, and IL-10 in the development of pulmonary tuberculosis. Pulmonary Medicine. 2012;**2012**:745483. DOI: 10.1155/2012/745483

[72] Dinarello CA. Biologic basis for interleukin-1 in disease. Blood. 1996;**87**(6):2095-2147

[73] Echeverry S, Shi XQ, Haw A, Liu H, Zhang ZW, Zhang J. Transforming growth factor-beta1 impairs neuropathic pain through pleiotropic effects. Molecular Pain. 2009;**5**:16. DOI: 10.1186/1744-8069-5-16

[74] Zhao B, Zhang X, Han W, Cheng J, Qin Y. Wound healing effect of an Astragalus membranaceus polysaccharide and its mechanism. Molecular Medicine Reports. 2017;**15**: 4077-4083. DOI: 10.3892/mmr.2017.648

[75] Thorey IS, Hinz B, Hoeflich A, Kaesler S, Bugnon P, Elmlinger M, et al. Transgenic mice reveal novel activities of growth hormone in wound repair, angiogenesis, and myofibroblast differentiation. The Journal of Biological Chemistry. 2004;**279**:26674-26684. DOI: 10.1074/jbc.M311467200

[76] Zhu Y, Colak T, Shenoy M, Liu L, Mehta K, Pai R, et al. Transforming growth factor beta induces sensory neuronal hyperexcitability, and contributes to pancreatic pain and hyperalgesia in rats with chronic pancreatitis. Molecular Pain. 2012;**8**:65. DOI: 10.1186/1744-8069-8-65

[77] Voigt J, Driver VR. Hyaluronic acid derivatives and their healing effect on burns, epithelial surgical wounds, and chronic wounds: A systematic review and meta-analysis of randomized controlled trials. Wound Repair and Regeneration. 2012;**20**:317-331. DOI: 10.1111/j.1524-475X.2012.00777.x

[78] Mason S, Clarke C. A multicentred cohort evaluation of a chitosan gelling fiber dressing. British Journal of Nursing. 2015;**24**:869-876. DOI: 10.12968/bjon.2015.24.17.868

[79] Ausili E, Paolucci V, Triarico S, et al. Treatment of pressure sores in spina bifida patients with calcium alginate and foam dressings. European Review for Medical and Pharmacological Sciences. 2013;**17**(12):1642-1647

[80] Daamen WF, van Moerkerkn HT, Hafmans T, Buttafoco L, Poot AA, Veerkamp JH, et al. Preparation and evaluation of molecularly-defined collagen-elastin-glycosaminoglycan scaffolds for tissue engineering. Biomaterials. 2003;**24**:4001-4009. DOI: 10.1016/S0142-9612(03)00273-4

[81] Lamberg SI, Stoolmiller AC. Glycosaminoglycans. A biochemical and clinical review. Journal of Investigative Dermatology. 1974;**63**:433-449. DOI: 10.1111/1523-1747.ep12680346

[82] Ma L, Gao C, Mao Z, Zhou J, Shen J, Hu X, et al. Collagen/chitosan porous scaffolds with improved biostability for skin tissue engineering. Biomaterials. 2003;**24**:4833-4841. DOI: 10.1016/S0142-9612(03)00374-0

[83] Price RD, Berry MG, Navsaria HA. Hyaluronic acid: The scientific and clinical evidence. Journal of Plastic, Reconstructive & Aesthetic Surgery. 2007;**60**:1110-1119. DOI: 10.1016/j.bjps.2007.03.005

[84] Vats A, Tolley NS, Polak JM, Gough JE. Scaffolds and biomaterials for tissue engineering: A review of clinical applications. Clinical Otolaryngology and Allied Sciences. 2003; **28**:165-172. DOI: 10.1046/j.1365-2273.2003.00686.x

[85] West DC, Shaw DM, Lorenz P, Adzick NS, Longaker MT. Fibrotic healing of adult and late gestation fetal wounds correlates with increased hyaluronidase activity and removal of hyaluronan. The International Journal of Biochemistry & Cell Biology. 1997;**29**:201-210. DOI: 10.1016/S1357-2725(96)00133-1

[86] Zhong SP, Zhang YZ, Lim CT. Tissue scaffolds for skin wound healing and dermal reconstruction. Wiley Interdisciplinary Reviews. Nanomedicine and Nanobiotechnology. 2010;**2**:510-525. DOI: 10.1002/wnan.100

[87] Chansiripornchai P, Pramatwinai C, Rungsipipat A, Ponsamart S, Nakchat O. The efficiency of polysaccharide gel extracted from fruit-hulls of durian (*Durio zibethinus* L.) for wound healing in pig skin. Acta Horticulturae. 2005;**679**:37-43. DOI: 10.17660/ActaHortic.2005.679.5

[88] Winter GD, Scales JT. Effect of air drying and dressing on the surface of a wound. Nature. 1963;**197**(5):91-92. DOI: 10.1038/197091b0

[89] Suzuki Y, Nishimura Y, Tanihara M, Suzuki K, Nakamura T, Shimizu Y, et al. Evaluation of a novel alginate gel dressing: Cytotoxicity to fibroblasts in vitro and foreign-body reaction in pig skin in vivo. Journal of Biomedical Materials Research. 1998;**39**:317-322. DOI: 10.1002/(SICI)1097-4636(199802)39:2<317::AID-JBM20>3.0.CO;2-8

Chapter 7

From Tissue Repair to Tissue Regeneration

Aragona Salvatore Emanuele, Mereghetti Giada,
Ferrari Alessio and Giorgio Ciprandi

Additional information is available at the end of the chapter

http://dx.doi.org/10.5772/intechopen.81291

Abstract

In Regeneration 3.0, the priority is to combine the anti-inflammatory activity of the nine proteins acting as growth factors in the bovine colostrum, the homeostatic, angiogenic and reorganizational activities of the matrix, the modulation of collagen synthesis and the remodeling of the epithelium. The choice of bovine colostrum and its associated properties was the basis for the design of devices that could also offer those properties: barrier action, anti-inflammatory action and pain reduction, reduction and absorption of exudates, combating of bacterial and fungal proliferation, antioxidant action and hydration and protection against skin diseases and dermatosis. We now know the key players in the wound healing process and we have new molecules available to act on them, but the future must necessarily lie in the transfer of molecules and information between the endothelium, ECM and cell membrane, which can be directed toward tissue regeneration if the resident stem cells have the chance of communicating and interacting with new therapeutic models, all this without forgetting that the human being is at the center of research and scientific evolution.

Keywords: wound healing, tissue regeneration, bovine colostrum, stem cells, aimed protocol

1. Introduction

The complexity of the wound healing process is increasingly understood and characterized. Until recently, the wound healing mechanism was interpreted as a fibroproliferative response with the aim of producing a cicatricial reaction (repair), with different mechanisms than those seen in a fetal environment, in which the scope of the healing process is tissue regeneration. However, recent awareness of the biological pathways and cell classes characterizing the various phases of the wound healing process and current attention toward biomaterials and possible new applications for stem cells, together with the use of bioengineered tissues, have led to a reinterpretation of this process from the perspective of regenerative medicine, intended as the possibility of recreating a tissue as similar as possible to the original.

Current understanding of some of the tissue repair mechanisms enables the application of therapeutic models that have become an established part of everyday practice. The healing process takes place over three complex phases: management of the inflammatory process, cell proliferation (excessive or impaired), and extracellular matrix (ECM) remodeling. Wound repair is characterized by the incomplete regeneration of the original tissue with hyperproduction of organized collagen, which can lead to the production of new tissue with an 80% similarity to the original tissue. Impaired host management of this process leads to an abnormal fibroproliferative response, causing the production of hypertrophic or keloid scars. While some of the mechanisms are already known, new discoveries in the field of molecular and cellular mechanisms enable us to hypothesize other tissue healing management mechanisms and to apply new therapeutic models to achieve results beyond those currently possible. As far back as 2013, Aragona and Marazzi and colleagues [1] published an article in the Italian edition of Surgical Tribune discussing new research in the treatment of skin lesions in regenerative medicine, establishing the bases for the interpretation of the inflammatory process that directly involve some of the cell classes naturally involved in the inflammatory process underlying wound regeneration.

Current gains in knowledge of tissue regeneration, and above all of stem cells and their behavior, open new ground and suggest new future therapeutic models. Research into the effects of electromagnetic fields on stem cells in particular indicates that a paradigm shift is within our grasp. With a little imagination, we can visualize ourselves as an avatar observing nature and the universe: we can close our eyes and listen to the sounds and energy emitted by cells, or open them to observe phenomena that yesterday, we thought a world away. We begin this journey through the study of the inflammatory process by taking a look at in-vitro experimental models, fundamental above all in understanding the molecular, genetic and cellular patterns of the various tissues.

2. The inflammatory model of skin lesions. From experimental model to humans

> *"Why, sir, his hide is so tanned with his trade that he will keep out water a great while, and your water is a sore decayer of your whoreson dead body."*
>
> *W. Shakespeare, Hamlet, Act 5, Scene 1.*

Understanding the inflammation process is enabled by the design and creation of in vitro and in vivo cellular models, with the primary objective of establishing the effect of the molecules of biological agents on the inflammatory process associated with the tissue repair and regeneration process. This innovation over animal models makes it possible to establish the role and concentration of all the humoral factors (cytokines and growth factors), genetic factors (genes expressed in the various phases of the process), cellular factors and, above all, the fibroblasts and collagen associated with the role of matrix metalloproteinases (MMPs) and tissue inhibitors of metalloproteinases (TIMPs), fundamental for extracellular matrix (ECM) remodeling. It also enables the concept of tissue regeneration to take over from tissue repair as the primary objective of research and clinical practice.

The literature is full of studies meticulously describing the inflammatory process of wounds. It should be remembered that modulation of this process and its impact on the proliferation, differentiation and function of inflammatory cells is aimed at controlling that very inflammation. Our research had the objective of framing all these observations and this scientific knowledge in the biological context in which the process takes place, within its specific individual reactivity.

The shift of perspective from inflammation to regeneration involves the systemic treatment of patients with skin and mucosal wounds and local anti-inflammatory treatment involving modulation of the endothelial and ECM inflammation, the anti-inflammatory cytokines and the MMPs.

Figure 1 highlights the switch between the wound repair and regeneration pathway and the chronic inflammation pathway that feeds the chronicity of the skin lesions. Initially, platelet activation leads to the release and activation of TGF-beta 1, PDGF, TNF-alpha and IL1, with the recruitment of neutrophils deputized to natural debridement and to regulation of the expression of the adhesion molecules. The neutrophils are followed by macrophages, the cell population now at the center of attention in wound healing research. These ensure sustained debridement, the release of proinflammatory cytokines, and the potentiation of the fibroproliferative response in the context of chronic inflammation.

The role of macrophages deserves a chapter of its own in relation to their division into the M1 population, which can eliminate invading microorganisms and promote the inflammatory response during the initial inflammatory process, and subsequently the M2 population, during the resolution of the inflammatory process. By losing its reactivity to inflammatory stimuli, the increasingly studied M2 population becomes capable of eliminating damaged cells and tissues, promoting neoangiogenesis and tissue remodeling.

This all takes place within the dynamic structure of the ECM, which can be defined as "the submerged world where everything is possible" thanks to the equilibrium between the glycoprotein, molecular and cellular components assured by the aqueous component that, in light of the latest knowledge, seems to enable communication between the cells and the ECM and could explain some amplification mechanisms of the healing process. The authors had the opportunity to test an in vitro model on both epidermal and Dry Eye Syndrome cell cultures. In both trials, the primary objective was to have a cellular, ultrastructural and biochemical model similar to real life in which to cause an injury similar to that under investigation. The biological injury, whether damage to the epidermis and dermis or creation of an area of dehydration on the eye surface, recreated the natural pathophysiological environment, and the in vitro model offers a faithful reflection. *"Efficacy of a New Ocular Surface Modulator in Restoring*

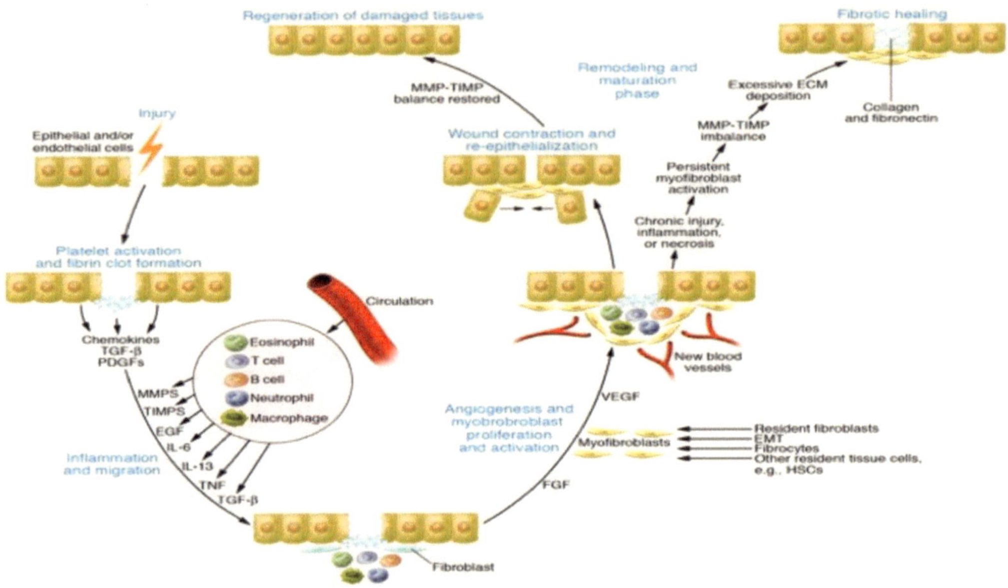

Figure 1. Highlights the switch between the wound repair and regeneration pathway and the chronic inflammation pathway that feeds the chronicity of the skin lesions (M. Meloni- Vitroscreen Milano Italy 2017).

Epithelial Changes in an in Vitro Model of Dry Eye Syndrome" Barabino and colleagues, Current Eye Research, in press [2].

The process of learning about the biological reality examined in vitro and the scientific observation necessary to recreate the metabolic, structural and ultrastructural conditions of a cell/tissue/organ model make it possible to understand and reproduce the biological mechanism involved. Above all, however – and this is the revolutionary part for the translation of research to clinical practice – they make it possible to predict quantitatively the model's response, and hence the natural response of the disorder under study, following treatment with a given biological substance. This means understanding if that biological substance – that drug – actually works.

For skin lesions, the in vitro model has an absolute value, because animal models suffer from important biological interferences. For investigation of the mechanism of action, the in vitro method opens up:

"the marvelous opportunity to discover something different, something unknown before now, because using a biological model guarantees the predictive value of the generated data and permits us to measure what cannot or should not be measured in vivo.

> *"Measure what can be measured, and make measurable what cannot be measured"* (Galileo).

"The in vitro model, therefore is not a test, but an experimental model, and in skin lesions it enables a better understanding of the mechanisms of action, the collection of quantitative information that could not be obtained in any other way, and the creation of a body of evidence, case by case." Marisa Meloni, CEO Vitroscreen, Milano, Italy.

It enables us to approach the real target and model, human beings (relevance), and to determine and distinguish between differences in the response (reliability) and to reproduce the response in vivo (predictivity). The model is reproducible (the tests can be repeated with similar results) and the biological response of the trial products can be confirmed at different times (reproducibility).

For researchers working with skin lesions every day, the in vitro experimental model makes it possible to develop a clinical intuition and investigate the hypothesized role of a therapeutic substances or agents, while the use of data from in vitro models and the testing of potential medications enables a decision on whether or not to develop them and use them in subsequent in vivo studies to add substance and support to the clinical studies.

As noted above, the repair and regeneration process consists of three phases (modulation of the inflammatory process, modulation of cell proliferation, and modulation of extracellular matrix remodeling), and regenerative medicine must be based on cell therapies, engineered tissues and biological products formulated by clinical research and able to mimic and reproduce the natural repair and regeneration process.

Before entering into the merit of the in vitro model, it is worth asking what diagnostic factors are predictive of an evolution toward healing. Clinical factors are the first to be considered: underlying conditions, comorbidities, nutritional status, and medical treatments. In relation to humoral factors, can proinflammatory cytokines, MMPs, growth factors and macrophages be measured or tested in a recalcitrant skin ulcer? Can they be made the diagnostic target of an inflammation that develops toward healing or toward chronicity? All these targets may be measurable and are – or could be – predictive, but we are still far from their use in clinical practice to establish the most suitable treatment.

In the author's opinion, it should not be forgotten that humans are variable individuals: we know more than ever how humans become ill, but we also know that the repair, regeneration and healing process is highly individual.

In vitro models of skin lesions enable us to establish the behavior of the innate immune system in the first, inflammatory phase, which lasts from 2 hours to 5 days. Cell migration and inter-cellular and cell–cell matrix adhesion have been observed (and are discussed below), and the following markers have been quantified: IL-1a, IL-8, TNF-alpha, IFN-A1, HSP-70 (Heat protein shock 70), MAP3K8, NK, CD68, MMP-2, MMP-9, ADAM15, ADAMTS8, ITGA1, ITGB2, and RPSA.

After 1 week, in both the experimental model and in vivo, the cell proliferation phase begins. This involves granulation of the newly formed tissue and modulation of the cell population (transition from M1 to M2, blockage of monocytes, increase in fibroblasts and deposition of type III and VII collagen), with a process defined as wound retraction and re-epithelialization. In this phase we can measure VGEF-C, CTNNB1 (gene expression of cadherin production), FLNB, TMP2, BPI, FN1, and DECORIN.

The remodeling phase involves an increase in collagen deposition and in its tensile strength, with the substitution of collagen type III by type I; this should not necessarily be encouraged, as it leads to cicatricial retraction and repair rather than regeneration of the original tissue.

We can thus determine the presence and role of IL-1a, IL-8, HPS70, NK and BPI in the injured tissue in the inflammatory phase, of IL1a-IL-8, TNF-alpha, MMP2, MMP9, ADAM15 and ADAMTS8 in the re-epithelialization phase, of ITGA1 and ITGbeta2 in the cell migration and adhesion phase, and of VEGF-C, CTNNB1, DNAI1, FLNB, and TPM2 in the subsequent phase, in which remodeling begins.

The biological processes involved in the various phases of cicatrization are complex and often concomitant. The inflammatory phase, the keratinocyte migration phase, the proliferation phase, the formation of new tissue, and remodeling are all associated with a number of morphological and biochemical changes that can be quantified in the various skin layers through the choice of relevant markers.

The observation of these pathophysiological phenomena and processes in nature leads us to hypothesize new therapeutic procedures. The ability to detect and quantify the biological agents involved in the process, and to study their behavior, could enable the development of new therapeutic strategies.

Innovation means searching and researching.

Researching means having intuitions that can be tested.

Testing means using scientific processes that can validate the research.

Skin lesions, precisely because they are an expression of a systemic pathological status, lead us to use the experimental model to validate future therapies based on awareness of the fine molecular and cellular mechanisms. Understanding the phenomena inherent to the acute and chronic inflammatory process as a defense mechanism activated by the body leads to an understanding of how people can become ill and recover. Reproducing these phenomena in vitro and validating them and comparing them with in vivo data enables the evaluation of any identified therapeutic agent and its possible use in clinical practice.

It can today be asserted that the skin is a sophisticated immune surveillance system acting through its network of epithelial cells, lymphocytes and AgP cells as well as its resident microbiota, the alteration of which can trigger serious consequences. Future experimental models will be characterized by studies in this sense, with great benefits for medical research, pharmaceuticals and cosmetics.

3. The inflammatory process in healing tissue in vivo. Molecular and cellular components involved

3.1. Changes in the healing process

Wound repair involves the partial regeneration of the original tissue, with hyperproduction of organized collagen, which can lead to the production of new tissue with an 80% similarity to the original tissue. Abnormal host management involves a fibroproliferative response that causes the production of hypertrophic scars or keloids. New scientific knowledge in the fields of molecular and cellular mechanisms allows us to hypothesize other healing tissue process management procedures and apply new therapeutic models.

Chronic non-responding skin lesions are incurred by a defect in ECM remodeling (third stage of the regeneration process). Abnormal collagen deposition blocks the action of fibroblasts and re-epithelialization is halted, resulting in an inflammatory process that becomes chronic due to the humoral (cytokines) and cellular components present that prevent the lesion from healing. The proinflammatory cytokines produced by the cell populations involved in wound healing trigger, promote and regulate the process by stimulating these cells (macrophages) to act. Any disruption of this combined and synergistic action between cytokines and M1 and M2 macrophages lays the basis for non-healing. In fact, M1 macrophages secrete IL1, IL6, IL12, TNF-alpha and MMPs, which in turn stimulate, amplify and regulate the proinflammatory phase preparatory to the next phase, where the switch to M2 produces TGF-beta and IL10.

In the chronic lesion, proteases alter the granulation tissue, stopping cell migration for the purpose of scarring. Histologic data demonstrating the altered regulation of synthesis and collagen synthesis is salient.

3.2. Scientific background of the operating rationale

Under the microscope, the endothelium-ECM-cell complex resembles a dynamic world in continuous movement, with genetically encoded interactions and biological pathways aimed at recovering the normal physiology of the damaged tissue (ES Aragona). This is the basis for the work method studied and applied in our Centre.

Attention is given to the role of MMPs, the enzymes that degrade the extracellular matrix, and to their balancing by their inhibitors (TIMPs) and cytokines, especially in local arterial and venous diseases. The cytokine TNF-alpha and gelatinase MMP-9, which are significantly over-expressed in both endothelial inflammation conditions and damaged venous vascular walls, are investigated in particular.

Endothelial cells play an important role in early wound repair, thanks to their ability to stimulate the inflammatory process. They produce large amounts of TNF-alpha, which can be quantified through intracellular mobility receptors for hyaluronic acid (ICAM). At the same time, endothelial function restoration begins with the restoration of endothelial glycosaminoglycans linked to the reduction of MMP9 and the block of MMPs through the action of natural or organic derivatives of the hydrodynamic substance hyaluronic acid. This increases the water level, thus enabling the zinc at the core of the MMPs to be blocked, triggering phase repair and regeneration.

TNF-alpha is an important mediator during the inflammatory phase and, with TGF-beta, activates the expression of MMP9. In in-vitro cell cultures, TNF-alpha is over-produced in the first 24 hours, and the proinflammatory function is preparatory to the repair process. TNF-alpha inhibits the collagen-alpha-1 gene in fibroblasts, stimulates the fibroblasts to produce collagen and promotes angiogenesis. (**Figure 2**).

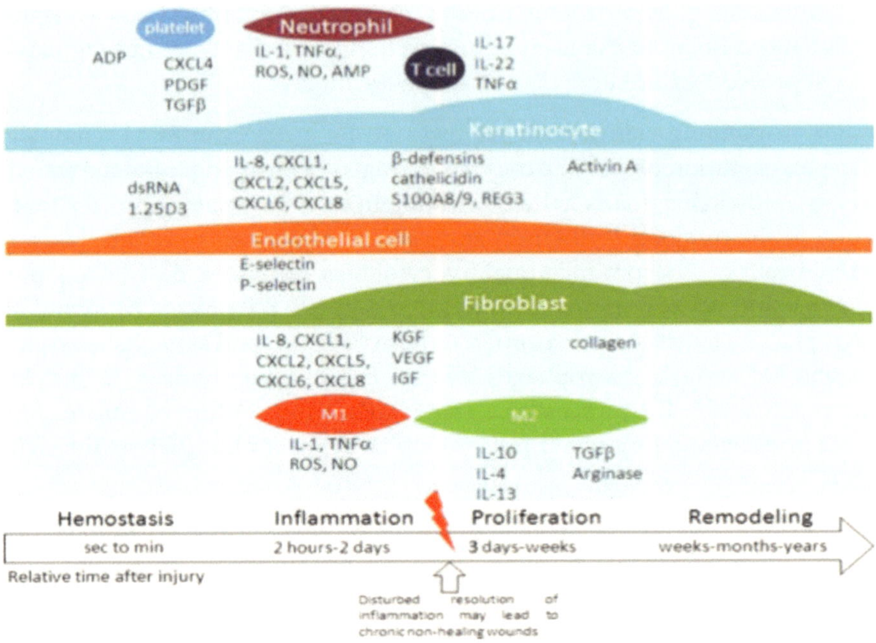

Figure 2. The phases of tissue regeneration and the involvement of cell types, micromolecules and extracellular matrix proteins.

The reduction in M1 macrophages and hence in TNF-alpha, associated with the block of monocytes and the increased production of fibroblasts and hence of collagen, creates the foundation for the M1-M2 switch and the start of the repair and regeneration process in an ever-dynamic and constantly changing cytokine and cellular pool (ES Aragona).

4. Macrophage regulation in wound healing

The role of M1 macrophages in the inflammatory process and of M2 macrophages in the repair and regeneration process is still debated, especially in the event of a disrupted M1/M2 ratio, which produces various pathological effects related to the chronification of inflammation and associated disorders. Naturally, in this case our focus is on non-healing.

It is worth repeating that M1 macrophages are proinflammatory cells to all effects, producing proinflammatory cytokines (IL1, IL6, IL12, TNF-a and oxidative metabolites (NO and SAD) (3, 4) which are involved in defense of the host and in the debridement process. (**Figures 3 and 4**).

The M2 population is stimulated above all by the drop in M1, IL4 and IL13; this is the key for the remodeling process, which follows or accompanies the switching-off and termination of the inflammatory process.

http://dx.doi.org/10.5772/intechopen.81291

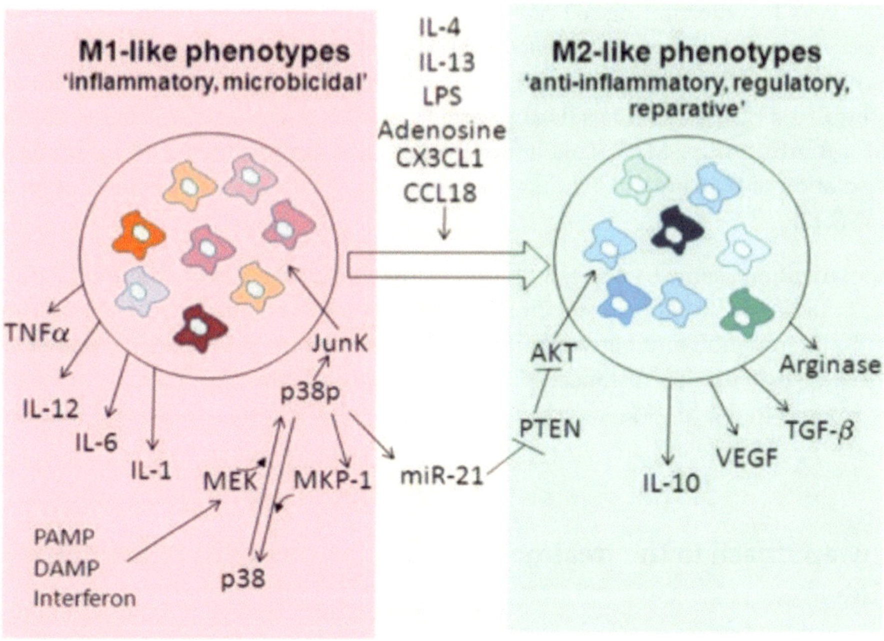

Figure 3. Cytokines pathways in M1-like and M2-like phenotypes.

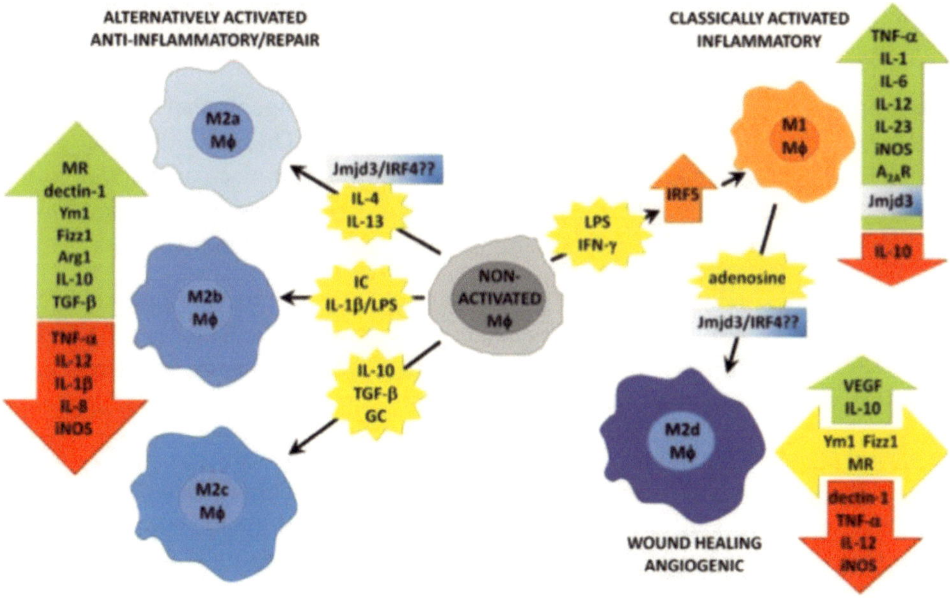

Figure 4. The type of macrophages, their differentiation and the role in tissue repair.

One of the keys for interpreting M1/M2 switching is the genotyping and receptor typing of the two populations and how they react to both chemical and energy stimuli, a concept we will return to below. The M2 population is divided into three subclasses, M2a, M2b and M2c. M2a is stimulated by the cytokines Il4/IL13 and IL4Ra. Leibovich and colleagues [3] also characterized a fourth group, M2d. This is involved in the diminishment of inflammation and the upregulation of IL10 and VEGF, like subtype M2a, which is associated with low levels of TNFa and IL12.

M1/M2 polarization seems to depend on two transcription regulators, the interferon regulatory factors IRF5 and IRF4. A correlation has been demonstrated between IFR5, high levels of M1 and inflammation and between IRF4 and M2, both linked to specific gene expressions and modulated by various substances. The latter include adenosine, which modifies the membrane's response to the M1-M2 switch, hence modifying the intracellular and ECM information signal [3].

5. A new approach to the treatment of skin lesions with regenerative medicine

5.1. The anti-inflammatory regenerative medicine (AIMED) protocol: the importance of inflammatory process modulation in triggering the tissue regeneration phase

The care and treatment of non-healing wounds is a major challenge for specialized centers. These wounds have a significant impact on health expenditure and a profound effect on the wellbeing of both patients and their families.

The skin is an important barrier. It protects us from numerous agents that would otherwise cause more frequent and more severe damage to our bodies. The skin system is a defense mechanism that aims to maintain a balance and involves various molecular, cellular, immune, endocrine, and neurological mechanisms. The understanding of these mechanisms has led to the development of numerous new drugs and medical devices for skin diseases.

Numerous authors have investigated the phases of wound repair processes and regeneration. The perfect picture is that of a complex system of humoral, cellular, molecular and ultrastructural regulation, described as a cohesive orchestra. This is the basis of the regeneration process, but it often stalls and impairs healing.

The Centre for Regenerative Medicine (now RMC) was set up by the Istituto Clinico Humanitas Mater Domini in July 2015 to focus on chronic wounds and high morbidity (infections, pain, complications), given their social implications. It has created a working group, now promoted by the Multidisciplinary Association for Wellbeing and Regeneration (AMbeR), involving numerous professionals working on the treatment and care of people with chronic skin and mucous membrane diseases. The team's research was the first step in collaboration and cooperation with other specialized centers, universities and organizations throughout Italy. Its attention is focused on the most important and decisive area of skin lesion management: modulation of the inflammatory process.

http://dx.doi.org/10.5772/intechopen.81291

The RMC's data on the etiological causes of skin lesions confirm the etiology of such a lesion, as reported in the studies provided by the various centers involved. The success of the guidelines and protocols will only be maintained if we carry on managing the inflammatory process with a view to regeneration (**Picture 1**).

The chronic skin wound outpatient clinic involves experts in various disciplines for the treatment of:

Vascular lesions; (**Picture 2**)

Pressure lesions; (**Picture 3**)

Diabetic foot lesions; (**Picture 4**)

Autoimmune and rheumatic lesions; (**Picture 5**)

Post-surgical skin lesions; (**Picture 6**)

Burns and scars. (**Picture 7**)

Current knowledge of gross and ultrastructural skin anatomy enables the stages of the regeneration process to be followed and highlights the importance of the extracellular matrix. This

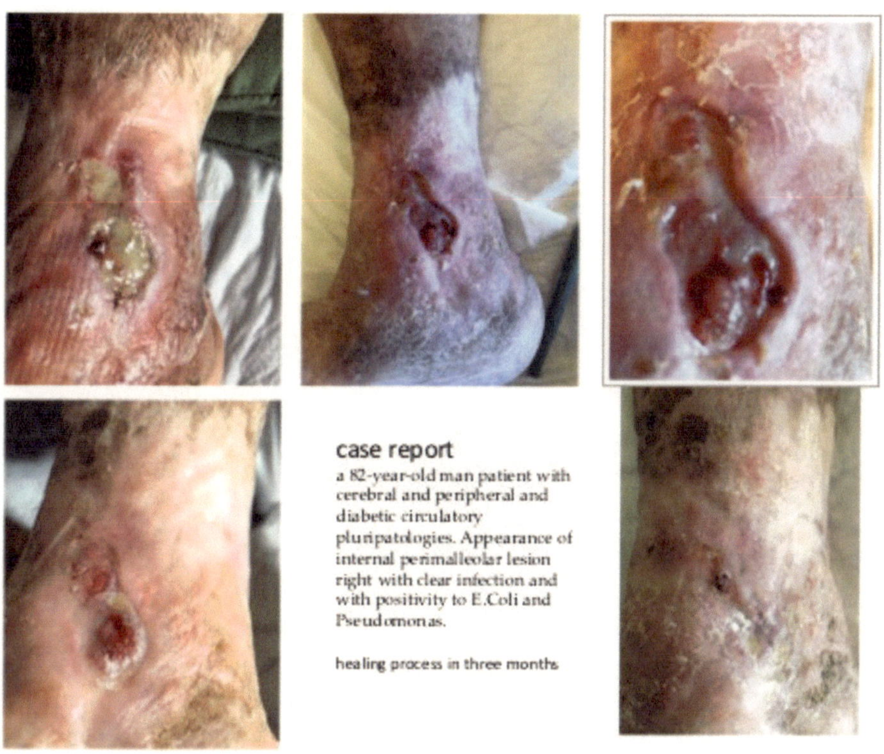

Picture 1. Case report. A 82-year-old man patient with cerebral and peripheral and diabetic circulatory pluripatologies. Appearance of internal perimalleolar lesion right with clear infection and with positivity to E. Coli and Pseudomonas healing process in 3 months.

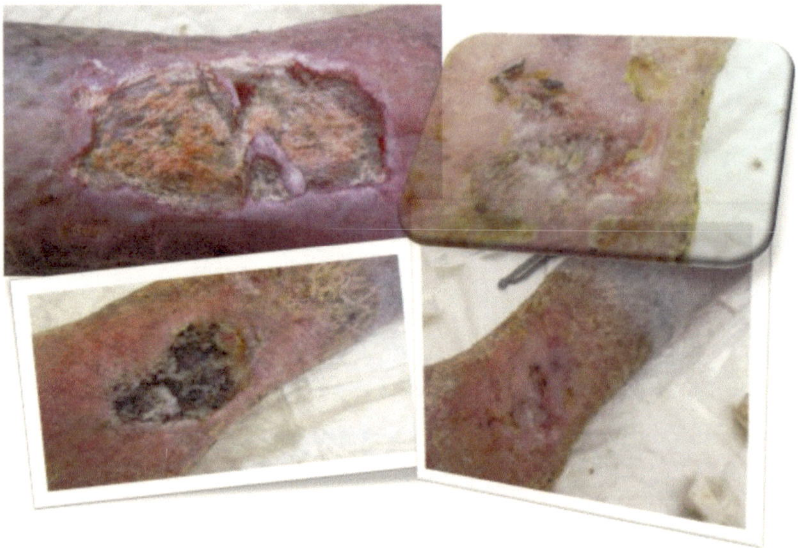

Picture 2. Case report. A 71-year-old man patient with vascular lesion present for 6 years and resistant to therapies. Healing process in 5 months.

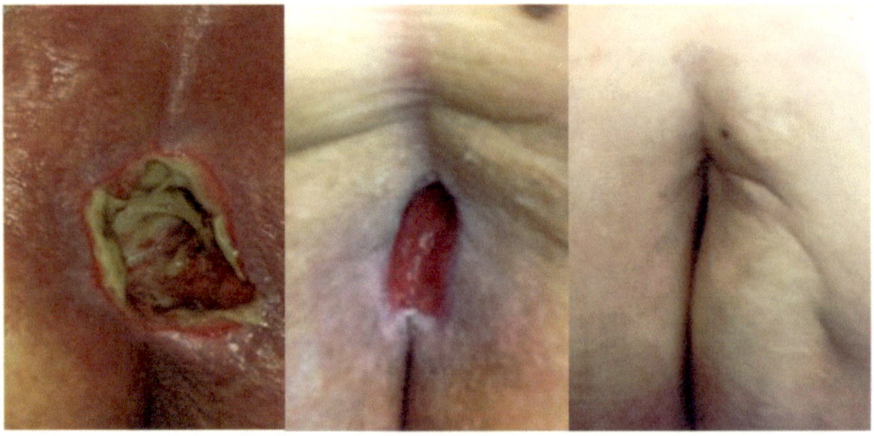

Picture 3. Case report. A 69-year-old patient with IV stade decubitus injury. Healing process in 35 days.

has the appearance of a semi-fluid gel, and contains enzymes, hormones and vitamins and a dense network of macromolecular complexes (GAGs, proteoglycans and glycoproteins). The cells are immersed in this active substance, whose electromagnetic properties are fundamental for the life of the cells themselves as well as the water in the human body. The coherence of the electromagnetic diffusion is essential for correct intercell and cell-ECM harmony.

The other aspect highlighted by research into the modulation of the inflammatory process is that the ECM determines the process of differentiation, proliferation and cell migration,

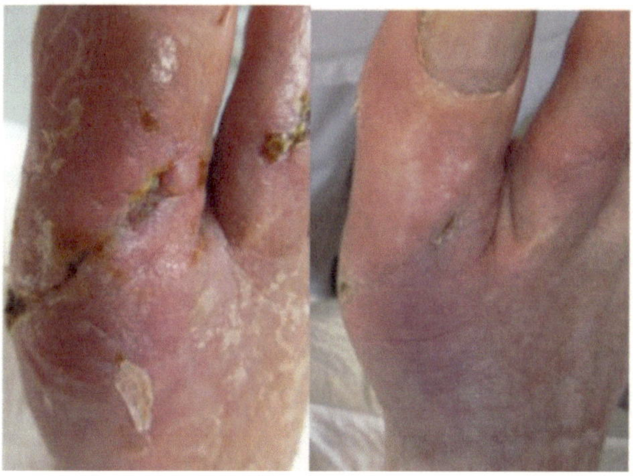

Picture 4. Case report. A 63-year-old patient with infected diabetic food. . Healing process in 2 months.

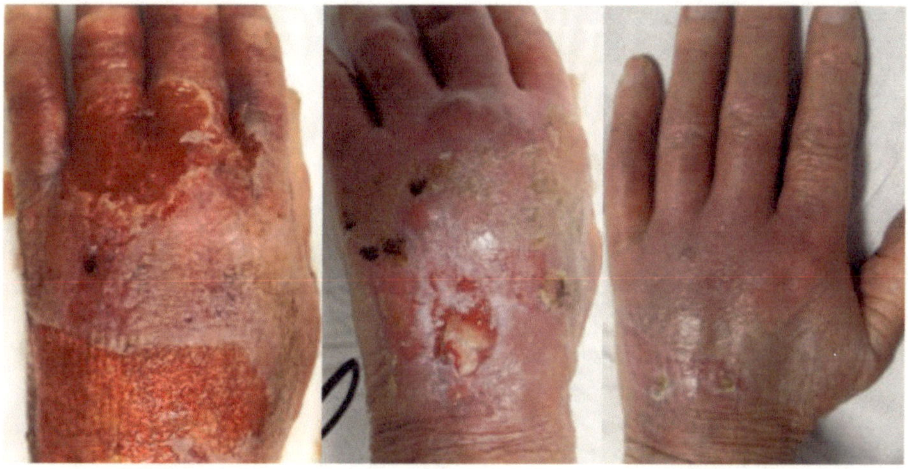

Picture 5. Case report. A 78- year-old patient with arthritis, left hand with inflammationand abscess. Healing process in 3 months.

ensuring the balance of all the components involved in the life cycle of the regenerative phase. The regeneration of skin that has been damaged by multiple etiological factors is made possible by its ability to interact with the outside, and especially the essence of the tissue, that is constantly renewed and capable of repairing and reacting to lesions due to the presence of epidermal stem cells in the dermis and epidermis. In patients with recalcitrant skin lesions, the presence of comorbidities such as chronic disease, diabetes, vascular insufficiency, peripheral edema secondary to heart failure, malnutrition, bedsores, and infections can affect the body's ability to respond to treatment, but can also have a negative effect on the inflammatory modulation process itself, triggering a chronic phase that feeds the non-healing of the lesions.

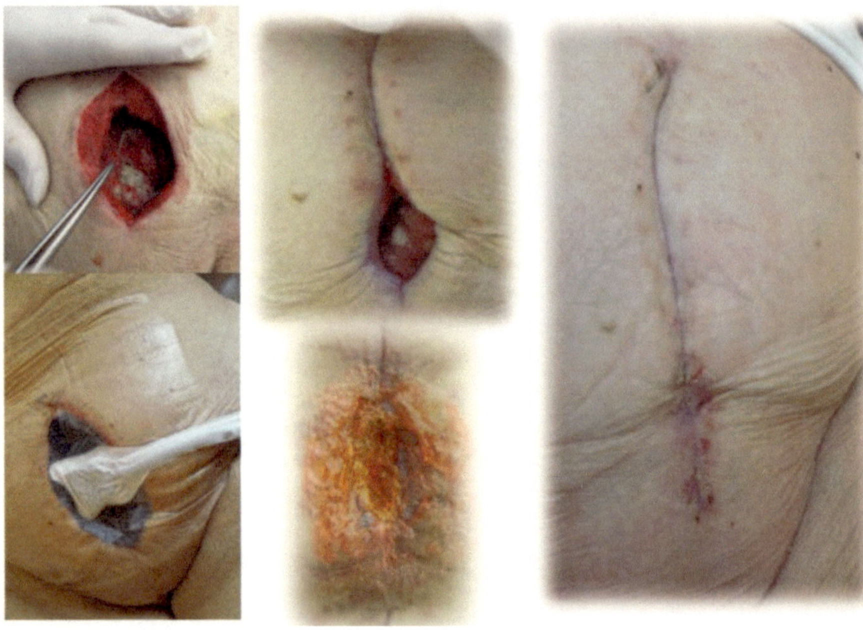

Picture 6. Case report. A 57-old-patient with dehiscence of the surgical wound. Application of NPWT therapy and Healing process in 2 months.

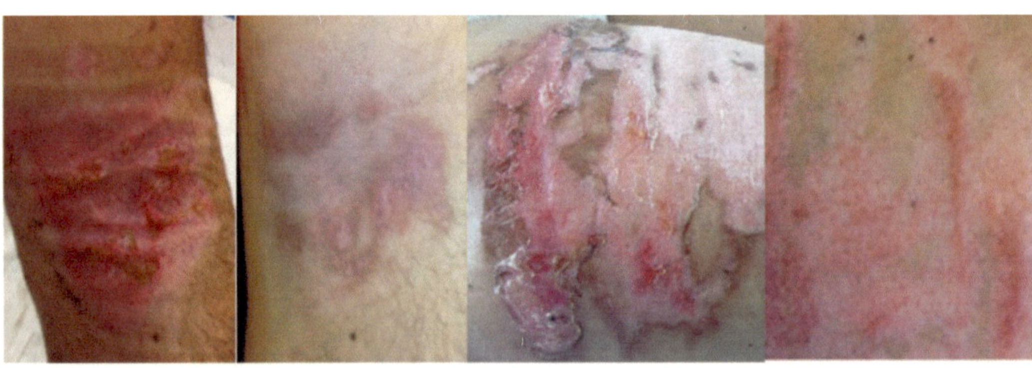

Picture 7. Case report. A 24 old-patient with II and III degree burns on the face and upper limb.

These stages are always present in all types of lesions and physiological process phases, and their timescales, interaction, genetic, humoral, cellular, and ultrastructural mechanisms (which are the basis for the regeneration of injured tissues, in both in vitro models and live models) are all understood. In this article, the authors underline some aspects of the repair and regeneration process in relation to the rationale of the proposed AIMED Model and cohesion between clinical research activities and their translation to methodology. Key roles are played by fibrin deposition and hydration of the matrix by hyaluronic acid, stimulating the production of fibroblasts, while other cell types (granulocytes, monocytes, M1 macrophages and cytokines) play a role in the shutdown of the inflammatory proliferative phase (endothelial cells, fibroblasts and keratinocytes) and the ECM remodeling phase.

http://dx.doi.org/10.5772/intechopen.81291

5.2. Personal experience; materials and methods

The regenerative medicine outpatient clinic (RMC) for the treatment of recalcitrant lesions was established in Castellanza in the summer of 2015. In 2017–2018, 869 patients (286 men and 583 women) were treated at the RMC, for a total of 1718 treatments. Even before applying national and international guidelines on the management of acute and chronic wounds the main activity was the formation of a multidisciplinary team sharing the same philosophy of care: to put patients, their inner world and their families at the heart of the process. The clinical research already practiced by some members of the RMC team was the driving force for the development of hospital treatment and home care models as a therapeutic continuum and for the transferral of the results of this research to clinical practice.

5.3. The foundation of the RMC

> *"There are skills and abilities, and then there's a subtle strength that the patients transmit to you, to say that everything we are doing has given them a better quality of life (Giada Mereghetti, RMC Coordinator).*

The Regenerative Medicine Centre (RMC) was set up in June 2015 in Castellanza, a town in the province of Varese in Lombardy, near the border with the province of Milan, on the basis of the skills and motivation of a group of professionals with a common objective. The RMC forms part of a much larger project, which aims to create a close-knit network of professionals to act as national and international spokespersons for a new way of looking at skin wounds. This ambitious project initially brought together professionals with different skills but who were united by a single mission: to confront and photograph the world of difficult wounds, broadening the objective beyond the usual common goal of mere treatment, and involving patients and their families.

Motivation is the main characteristic common to all project members: the same members who (initially only through ideological discussions) later actively contributed to the RMC's construction, putting an ideal and an objective into practice. Each of the individual professionals, with their important personal experience of the medical world and with years upon years of study in their various scientific disciplines, decided to contribute their knowledge, experience and abilities to the construction of a new organizational model and the creation of a close-knit network of activities, which they hope will spread through the entire country. Each of the members has embraced the philosophy of caregiving, associating respect for the clinical priorities of the patients and their families with the use of national and international methods and guidelines for clinical research and the continuous evolution of the field of wound management. From this perspective, all the professionals making up the RMC outpatient team, with their individual duties and respect for the shared guidelines and protocols, have opened up their perspective of wounds in relation to constant interaction with the university and hospital research institutes with which they work.

The RMC is close to achieving its main research objective in relation to the treatment of wounds: namely, gaining knowledge of the inflammatory process resolution mechanisms in tissue repair and regeneration. Its ambition is an organizational model which takes its professionals outside the hospital walls to enable their scientific and human knowledge to be transferred to and shared with the key players in this project: the patients and their families.

5.4. Main objectives of the RMC

- To respect the mission of managing patients with any acute or chronic lesion affecting the skin or mucous membranes of any etiology (vascular, diabetic, rheumatological, traumatic) while respecting their humanness as a whole.
- To standardize the mechanisms for stimulating regenerative and reparative biochemical and cell processes leading to the healing of lesions, making use of the abilities of the team's clinicians alongside the public and private institutes with which RMC works.
- To create new therapeutic models at the base of regenerative medicine to exploit synthetic biological molecules, engineered tissues and cell therapies that could reproduce the body's own wound repair mechanisms in everyday clinical practice.
- To remain part of a much wider project that focuses attention on skin, cartilage and mucous membrane lesions and places patients at the center of an innovative, barrier-free patient journey.
- To take care of the patient from diagnosis through treatment and follow-up, providing services as needed on the basis of clinical indications and integrating them with innovative complementary treatments.

5.5. Clinical care journey at the RMC

The patient journey in the RMC thus requires careful management involving numerous professionals with distinct areas and responsibilities. Patients go through a well-defined process that should give them a sense of competence, humanity and harmony, making them feel an active part of the group alongside the medical workers treating them. These workers act through the application of protocols and guidelines detailing the treatment and use of the main advanced dressings in relation to the different wound types, which are drawn up on the basis of the main clinical studies found in the literature and others, published more recently, followed directly by the RMC. The RMC makes use of both its own professionals and those employed by the institutes in which it works, as well as of partners and disciplines whose goal is to channel their energies toward the better treatment of patients with skin, cartilage and mucous membrane lesions.

5.6. Care and assistance in the RMC

Given the main objective and mission of the RMC, which can be summarized as the management of patients with any acute or chronic lesion affecting the skin or mucous membranes and who have non-healing ulcers or wounds of different etiologies (vascular, diabetic, rheumatological, traumatic), the RMC's activities can be classified in the following areas:

- Assessment of the lesion;
- Overall assessment of the patient;
- Management and removal of the cause leading to the formation of the lesion;
- Application of validated, shared protocols;

- Prevention and management of complications;
- Ultrasound treatment of skin lesions to remove necrotic and fibrinous tissue, acting as a bactericide and stimulus for tissue regeneration;
- Surgical procedures for biopsies, surgical debridement, and removal of lesions with reconstruction and/or skin grafts;
- Documentation of the assessments and procedures through shared records;
- Creation of protocols on the basis of technological innovations and monitoring of markers;
- Consultancy and cooperation with all in-house services (Inpatient wards and Accident & Emergency Department);
- Consultancy and cooperation with community services (GPs, integrated home care (ADI), residential care homes (RSA));
- Cooperation with the training department to create a network of consistent, competent professionals;
- Promotion of community outreach initiatives;
- Health education.

The Castellanza RMC has a 360° structure, in which the specialists taking charge of care injuries collaborate in important phases of patient assessment and management of both the injuries and the patients as a whole. After this phase of diagnostic classification, the patients are provided with multilevel treatment that applies all the steps detailed in international guidelines,

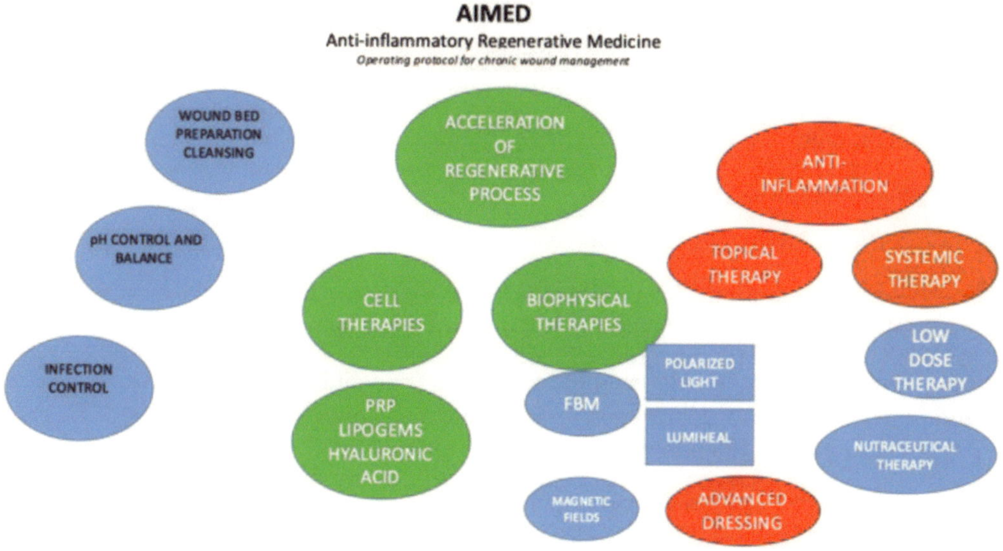

Figure 5. AIMED - Anti Inflammaging regenerative medicine: operating protocol for chronic wound management (E.S. Aragona – 2017).

but with an additional, innovative perspective that gives importance to anti-inflammatory and regenerative activity.

The AIMED operating protocol provides local treatment of skin lesions and a general evaluation of the patient, with particular attention to the preliminary assessment of the causes of lesion). (**Figure 5**). The model enables the dynamic partnership of all professionals working with RMC specialists to ensure a simple, interruption-free patient journey in the Institute. An example of this is the in-house cooperation with the Cardiology and Hemodynamics Dept. for vascular lesions of arterial origin, which are evaluated within a multidisciplinary team where, from their first visit to the clinic, patients are guided through a diagnostic angiography journey involving a vascular rehabilitation process. In these revascularized patients the care model also focuses on the risks of reperfusion and the production of a proinflammatory state with increased peripheral oxidation and potential necrosis of the tissues affected by the critical ischemia.

6. Description of the lesion model under the AIMED protocol

The lesions are classified by type and stage in accordance with international guidelines, and the various types of advanced treatment are assessed and selected in relation to the type of lesion and the operating protocol, with attention to pharmacoeconomics.

Five basic operating protocol steps.

Step 1: Preparation of the lesion for treatment. This includes cleansing and combating infections using current methods [4].

Step 2: Topical and systemic treatment protocols to modulate the inflammatory phase and trigger the regenerative phase.

Step 3: Biophysical therapies to stimulate regeneration.

Step 4: Cell therapies.

Step 5: Surgical therapies.

These steps are discussed below in detail.

STEP 1—Wound Preparation

The first step is deep cleansing of the wound and modifying its pH. This important step requires careful management: cleaning the wound of nonviable tissue, fibrin, protease, bacteria and biofilm or cellular debris can eliminate potential causes of non-healing. This is followed by modification of the lesion's pH.

The pH value within the microenvironment of the wound directly and indirectly influences all biochemical reactions that take place in the healing process. It has been shown that the pH of the surface of a wound plays an important role in wound healing and helps to control the infection and increase antimicrobial activity, the release of oxygen, angiogenesis, protease activity and bacterial toxicity. The pH value influences cellular events that regulate the healing process of wounds. It was observed that the acute and chronic wounds with an alkaline pH have a lower rate of cure than the wounds with a pH close to neutral. The wound healing process slows down when the pH is high, under alkaline conditions. (Levine).

Intact skin has a pH between 4.8 and 6, depending on the area in question. The pH of wounds cannot be easily measured, but literature data demonstrate that a wound pH of around 4 can trigger a more rapid wound healing process.

In *The effects of pH on wound healing, biofilms, and antimicrobial efficacy* published in Wound Repair Regen. 2014 (March) [5], Percival et al. attribute wound pH with an important role in the activity of MMPs, TIMPs and fibroblasts and in collagen production. pH also interferes with bacterial proliferation and the patient's immunological response, and its monitoring and control is one of the strategies used to trigger the healing process. In *The effect of pH on the Extracellular Matrix and Biofilms,* published in Adv. Wound Care, Jul 1,4 [6], Jones, Cochrane and Percival provide an overview of the role of pH and its effect on the ECM and biofilm in connection with wound healing. Chronic lesions have an alkaline pH, while the pH tends toward acidity during the healing process.

The model involves the use of commercially available products chosen on the basis of their properties, their contact time and the duration of their action on the wound.

Polyhexanide with betaine surfactant.

Hypochlorous acid.

The authors of the present article have started an observational study of a class III medical device following a study of the bacterial load of the lesion and of certain bacterial strains (*Staphylococcus aureus, Staph. epidermidis, Escherichia coli* and *Pseudomonas aeruginosa*) that associated a pH of 4.5–5.00 with the mechanical removal of bacteria and protease due to the presence in its composition of d-mannose, copper sulfate, zinc and other components that are part of the authors' know-how.

STEP 2A—Topical Treatment

The topical treatment involves two phases. The first, enzymatic and mechanical debridement (the technique preferred by the authors), is the crucial moment in wound management, eliminating the mechanical and biochemical causes that can perpetuate the inflammatory process and preparing the wound for the action of biological and physical substances that can trigger a local anti-inflammatory action and catalyze the proliferation of cell populations, ensuring good hydration in the wound bed.

The lesions are always treated with the local application of medical devices, biophysical therapies and cell therapies.

STEP 2B—Systemic Treatment

Even though it is described as part of step 2, systemic treatment is applied from the very start of the wound's management under a 360°, polyvalent protocol depending on the type and severity of the lesion.

Administration of a dietary supplement containing a well-balanced mix of serratio-peptidase, escin, bromelain and selenium. This supplement has proteolytic, fibrinolytic, anti-edema and draining properties, as well as an antioxidant action.

The rationale for the prescription of this supplement is:

- Anti-inflammatory action (proteolytic and fibrinolytic);
- Bacteriostatic action in uninfected lesions and antibiotic therapy in infected lesions;
- Anti-edema and draining action;
- Reduction of secretions;
- Pain relief;
- Promotion of healing [7].

Administration of low-dose cytokines to combat the inflammatory process.

Patients are prescribed with 3–6 months of treatment with low-dose cytokines, formulated with a kinetic system called Sequential Kinetic Activation (SKA), and containing:

1. Anti IL-1 - regulation and suppression of the inflammatory response.
2. IL-10 - adjustment of the anti-inflammatory process in chronic diseases with reduction of IL-6.
3. IL-4 - Th1-Th2 switch control.

Low dose therapy is an important part of wound management because it introduces into clinical practice a strategic concept for future therapies: the disease may be the result of an altered concentration of messenger or signal molecules (hormones, cytokines, neurotransmitters) for cellular activity, and in this case the modulation of these molecules can restore the disrupted balances, enabling healing [8].

STEP 3—Biophysical Therapies

Photobiomodulation

During the process the wound is subjected to dual-type light frequencies for 8–20 minutes.

1. Polarized light

RMC is the first center in Italy to use a unique light source that is:

- Polarized, propagating in parallel planes;
- Polychromatic, with a wavelength ranging from 480 to 3400 nm;
- Incoherent, with out-of-phase waves delivering low-intensity light;
- Low-energy, reaching the wound with a constant intensity, producing bio-stimulating effects.

It has been demonstrated that polarized light at 590 nm stimulates angiogenesis and growth factors, while at 830 nm it activates the cells involved in wound healing; a dose of 20 J/cm^2 stimulates increased collagen deposition, an increase in myofibroblasts and a better ultra-structural organization of the wound healing process [9–14].

2. LumiHeal

The Lumiheal protocol involves the use of broadband wavelengths (blue, green, yellow/orange from 450 nm to 610 nm) from a light emitting diode to amplify the physical effect of stimulation of the regenerative processes in the injured area due to the emission of photons in the form of fluorescence. The LumiHeal Protocol has been applied over the last 3 months in 8 patients with complicated treatment-resistant infected wounds. The improvement in the wounds is documented by photographic evidence [15–20].

Pulsed electromagnetic fields (PEMF)

High intensity, variable frequency magnetic fields for outpatient and home treatment. As already demonstrated in our first patients, they:

- Are anti-inflammatory, through modulation of the profile of cytokines produced by proinflammatory cells (IL-1, NGF, ROS, IL8);
- Are angiogenic, with increased proliferation of endothelial cells and FGF-2 (fibroblast growth factor), improving microcirculation;
- **Improve the microcirculation**, with increased collagen production [21, 22].

STEP 4—Cell Therapies

Platelet-rich plasma (PRP)

PRP is a powerful concentrate of growth factors that stimulate tissue regeneration and is used to treat damaged tissues. Under current Italian legislation, the PRP used by the RMC must be prepared in a local transfusion center (**Picture 8**) [23–26].

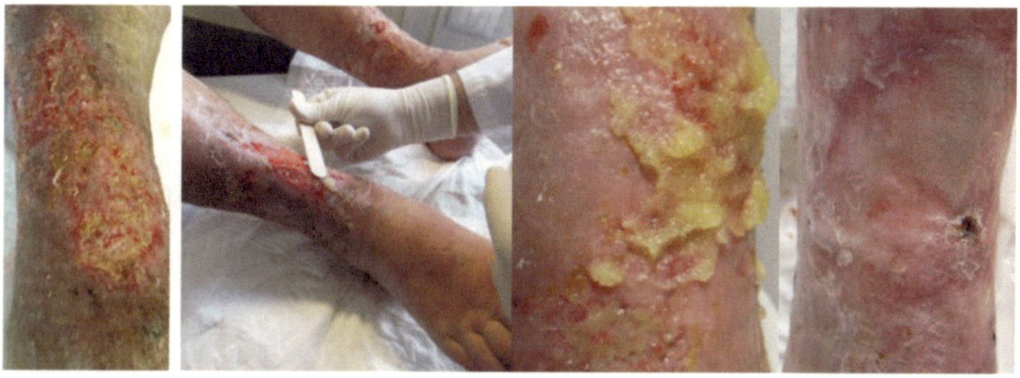

Picture 8. Case report. A 74-old-patient with vascular ulcers of the lower limbs treated with PRP.

Lipogems

Method for obtaining, through adipose liposuction, micro-fractured tissue for autologous use, which is reapplied to patients with skin lesions to further stimulate the cell regeneration process [27–30].

STEP 5—Surgical Therapies

At the RMC, surgical therapies for the repair of skin lesions are standardized. They involve the use of skin substitutes that promote the production of a structured collagen matrix, enabling better angiogenesis. When monitoring the application of skin substitutes, the focus is on the skin's reparative capacity as well as the risk of tissue rejection. The removal of any necrosis when cleaning the wound is essential to prepare it for autologous or heterologous grafts that fully integrate into the patient's dermis, and signs of rejection must be managed promptly.

7. From repair to regeneration: Regeneration 3.0

7.1. The Prometheus project

The RMC's clinical experience in cell therapies is based on the traumatic extraction methods that underlie the preparation of platelet-rich plasma and the extraction and centrifugation of adipose tissue (lipoaspiration) with the aid of modern technology. The results of their use in a treatment pathway that accompanies patients in their management are remarkable.

In relation to the use and performance of mesenchymal cells (immunomodulatory, paracrine and regenerative activity) in the RMC's clinical research, the multidisciplinary team were united by the realization that mesenchymal cells cannot be used in therapy and there is a need to optimize a daily therapy that has a similar effect on cell and tissue biostimulation. The Prometheus Project - Alfakjn Wound Care has been embraced by the RMC because it is *innovative* and because it anticipates the next frontier for regenerative medicine: *specific, individualized cell therapies.* Growth factors have made an explosive breakthrough into clinical practice, and the decision to focus on the quality and efficacy of the therapies containing them is strategic for the near future.

A careful analysis of the components of and claims made for the medical devices trialed by the RMC for the treatment of superficial and deep wounds and lesions through a clinical research joint venture has highlighted the need for a scientific value to be attributed to the rationale for using these devices, within the framework of a multidisciplinary activity intended to give added value to the device's action in regenerative medicine. The objective of the RMC's study was to offer an innovative solution to the current difficulties in managing nonhealing skin lesions. To do this, we first tried to answer a question: Do difficult wounds exist, or is it simply that we do not know how to treat them?

Our research is based on two articles, published in 2016 (Zhao R et al.: Inflammation in Chronic Wounds. Int J Mol Sci) and 2017 (Han G et al.: Chronic Wound Healing: A Review of current Management and Treatments. Adv. Ther) [12, 13].

These articles affirm what we wrote in the introduction: inflammation has a major role in the wound healing process, in which disabling chronic diseases add to local systemic effects such as tissue hypoxia and pH changes, post-revascularization damage, cell aging and infections. Therapeutic resources take account of the numerous techniques and resources available, with particular attention to growth factors.

In this research process we began with a definition: **Repair 1.0**, signifying a dressing process involving the use of advanced dressings. This type of dressing is required to maintain an adequate wound moisture level, to be partly or totally occlusive, and to passively absorb the exudate, with a function determined by the patient's metabolism and biological "performance".

Repair 2.0, in contrast, involves the use of bioactive dressings with a biological action on the wound (hyaluronic acid, collagen, silver, etc.). From this perspective, the RMC investigated a sterile gauze dressing in which the role of the bioactive substances (hyaluronic acid, carnosine) is specifically defined in the literature, and involves mechanical protection of the lesion (gauze) combined with a direct anti-inflammatory action.

Zhao et al. examine the causes of nonhealing wounds, and attribute the greatest responsibility to the inflammatory process. That study's relevance to the present article is its affirmation of the role of nitric oxide in the repair process and the well-known harm caused by ROS that, through systemic or topical treatment with antioxidants (carnosine), can be turned around in non-responding lesions [31].

In this context, we began working with bioactive substances with innovative properties (in relation to both composition and biological action) in comparison with their competitors. This potential innovation lies in the use of bovine colostrum, that, when stabilized through industrial processes to a pH of 6.8, assures the compound's stability and its action against the tissue acidosis found in damaged tissues. This has positive consequences for the modulation of the inflammatory process and the tissue repair process as well as on the ability to stimulate the cellular and ultrastructural regenerative process. (Bagnara G: *Le cellule staminali*, Cap 11. Ed Esculapio 2017).

In **Regeneration 3.0**, the priority is to combine the anti-inflammatory activity of the nine proteins acting as growth factors in the bovine colostrum, the homeostatic, angiogenic and reorganizational activities of the matrix, the modulation of collagen synthesis and the remodeling of the epithelium. The choice of bovine colostrum and its associated properties was the basis for the design of devices that could also offer those properties: barrier action, anti-inflammatory action and pain reduction, reduction and absorption of exudates, combating of bacterial and fungal proliferation, antioxidant action and hydration and protection against skin diseases and dermatosis.

This is the culmination of an in-vitro and an in-vivo test.

7.2. In Vitro comparative evaluation of wound healing activity of medical

The purpose of this test is to compare the efficacy of two medical devices in the repairing of wounds simulating this situation in vitro by making a cut on cell monolayer of human

Campione/*Sample*	Controllo negativo/*negative control*	Pr 1 mg/ml	Pr 0,25 mg/ml	Pr 0,15 mg/ml
O.D. Valore medio / *Mean value*	1,9	1,292	1,659	1,755
pg/ml Valore medio / *Mean value*	3064,727	1959,970	2627,693	2838,670
% IL8	100	63,95	85,74	92,62
% riduzione IL8/ *% reduction of IL8*	0	36,05	14,26	7,38

A % of reduction of IL8 is observed at tested concentrations of 1 and 0.25 mg/ml

Campione/ *Sample* mg/ml	1	0,25	0,15	Controllo negativo/ *Negative control*	CQ
O.D. Media /*Medium*	1,419	1,473	1,648	1,586	2,566
% Vitalità cellulare/ *% of cell vitality*	89,50	92,87	103,89	100,00	161,78

The viability of fibroblasts in the plates treated with PP003 AIM Gel Herpes (AI13-003D) Lotto 11/2014 has proved to be comparable to that of untreated cells, indicating the total absence of cytotoxicity of the tested medical device and to demonstrate a modulation of the metabolism of the cells that resulting healthy and viable and able to reconstruct the monolayer where we have made the cut

Figure 6. In vitro comparative evaluation of wound healing activity of medical devices, Alfakjn ResearchCenter Milano 2018 by Bio Basic Europe SRL. Via A. Panizzi,10 Milano Italy.

fibroblasts (Hude) and then evaluating the approximation of the edges of the cut in cells treated with the two medical devices, in comparison to untreated cells. In order to select the concentrations of 2 medical devices to be used for the test r (not cytotoxic concentrations for the cells), a preliminary MTT cell cultures of fibroblasts was performed. The cells were treated with scalar concentrations of the two medical devices (as low as 1 mg/ml and subsequent dilutions 1: 2) and untreated cells were used as negative control. Based on the obtained results concentrations of 2 medical devices of 1–0.25–0.15 mg/ml were chosen to continue the test. After making a cut on the cell monolayer of confluent fibroblasts (simulation of a wound), the cells were treated with the chosen concentrations of the two medical devices, as negative control untreated cells were used and, as internal quality control one standard with known activity of wound healing activity. Therefore, we have performed a morphologic evaluation of the monolayer by microscopy and a measurement of IL-8 levels. From the morphological evaluation a net approach of the flaps of the monolayer was observed in the plates treated with the various concentrations of Colostrum Gel. The dosage dell'IL8 showed significant decrease in the% of IL8 to concentrations of 1 and 0.25 mg/ml by both tested medical devices, showing therefore a comparable anti-inflammatory action on fibroblasts (**Figure 6**). These results indicate that the effectiveness of the active ingredients present in the product have a different target than the reduction of the inflammatory response. The obtained results have showed the effectiveness in wound healing of the medical device Colostrum Gel, compared to the medical device Gel no active. The medical device Gel Herpes no active is in fact shows a "nutrient" activity on cells but it is not able to stimulate the repair of the damage (cutting), this latter activity is due to the presence of actives ingredients present in the formula of Colostrum Gel. Colostrum Gel reduced IL8 production by fibroblasts and contains active ingredients. Those stimulate wound healing (simulation in vitro by cutting the monolayer of cultured fibroblasts and evidence of the approximation of the edges of the cut and almost total closure of the same) (**Figure 7**).

7.3. Topical use of Colostro AIM 4% fluid cream in a murine model of pressure ulcers

This study reports the development of a murine model of pressure ulcers by using externally placed magnets to create the ischemic events of ischemia reperfusion (IR) injury.

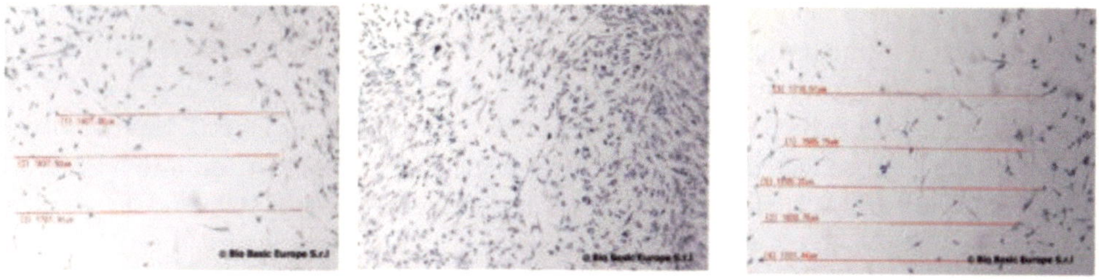

Any approximation of the edges of the cut are observed

An evident approximation of the edges of the cut with almost total closure of the same is observed

Any significant approximation of the edges of the cut are observed

Figure 7. In vitro comparative evaluation of wound healing activity of medical devices - Cell Growth . Alfakjn ResearchCenter Milano 2018 by Bio Basic Europe SRL. Via A. Panizzi,10 Milano Italy.

The animals were individually housed, their backs have been shaved, cleaned with alcohol, the skin has been gently pulled up and placed between two round ceramic magnetic plates which have a 12-mm diameter (113 mm^2) and are 5 mm thick, with an average weight of 2.4 g and 1000G magnetic forces; this process creates a compressive pressure of 50 mmHg between the two magnets. Then the animals have been divided into two groups as follows:

Control group: three IR cycles have been performed in 3 mice to initiate decubitus ulcer formation. A single IR cycle consists of a 12-hour period of magnet placement, followed by a release of rest period of 12 hours. After the 3 IR cycles, the animals have been sacrificed.

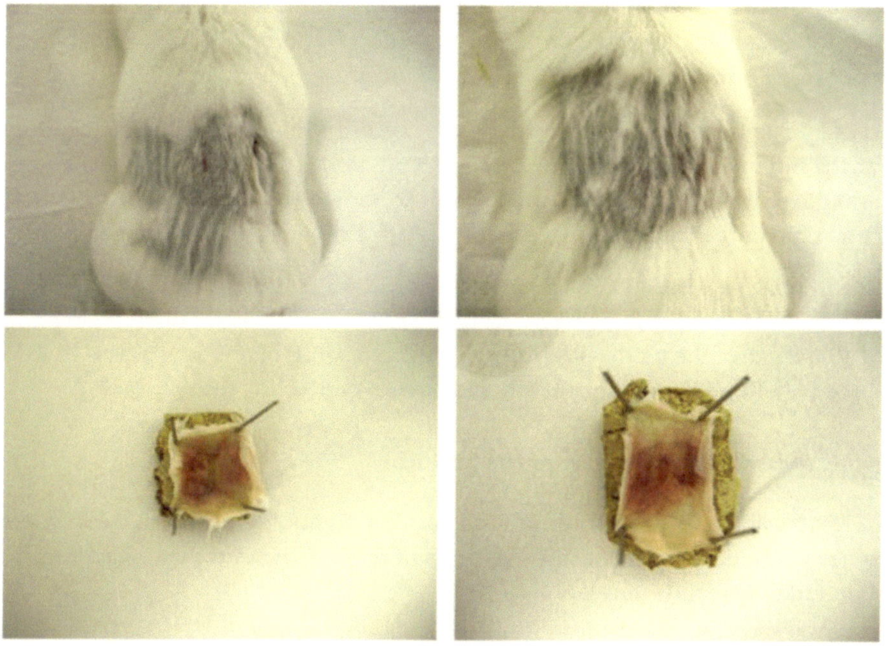

Picture 9. Initiate decubitus ulcer formation in mice to test colostrum derivative therapy.

Group B: three IR cycles have been performed in each mouse to initiate decubitus ulcer formation. A topical administration of 200 mg of AIM LIFEIN- SIDE 4% (AI13–002-B) has been applied on the backs of each mouse the day before the first IR cycle and at the end of each compressive cycle. After the 3 IR cycles, the animals have been sacrificed. Skin samples of each mouse have been collected from the treated area, fixed in 10% phosphate-buffered formalin and wax embedded. 2 μm thickness sections were obtained and collected on silanizated slides and stained by hematoxylin- eosin. The samples were then observed with an optical microscope Nikon 80i, fitted with a digital camera (**Picture 9**).

8. Results

1. Control group: 3 IR cycles Skin macroscopic analysis Macroscopic analysis of dorsal skin revealed the presence of mild skin lesions, edema and signs of necrosis of the epidermis. (Photo 10). Histological analysis of dorsal skin samples stained by hematoxylin–eosin showed: wide ulcerative area of the epidermis; marked spongiosis of basal layer (intercellular bridges appear very prominent); marked diffuse inflammatory infiltrate; conjunctival edema; vascular hyperemia; presence of extravasal erythrocytes (**Picture 10**).
2. Group B: 3 IR cycles+Colostro AIM at the end of each compressive cycle and the day before the first IR cycle. Skin macroscopic analysis. Macroscopic analysis of dorsal skin revealed: skin ulcers with necrosis areas and edema (**Picture 11**). Histological analysis of dorsal skin samples stained by hematoxylin–eosin showed: wide ulcerative area of the epidermis; when present epidermis is hyperplasic, with not regular thickness, marked spongiosis of basal layer and presence of lymphocytes; marked diffuse inflammatory infiltrate; conjunctival edema; vascular hyperemia; presence of extravasal erythrocytes (**Picture 12**).

The most significant aspect with a view to new tissue regeneration therapies and hence the control of the inflammatory process were the results in relation to the disappearance of the wound and the reduction of the inflammatory process. This requires the future consideration of the action time of the medical device and its contact time with the damaged tissue.

The results in relation to clinical healing take account of chronic conditions defined as non-responders and their good management from the time of diagnosis. The data on patient compliance with the use of the medical device reveal the absence of any symptoms or side effects, ensuring the patient's safety and boosting the device's reliability and efficacy.

8.1. Analysis of results and validity of the protocol

The RMC treats patients with chronic wounds of various etiologies. The AIMED model treatment has been applied in 85% of cases. Analysis of the 360° wound management process has revealed remarkable results in relation to:

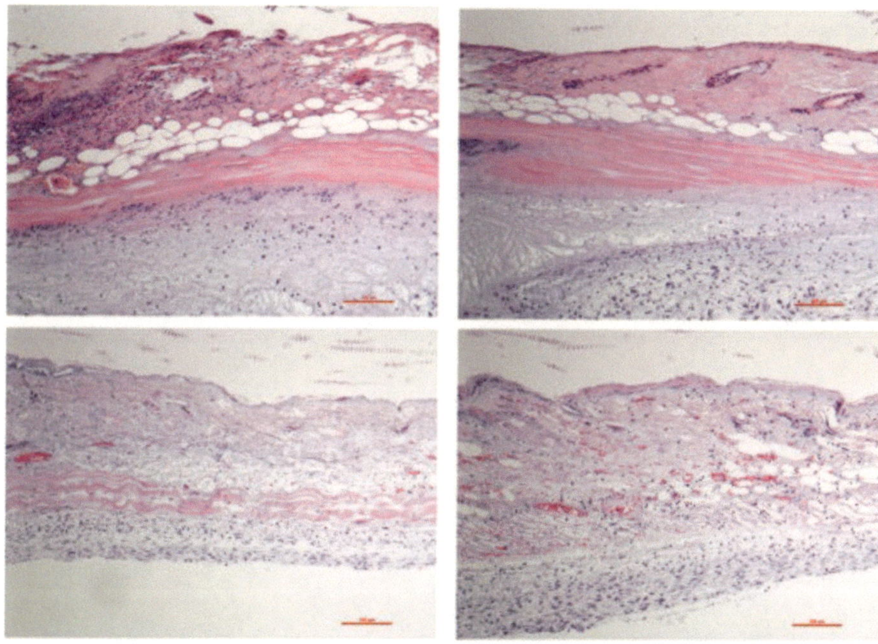

Picture 10. Wide ulcerative area of the epidermis; marked spongiosis of basal layer (intercellular bridges appear very prominent); marked diffuse inflammatory infiltrate; conjunctival edema; vascular hyperemia; presence of extravasal erythrocytes.

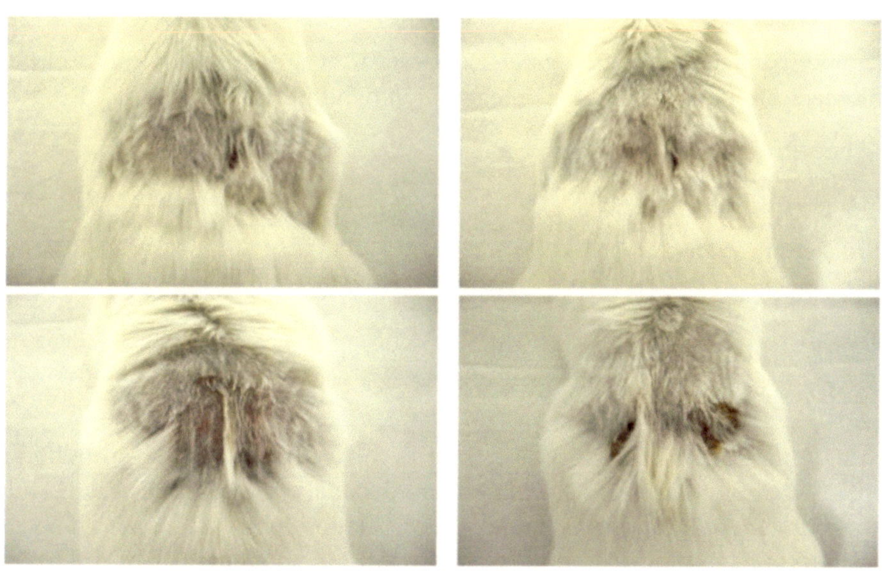

Picture 11. Macroscopic analysis of dorsal skin revealed: skin ulcers with necrosis areas and edema.

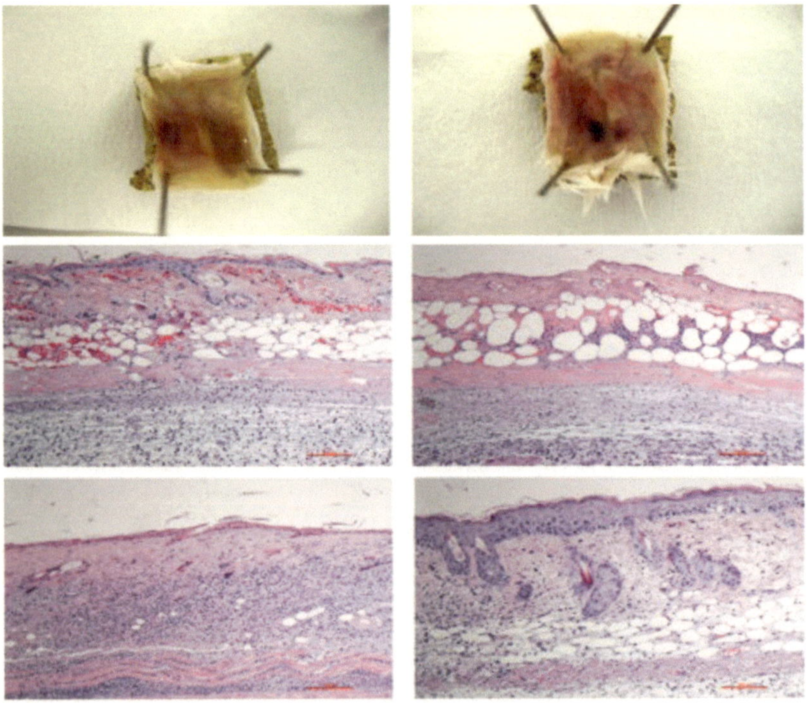

Picture 12. Wide ulcerative area of the epidermis; when present epidermis is hyperplasic, with not regular thickness, marked spongiosis of basal layer and presence of lymphocytes; marked diffuse inflammatory infiltrate; conjunctival edema; vascular hyperemia; presence of extravasal erythrocytes.

- Best wound management with a greater awareness of dressing protocols and the use of existing medications on the market, integrated into the AIMED model;
- Rapid healing;
- Pain reduction;
- Reduced complications and signs of comorbidity;
- Reduced health expenditure;
- Better compliance and patient and family satisfaction;
- Reduced rate of recurrence.

Another important aspect of the RMC's activity is the constant back-and-forth between the results obtained through clinical observation and the analysis of the collected data through clinical research, in the light of a possible reinterpretation in a future scenario focusing on two key aspects of the healing of chronic wounds: anti-inflammatory action and regenerative action [31, 32].

In this article, the authors lay down the scientific basis for a chronic wound healing process involving an appropriate sequence of the modulation of the inflammatory and proliferative

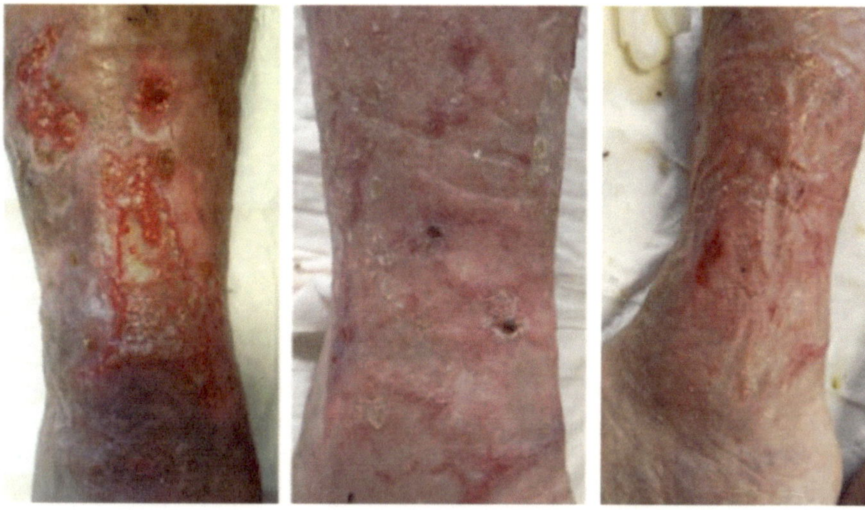

Picture 13. A 73-year-old patient with heart failure and lower limb ulcers. Healing process with the AIMED method in 3 and a half months.

processes and remodeling of the ECM. At the same time, they highlight how the abnormal evolution of the inflammatory process to a chronic condition involves abnormal cellularity, inappropriate collagen deposit and the presence of protease, preventing re-epithelialization and regeneration of the lesion. (**Picture 13**).

Knowledge of the biological pathways at an ultramolecular and cellular level enables the identification of various areas where clinical research could intervene with biological drugs or biophysical therapies to influence the healing pathways of non-responding chronic wounds or stimulate the metabolic or regenerative processes, blocking the mechanisms leading to chronicity and, in particular, intervening in the chronic inflammatory process. In this case, in vitro tests could help by enabling new biological compounds to be tested on cellular models of skin damage. We have demonstrated that colostrum is paradigmatic of the therapeutic philosophy adopted by the RMC, in the sense that it is capable of reducing levels of proinflammatory cytokines and protease (MMP-9), blocking M1 activity and stimulating the activity of fibroblasts, resulting in the production of type III and VII collagen to aid regeneration.

Analysis of the results obtained with low dose therapy and the effects of biophysical therapies (photobiomodulation and PEMF) could provide guidance on aspects that the authors consider to be of current and future interest: modulation of nitric oxide in vasodilation and the provision of regenerative molecules (PEMF), and the reduction of the inflammatory component (IL-6 and C-reactive protein). Analysis of the current literature suggests that reduction of the inflammatory component is the key to regenerative recovery of chronic nonresponding wounds, now that we have a better understating of their pathogenesis and pathophysiological processes. The adoption of a 360° rather than sequential wound management model is based on the authors' choices and experience, and has a firm scientific basis. We believe that this model ensures that patients receive the best possible care and attention.

9. Conclusions

The molecular pond is in a state of constant agitation and turbulence, with the molecules spinning and vibrating and bouncing off one another…

Life on the Edge – J. McFadden and J. Al-Khalili

10. The future of regeneration

The study of biological molecules has enabled a glimpse of a possible new key for the interpretation of biological phenomena linked to management of the inflammatory process, and some such molecules could be prototypes for others still to come. The greater availability of water molecules around more hydrophilic molecules and the better organization of the body's water seem to produce a greater and better biological response.

> *"We could interpret the disease as a loss of some levels of cohesive hierarchy between the domains, with a consequent loss of the electromagnetic control exerted over the biomolecules" (E. Del Giudice).*

In the study of the hydrodynamic behavior of numerous molecules, it always comes back to the endothelium, the ECM and the cells themselves. The role of the cell membrane seems worthy of attention, as its structure enables substances to travel or be transported into the cell, but the functional properties of the membrane that we know today make it the protagonist of a new biological culture, in which chemistry meets anatomy and anatomy is subject to physical stimuli that can modify its essence [33–36].

The inner cell is packed with a thick, intricate network of microtubules formed by well-known proteins (tubulin). This network, called the **cytoskeleton**, has a complicated and constantly changing dynamic structure and function: some branches form, others break down and disappear, others extend in multiple directions.

Most intracellular metabolic reactions take place along the branches of the cytoskeleton. Its structure is thus fundamental for biochemical functionality (a new functional concept), which marks a continuum between the cell nucleus, the membrane and the outside of the cell, protected by another important structure, the glycocalyx. When the cell dies, its cytoskeleton breaks down. This highly dynamic behavior is difficult to understand, but there have been a number of studies of both the biochemistry involved and the energy and charge transport capacity along the microtubules (Davydov, 1982 and references reported therein).

The cytoskeleton is a system of canals (microtubules) in which substances are transported and information is transmitted. This is made possible because all its molecules, including water (which makes up 80% or more of the cytoskeleton by weight), have a dipole moment – in other words, an electrically charged spatial distribution involving a positively charged pole and a negatively charged pole. **All macromolecules become biologically active only if they are immersed in an aqueous matrix.** This demonstrates the predominant role of water in living beings. Intuition is transformed into scientific data and becomes reality.

Quantum medicine returns to that concept of electromagnetic fields, the energy of which can change the very essence of nature. The concept that emerges is that the cell can undergo a self-healing process if it receives the right information: this is the new advance.

Stem cells will be mentioned only briefly, as it will be left to other authors to present the latest data. Stem cells deriving from adipose tissue have now become part of everyday clinical practice. However, their results in the treatment of skin wounds are not yet unequivocal, as the greatest obstacle they encounter, directly after implantation, is the inflammatory reaction of the host. They have a migratory capacity that enables them to reach the target site through the blood, enabling rapid access to the entire body. They are then captured by the target organs through complex interactions with endothelial cells that enable them to leave the circulation for tissue regeneration.

Given this premise, stem cells could offer an opportunity for the regenerative treatment of skin lesions, but only if used according to holistic principles. The authors explain their view by returning to the concept of self-healing of the cell in a context such as tissue regeneration, where cell proliferation and differentiation are specific and fundamental processes. After transplantation, stem cells work only if they can communicate with the stem cells already resident in the tissue, acting as a starter and stimulating the existing cells through the cell membrane. In 2012, Yamanaka won the Nobel prize for a 2006 study on the induction of stem cells from fibroblasts through cell manipulation, observing that adult cells can be reprogrammed to become pluripotent. The limitation of this technique is the low efficiency of the differentiation process and the oncogenic risk caused by the use of viral vectors.

Today, stem cells can be incubated and stimulated with platelet lysate, which stimulates their proliferation, or with biological agents, but they can also be reactivated in vivo through low-intensity magnetic fields affecting the matrix, membrane and cytoskeleton. Following external stimulation from receptors, the microtubules immersed in the intracellular water vibrate and transmit information to and from the nucleus through signal molecules, just as a dipole transmits the signal beyond the point where it was generated, amplifying the response and turning the cell membrane into a center for signal processing and communication with the outside world. The microtubule is a "molecular cable" that enables the system to memorize information (*C. Ventura*). All this is made possible by the presence of water, which is essential to enable the humoral and cellular components to perform their roles and the microtubules to spread a dynamic network sensitive to even the slightest signal alteration: a "conscious" network that modulates recognition and communication through the signification of coded messages.

Pluripotent stem cells differentiate thanks to an epigenetic code comprising a molecular network that turns specific genes on and off. The information carried by the molecules is only a part of all the information that reaches the cells, of which a large part arrives with magnetic and sound fields. Ventura and colleagues differentiated embryonal stem cells from heart tissue cells by subjecting them to low frequency (50 Hertz), low intensity (0.6 mm tesla) electromagnetic fields.

> *"The cells communicate with each other using information carried by molecules, which act over a short range, or transported by electromagnetic waves and sounds transmitted over a long range and targeted precisely to the molecules" (Pier Maria Biava).*

Molecular information comprises a concerto that enables life to begin and maintain its balance. It is a chemical system governed by electromagnetic forces. The body's water enables this electromagnetic regulation of the biochemistry, as described in the studies of Emilio Del Giudice on the dynamics of water. Cohesive water (in which the molecules are held together by smaller energy forms) oscillates at a given frequency and attracts molecules that resonate at the same frequency. These molecules interact chemically and produce a new form of energy that, in turn, "reconditions" the magnetic field, modifying its frequency and causing the emergence of its information content of various levels of complexity, which tells the water molecules what to do.

"We could interpret disease as a loss, by the body's water, of some levels of cohesive hierarchy between the domains, with a consequent loss of the electromagnetic control exerted over the biomolecules (Emilio Del Giudice).

While awaiting the new frontiers and conquests that the use of stem cells will open up in the field of cell regeneration, today it is possible to introduce biological therapies tailor-made for each individual patient. The biological molecules used in the preclinical and clinical phase enable greater communication between the patient's biological components (endothelium, matrix, cell), thanks to their greater hydrodynamic capacity and the formation of cohesive, organized water, which modulates the components of the inflammatory process and directs it toward tissue regeneration and healing of skin wounds.

> *Later I looked again, and before my eyes a door stood open in Heaven, and in my ears was the voice with the ring of a trumpet, which I had heard at first, speaking to me and saying, "Come up here, and I will show you what must happen in the future."*

Revelation 3.4

In conclusion, this article has briefly presented our current knowledge of the modulation of the inflammatory process. It first discussed the possibility of following the process in in-vitro models – a valuable option, both for the knowledge they provide and for the possibility of learning more about the behavior of biological agents in relation to tissue regeneration. It then followed the process from a molecular perspective, delving into the "magma" of the pro- and anti-inflammatory cytokines and concentrating on what needs to be blocked in order to reduce the inflammatory process (TNF-alpha and IL1), without losing sight of the structure of the ECM, which remains the main target and the place in which the newly formed tissue is remodeled. It went on to discuss current results in relation to the possible clinical application of stem cells in regenerative medicine, highlighting the role of biological water as a transducer of molecular and energy information perceived by the stem cells, as well as the role of the cell membrane which, in the presence of water and in concert with the complex of molecular" cables" (the cytoskeleton), becomes a signal and information processing center involving receptors, adhesion molecules, the ECM structure and cell populations, with a "chimera" effect that is subject to both known and undiscovered physicochemical laws.

We would like to end with some practical considerations. The wound healing process is a complex process intertwined with the biological mechanisms causing individuals to become ill. Systemic and local factors combine to cause the process to become chronic and perpetuate itself in the skin wound, an expression of it all. Bacterial infections, which are difficult to combat due to antibiotic resistance, greatly complicate the roles of our innate immune system and lymphocytes. Reading between the lines of routine blood tests, the patient's discomfort can often be sensed through information on the nitrogen balance and the hemoglobin value. The lack of new antibiotics and the impossibility of treating patients at home with hospital medications mean that new, more biological and more physical pathways must be investigated to interact with and defeat bacteria. The results of Montagnier and colleagues suggest that exposing bacteria to electromagnetic fields and hence altering their genetic code or forcing their membranes to become more water permeable could lead to their implosion.

We now know the key players in the wound healing process and we have new molecules available to act on them, but the future must necessarily lie in the transfer of molecules and information between the endothelium, ECM and cell membrane, which can be directed toward tissue regeneration if the resident stem cells have the chance of communicating and interacting with new therapeutic models; all this without forgetting the human being, at the center of research and scientific evolution [37, 38].

Author details

Aragona Salvatore Emanuele[1]*, Mereghetti Giada[1], Ferrari Alessio[2] and Giorgio Ciprandi[3]

*Address all correspondence to: saadmaswood@gmail.com

1 Center of Regenerative Medicine—Humanitas Mater Domini, Castellanza, VA, Italy

2 Alfakjn Research Center, Valenza Po, Alessandria, Italy

3 Allergy Clinic, Casa di Cura Villa Montallegro, Genoa, Italy

References

[1] Aragona SE et al. La Medicina Rigenerativa: Le nuove ricerche per la cura delle lesioni cutanee. Surgical Tribune Ed Italiana. Gen-Feb 10-14. 2013;**1**

[2] Barabino S et al. Efficacy of a new ocular surface modulator in restoring epithelial changes in an in vitro model of dry eye syndrome. Current Eye Research. Mar 2017;**42**(3):358-363

[3] Ferrante CJ, Leibovich SJ. Regulation of Macrophage Polarization and Wound Healing. Advanced Wound Care. Feb 2012;**1**(1):10-16

[4] Shultz GS et al. Wound bed preparation a systematic approach to wound management. Wound Repair and Regeneration. 2003;**11**(suppl 1):S1-S28

[5] Percival SL et al. The effects of pH on wound healing, biofilms, and antimicrobial efficacy. Wound Repair and Regeneration. Mar-Apr 2014;**22**(2):174-186

[6] Jones EM, Cochrane CA, Percival SL. The effect of pH on the extracellular matrix and biofilms. Advances in Wound Care. 2015;**4**:431-439

[7] Aragona SE et al. Le Lesioni cutanee vascolari. Journal of Clinical Medicine and Therapy. 2017;**19**(2)

[8] Aragona SE et al. Chronic inflammation therapy combined with low dose cytokines in the treatment of chronic ulcers of lower limbs. Journal of Biological Regulators and Homeostatic Agents. 2017;**31**(2 Suppl):193-200

[9] Dreifke MB et al. Current wound healing procedures and potential care. Materials Science & Engineering, C: Materials for Biological Applications. 2015;**48**:651-662

[10] Khan I et al. Biophysycal approaches for oral wound healing: Emphasis on photobiomodulation. Advances in Wound Care. 2015;**4**(12):724-737

[11] Aragona SE et al. Photobiomodulation with polarized light in the treatment of cutaneous and mucosal ulcerative lesions. Journal of Biological Regulators and Homeostatic Agents. 2017;**31**(2 Suppl):213-218

[12] Lipovsky A, Nitzan Y, Lubart R. A possible mechanism for visible light-induced wound healing. Lasers in Surgery and Medicine. 2008;**40**:509-514

[13] Corazza AV, Jorge J, Kuraci C, Bagnato VS. Photobiomodulation on the angiogenesis of skin wounds in rats using different light sources. Photomedicine and Laser Surgery. 2007;**25**:102-106

[14] Yadav A, Gupta A. Noninvasive red and near-infrared wavelenght-induced photobiomodulation: Promotin impaired wound healing. Photodermatology, Photoimmunology and Photomedicine. 2017;**33**:4-13

[15] Aragona SE et al. Photobiomodulation in the treatment of chronic non–responding wounds. Journal of Biological Regulators and Homeostatic Agents. 2017;**31**(2 Suppl):201-205

[16] Kuffler DP. Photobiomodulation in promoting wound healing: A review. Regenerative Medicine. 2016;**11**:107-122

[17] Peplow PV, Chung TY, Baxter GD. Photodynamic modulation of wound healing: A review of human and animals studies. Photomedicine and Laser Surgery. Mar 2012;**30**(3):118-148

[18] Ranjbar R, Takhtfooladi MA. The effects of photobiomodulation therapy on staphilococcus aureus infected surgical wounds in diabetic rats. A microbiolgical, histopathological, and biomechanical study. Acta Cirúrgica Brasileira. Aug 2016;**31**(8):498-504

[19] Medeiros JL, Nicolau RA, Nicola EM, dos santos JN, Pinheiro AL. Healing of surgical wounds made with lambda 970-nm diode laser associated or not with laser phototherapy (lambda 655 nm) or polarized light (lambda 400-2000 nm). Photomedicine and Laser Surgery. Aug 2010;**28**(4):489-496

[20] Houreld NN, Ayuk SM, Abrahamse H. Expression of genes in normal fibroblast cells(WS1) in response to irradiation at 660 nm. Journal of Photochemistry and Photobiology. 2014;**130**:146-152

[21] Aragona SE et al. Electromagnetic field in control tissue regeneration, pelvic pain, neuro-inflammation and modulation of non – neuronal cells. Journal of Biological Regulators and Homeostatic Agents. 2017;**31**(2 Suppl):219-225

[22] Costin GE, Birlea SA, Norris DA. Trends in wound repair repair: cellular and molecular basis of regenerative therapy using electromagnetic fields. Current Molecular Medicine. 2012;**12**:14-26

[23] Everts PA, Knape JT, Weibrich G, Schonberger JP, Hoffmann J, Overdevest EP, et al. Platelet-rich plasma and platelet gel: A review. The Journal of Extra-Corporeal Technology. 2006;**38**:174-187

[24] Christgau M, Moder D, Hiller KA, Dada A, Schmitz G, Schmalz G. Growth factors and cytokines in autologous platelet concentrate and their correlation to periodontal regeneration outcomes. Journal of Clinical Periodontology. 2006;**33**:837-845

[25] Marx RE. Platelet-rich plasma (PRP): What is PRP and what is not PRP? Implant Dentistry. 2001;**10**:225-228

[26] Alio JL, Arnalich-Montiel F, Rodriguez AE. The role of "eye platelet rich plasma" (E-PRP) for wound healing in ophthalmology. Current Pharmaceutical Biotechnology. 2012;**13**:1257-1265

[27] Bagnara G. Le Cellule Staminali, Cap 11. Ed Esculapio. 2017

[28] Otero-Vinas M, Falanga V. Mesenchymal stem cell in chronic wounds: The spectrum from basic to advanced therapy. Advances in Wound Care. 2016;**5**:215-222

[29] Gaur M et al. Mesenchimal stem cellfrom adipose tissue in clinical application for dermatological indications and skin aging. International Journal of Molecular Sciences. 2017;**18**(1):208

[30] Carlo T, Valeria C, Carlo V. Adipose tissue and mesenchymal stem cells: State of the art and lipogems® technology development. Current Stem Cell Reports. 2016;**2**:304-312

[31] Zhao R et al. Inflammation in chronic wounds. International Journal of Molecular Sciences. 2016;**17**:E2085

[32] Han G et al. Chronic wound healing: A rewiew of currente management and treatments. Advances in Therapy

[33] Mario BP, Silvia C, Federica F, Eva B, Liza L, Domenico R, et al. Stem cell differentiation stage factors from zebrafish embryo: A novel strategy to modulate the fate of normal and pathological human (stem) cells. Current Pharmaceutical Biotechnology. 2015;**16**:782-792

[34] Ventura C et al. Melodie cellulari—Elettromagnetismo, musica e suono della voce per parlare alle dinamiche più profonde della nostra biologia la medicina biologica. 2017. vol. 3

[35] Montagnier L, Aissa J, DelGiudice E, Lavallee C, Tedeschi A, Vitiello G. DNA waves and water. Journal of Physics Conference Series. 2011;**306**:012007

[36] DelGiudice E, Preparata G, Fleischmann M. QED coherence and electrolyte solutions. The Journal of Electroanalytical Chemistry. 2000;**482**:110-116

[37] Ader R, Cohen N. Psychoneuroimmunology: Conditioning and stress. Annual Review of Psychology. 1993;**44**:53-85

[38] Ader R, Cohen N, Felten D. Psychoneuroimmunology: Interactions between the nervous system and the immune system. Lancet. 1995;**345**(8942):99-103

Chapter 8

Growth Hormone (GH) and Wound Healing

Diego Caicedo and Jesús Devesa

Additional information is available at the end of the chapter

http://dx.doi.org/10.5772/intechopen.80978

Abstract

Wound healing is complex and numerous factors overlap perfectly with the goal of wound closure. Among them, we will focus on a large amount of experimental and clinical evidence on the action of GH in wound repair. We will analyze how the physiological rhythm of GH secretion influences this process, and also one of the most important signaling pathways that mediate the effects of GH on tissue regeneration. The role of IGF-1 and the factors that stimulate GH secretion and that have also been shown to improve healing will also be reviewed. In addition, it will be analyzed the cellular senescence process, which plays a key role in nonhealing wounds associated with chronic diseases. The benefit of GH in this last circumstance is especially important. The lesions associated with catabolic states, mainly burns, are considered a delicate situation in which it is extraordinarily difficult to act with growth factors due to the fragile situation of these patients, often children. The positive action of GH in these states will also be described. In summary, we will analyze many evidences about the beneficial effects of GH and its main secretagogues in the healing of wounds.

Keywords: wound healing, growth hormone, tissue regeneration, IGF-1, cellular senescence, chronic diseases, catabolic states, secretagogues

1. Introduction

Wound healing represents a major challenge in medicine due to its complexity and potential severity. It is a sequential process that requires the perfect interaction of many factors and cell types. As is well known, the key aspects in wound healing are the growth of granulation tissue and the proliferation and migration of keratinocytes at the edges of the wound. For this, a series of cytokines and growth factors arriving from blood and others produced locally, act in an autocrine or paracrine manner, orchestrating the communication between cells and regulating the healing process [1–4]. In the normal repair of a tissue, the resident cells have the mission of producing these cytokines and growth factors that cooperate in their repair function. In fact, it has been discovered that some of them promote cell proliferation, angiogenesis, and synthesis of extracellular matrix (ECM) [5]. Therefore, the direct application in the wound of specific stimulating peptides is expected to increase the healing of chronic ulcers until now considered as incurable.

We currently know that growth hormone (GH) is a pleiotropic factor capable of acting positively in many organs and tissues. For years, the use of GH for wound healing has been investigated [6, 7]. For example, the use of recombinant human GH as an anabolic treatment in burns to accelerate wound healing is already classic [8, 9]. Patients with severe burns who were treated with systemic GH improved both their healing and their survival [10, 11]. More recently, a number or studies have shown that GH is a promising agent in the acceleration of wound healing [12, 13]. In addition to the stimulation of granulation tissue formation, GH increases collagen deposition, and facilitates epithelialization [14, 15]. This effect of GH has been seen in experimental models of undernourished rats, in which the administration of the hormone made the granulation tissue to grow in previously induced wounds [16]. Similar results have been found in GH-transgenic mice models [17]. Although contradictory data can be found in the literature on this particular action of GH, most studies support its benefit, and evidence of its positive effects (**Table 1**) will be described widely later in the text. It should be noticed that GH activation normally is produced in morbid conditions as catabolic or chronic diseases, and it may have no effect in healthy subjects. For example, when we artificially produce an injury in normal individuals, there are no differences about the speed of wound healing between GH-treated subjects and controls [18]. Furthermore, some data suggest that systemic GH treatment is detrimental for wound healing in healthy individuals [19]. The same is found in healthy people if we try to stimulate the immune system with GH [20]. There is much evidence to support an angiogenic effect of GH in patients with critical limb ischemia that suffer usually from ischemic ulcers; or its benefit in aging or in diabetes mellitus (DM) [21, 22]. The latter data show the specific role that the hormone can play depending on the morbid condition of the patient. **Figures 1–3** show the evolution of a patient with critical ischemia of the lower limbs, suffering from an ulcer, before and after 8 weeks of treatment with subcutaneous GH administration (0.4 mg/day).

The regulation of metabolic factors acting on wound healing is well known, albeit some aspects have still to be elucidated. Growth hormone-releasing hormone (GHRH) and Ghrelin are some of the most important factors controlling not only the synthesis and release of GH from the pituitary gland, but also regulating the GH receptor (GHR) and its function [23, 24]. As it will be detailed further, both hormones have also been described as having the ability to improve the healing process. Although this is not the aim of this review, at this point we cannot forget the association between Klotho and the GH/IGF-1 axis [22], especially during aging.

The key problem is to find the best way for the hormone to be administered, and the best vehicle to carry it out. However, while for GH both systemic and local administration have been demonstrated to be effective in the healing of wounds, in the case of IGF-1, the main mediator of GH actions, systemic, unlike local use, has no effect, probably because GH can have direct actions that are added to its indirect actions stimulating other growth factors involved in

http://dx.doi.org/10.5772/intechopen.80978

A. Inflammation phase

- Stimulates the recruitment of inflammatory cells: monocytes and T-lymphocytes by increasing MCP-1, without changing neutrophil count.
- Diffuse wound occupation of inflammatory cells.

B. Proliferation phase: granulation tissue formation (dose-dependent)

- Diffuse wound occupation of fibroblasts and myofibroblast.
- Increase fibroblasts proliferation along with total collagen deposition.
- Increase secretion of ECM: scaffold function.
- Increase proliferation and migration of keratinocytes, accelerating epithelization.
- Angiogenesis:
  - ◊ Boosts the formation of capillaries.
  - ◊ Directly, or indirectly: VEGF, FGF, or SDF-1.
  - ◊ Attraction of endothelial cells from the bone marrow.
- It could improve neurogenic response.
- High doses of GH can delay wound closure (overgrowth of granulation tissue).

C. Remodeling phase

- Accelerates the remodeling of the granulation tissue.

Table 1. Key points about evidence of GH and wound healing.

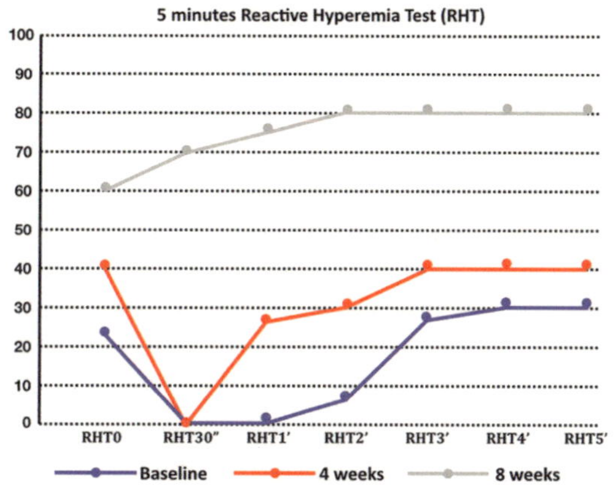

Figure 1. Five minutes reactive hyperemia test. Response to artificially induced ischemia in an affected limb with Chronic limb-threatening ischemia and a nonhealing wound. The limb is compressed until losing the flow for 5 minutes. Results after 8 weeks of systemic GH treatment. RHT: reactive hyperemia test; RHT0: ankle pressure at baseline; RHT30″: ankle pressure at 30 seconds; RHT1′-2′-3′-4′-5′: ankle pressure at 1, 2, 3, 4 and 5 minutes. y axis: mm Hg (data obtained from the GHAS trial).

wound healing. It has to be highlighted that the concentration of GH, when applied locally, and the dose, when a systemic administration is chosen, are also of importance and may determine the final effect and/or the appearance of complications. Systemic GH may increase the collagen production and mechanical strength of wounds [15, 25]. It has been reported

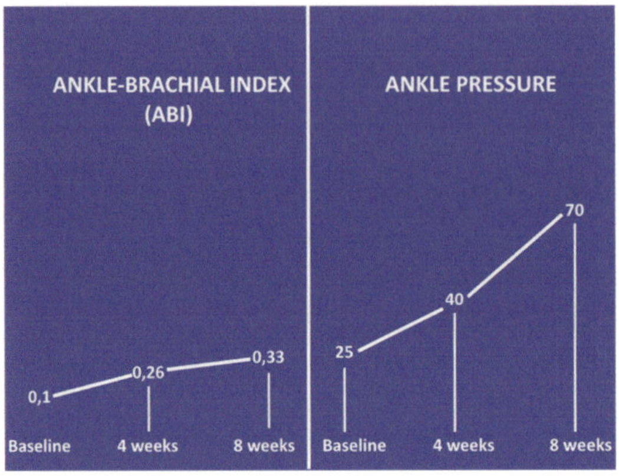

Figure 2. Evolution in the same patient that in **Figure 1** of the ankle-brachial index (ABI), calculated as the rate of the arterial ankle pressure divided by the arterial brachial pressure, and the arterial pressure at the ankle (measured in mmHg). Results show a positive evolution in angiogenesis, parallel to the wound evolution and the 5 minutes RHT (data obtained from the GHAS trial).

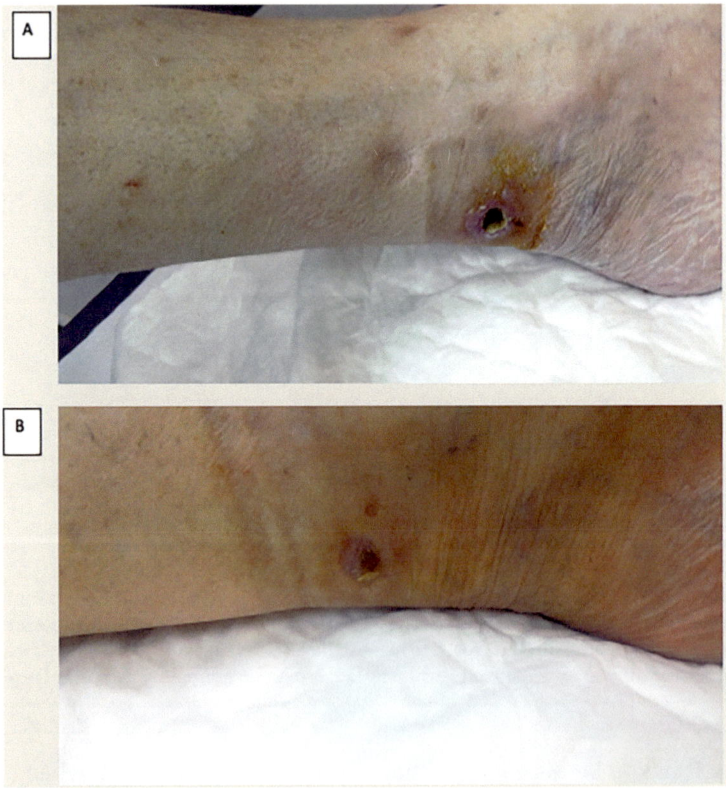

Figure 3. Picture of a nonhealing wound in the same patient as in **Figure 1** suffering from Chronic limb-threatening ischemia. Evolution after 8 weeks of systemic administration of GH: (A) baseline picture and (B) final picture (data obtained from the GHAS trial).

that systemic GH administration could accelerate the split-thickness skin defect in pigs [7]. However, systemic use of GH may induce side effects that must be considered when using this way. Such collateral effects are dependent on dose and time of administration. Although the topical use of GH seems to be better to reduce the possibility of side effects, unfortunately, this way of administration also present some deficiencies. Nevertheless, GH therapy has also the advantage of its relatively low cost. To produce growth factors for medical use in non-healing wounds is costly, and hence, increasing the production of these factors by local GH administration, could be more cost-effective.

2. Experimental and clinical evidences of GH action on wound healing

GH actions on wound healing have been evaluated in different studies from the macroscopic and microscopic points of view.

During the inflammatory phase of skin wounds in mice, GH stimulated the recruitment of inflammatory cells after 3 days of topical treatment, allowing to improve the degradation of the injured tissue [26]. Monocytes, monocyte chemoattractant protein-1 (MCP-1), and T-lymphocytes play a key role in the control of the healing process. GH is a strong inductor of these cells [27–29] and activates human monocyte chemotaxis and migration [29]. A low dose of exogenous GH administration induces the expression of MCP-1 mRNA up to eight-fold [28]. However, as it will be described further, the stimulation of these immune cells by GH not only benefits inflammatory phase, but also angiogenic and neurogenic responses [19]. After analyzing the areas of wounds in the inflammatory phase when GH is used topically in mice, GH-treated mice increased the number of macrophages by about 15%, and the number of lymphocytes by 50% without changing neutrophil recruitment [26].

The effects of GH on the immune system have been extensively analyzed. In a model of peritonitis, GH reduced bacterial counts in the peritoneal layer and increased the number of exudative neutrophils [30]. Furthermore, GH increases the thymic mass in patients infected with human immunodeficiency virus (HIV), and the number of CD4+ T-lymphocytes [31]. In these cases, GH was able to restore immune function.

A study in male mice in which an incision wound occurred showed that local administration of GH led to increased cellular infiltration in the wound area, mainly occupied by inflammatory cells, fibroblasts, and myofibroblasts, while in the control group (who did not receive the hormone) this type of cellular infiltration was only observed at the edges of the wound. This finding indicates that GH, directly or indirectly, had accelerated the migration and recruitment of cells, such as fibroblasts, to the site of injury [26].

Fibroblasts play a key role in all aspects of this process. In response to early injury signals, fibroblasts proliferate and migrate into the wound. They significantly contribute to the synthesis of the extracellular matrix (ECM), providing a scaffold for cellular ingrowth [32]. In addition, fibroblasts secrete various important cytokines with both autocrine and paracrine effects [33–36]. This concept is schematized in **Figure 4**.

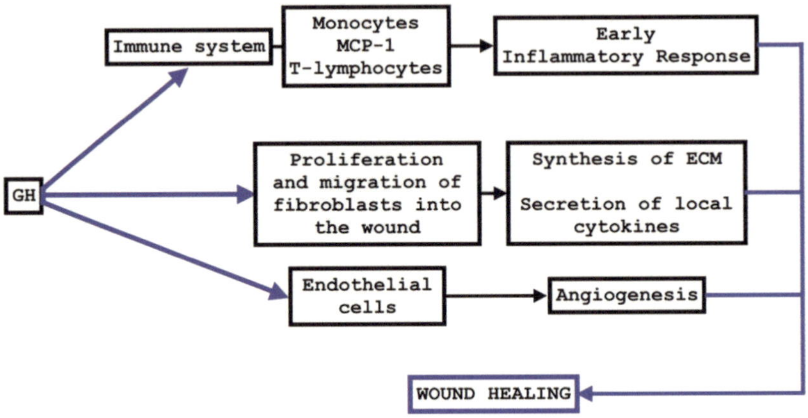

Figure 4. Schematic description of the effects of GH on a wound during the early inflammatory process and stages after it. Lastly, GH also induces the acceleration of the granulation tissue and the wound is healed. Blue arrows indicate stimulation.

The role of GH in accelerating the granulation tissue has been described in previous work [37]. The cell recruitment along with collagen deposition was also accelerated in response to GH during the phase of granulation tissue. An increased mitosis and migration of keratinocyte were found after 7 days of the incision in mice treated with the hormone, parallel to the secretion of ECM to give consistency to the aforementioned granulation tissue [26]. In this study, it was observed that GH accelerated the migration and proliferation of these cells already in the first week of treatment [26], but also the analysis of the samples showed that topical treatment with GH, regardless of the concentration used, increased the total collagen deposition after 7 and 14 days of treatment. That is, GH therapy not only accelerated the remodeling of the granulation tissue, but also the epithelization, with a more stratified epidermis. Another study showed that the systemic application of GH stimulated the formation of granulation tissue in wounds of malnourished rats [16].

In vitro studies on plates coated with Matrigel® with endothelial cells have shown that GH produces a mitogen effect, which affects cell morphology, increases ECM and boosts the formation of structures similar to capillaries [38]. Some data supporting the action of GH on collagen deposition have been described in patients with acromegaly, in whom the excess of GH determines severe cardiac damage with fibrosis [22].

The role of GH in fibroblast proliferation is crucial for the wound healing process [39]. In one study, when GH was applied topically, fibroblast proliferation increased significantly, as indicated by a tetrazolium-based colorimetric assay. However, the increase in proliferation differed according to the concentration of GH, being 2.5 IU/L the best dose to stimulate the proliferation of fibroblasts [40].

Angiogenesis plays a key role during the granulation phase and tissue remodeling, as new vessels are required for the progression of wound healing. Endothelial cells express the GHR [41], and the participation of GH in the latter process has been widely demonstrated and reviewed [21, 22, 42]. Moreover, GH-transgenic mice show an increase in blood vessels during tissue repair [19].

GH can act directly on endothelial cells through the GHR, or indirectly, by increasing others growth factors such as VEGF, FGF, or SDF-1; in this way, the hormone facilitates the proliferation, migration, and formation of endothelial cell tubes, as well as the attraction of that type of cells from the bone marrow through the CXCR4 receptor for SDF-1 [43].

The formation of blood vessels is already observed 7 days after the local administration of GH in mice. Again, the dose utilized is important, since at 10^{-7} M doses of GH a higher number of blood vessels was produced in the granulation tissue, compared to the control group and the group treated with GH 10^{-8} M [26]. A similar effect was also observed after 14 days of treatment, indicating that GH maintained its proangiogenic effect during the 2 weeks of application.

All these results point out that GH is a member of those molecules that have pleiotropic actions on skin cells, and confirm previous research showing that after an injury to the skin, the process of wound healing is accelerated in GH-transgenic mice overexpressing GH [19]. In the latter study, full-thickness incisional and excisional wounds developed a highly vascularized granulation tissue. However, the bursting strength of these injuries did not increase. In these injured mice, wound closure was even delayed as a result of increased granulation tissue formation, demonstrating that, on one hand, GH can grow this essential tissue for healing, but on the other hand, at high doses, the overgrowth of granulation tissue can even delay wound closure. The authors of this study also support the fact that this action of GH on healing is probably not mediated via IGF-1 [19], in contrast to previous studies that hypothesized a direct role of IGF-1, induced by GH, in healing wounds [44, 45]. Currently, many evidences support the fact that circulating IGF-1 does not affect the wound, but that IGF-1 produced locally by fibroblasts, macrophages, and endothelial cells is the responsible for wound healing [46, 47]. Nevertheless, topically applied GH also increases the concentration of IGF-1 mRNA in the granulation tissue in vivo [48]. In any case, if the effect of IGF-1 on wound healing occurs as a consequence of the local production of IGF-1, induced by GH within the wound, it is equally important the fact that the topical administration of GH can facilitate the healing of wounds.

Furthermore, as it will be described later, some of the hormones related to the control of GH secretion, as GHRH and Ghrelin, have also shown positive effects on wound healing, showing, once again, the strong influence of GH on wound healing.

2.1. Signaling pathways in wound healing

2.1.1. The JAK/STAT signaling pathway

The Janus kinase (JAK) signal transducer and activator of transcription (STAT) pathway is considered one of the most relevant intracellular signaling pathways utilized by hormones, growth factors, and cytokines to carry out their cellular actions [49], and it is also involved in wound healing [50]. Cell proliferation, migration, differentiation, and apoptosis are mediated by this pathway [51]. When its control is altered, this promotes chronic inflammation.

Basically, the regulation of the JAK/STAT pathway is carried out by various mechanisms such as tyrosine phosphatase, internalization-degradation of signaling molecules, receptor antagonists, and inhibitors such as inhibitors of activated STAT proteins (PIAS) or suppressors of cytokine signaling proteins (SOCS) [52].

Indirect examples of the implication of this pathway in wound healing are the relationship of the same with the immune system, the main actor during healing. Inhibitors of the JAK/STAT signaling pathway are currently used to treat autoimmune diseases, including psoriasis and rheumatoid arthritis [53].

GHR is a transmembrane protein belonging to the family of receptors of class I cytokines, which homodimerizes after its binding to the ligand and signals through the family of tyrosine kinases of JAK2 and the recruitment of transcriptional factors of the STAT type, in particular isoforms 3 and 5. Intracellular signaling involves the activation by phosphorylation of different intracellular proteins, including IRS-1, MAPK, and phosphatidylinositol 3-kinase (PI3-K) [54]. Intracellular signaling induced by GH is downregulated by the family of cytokine signaling suppressors (SOCS) [55].

Different members of this pathway have been described, but their main mission is to transmit extracellular information, via specific receptors binding of the ligand and phosphorylation, to the nucleus. To describe the functioning of the latter pathway is out of the scope of this review, and we will focus on those aspects related to wound healing.

2.1.1.1. Role of JAK/STAT in wound healing

Fibroblasts, endothelial cells, keratinocytes, and macrophages, are some of the cells in which cytokines and growth factors, using the JAK/STAT pathway, play a key role during the wound repair process. Pathological conditions can affect the normal functioning of this pathway, delaying the closure of the wound, and leading to the development of a chronic wound [56]. For example, Feng and colleagues studied the gene expression pattern of seven SOCSs members in tissue collected from chronic venous leg ulcer patients; they found significantly higher mRNA levels of SOCS3 and SOCS4 in chronic nonhealing ulcers as compared to healing/healed ulcers [57]. In chronic wounds, it is required that the JAK/STAT pathway be upregulated, especially in cases when its normal functioning has been compromised; more specifically in an environment of senescent cells or DM where there is a reduced growth factor/receptor signaling [53].

As known, GH is one of the growth factors using the JAK/STAT pathway as an intracellular signaling pathway for exerting its actions. In fact, the inhibition of this GH signaling by SOCS members has been defended as a key factor affecting GH effect along with vasoinhibins. Moreover, GH induces the expression of CIS and SOCS1–3, which suggests that these proteins may also play a physiological role in the regulation of GH secretion. SOCS2 seems to act downregulating GH activity [58]. In this sense, pro-inflammatory cytokines such as IL-1B or TNFα, and endotoxins, which are frequently increased in inflammatory states such as DM or in patients suffering from severe peripheral ischemia, may induce SOCS proteins which could lead to a GH insensitivity. Nevertheless, SOCS2 has been found that paradoxically may upregulate GH signaling at high concentrations in mice [58]. Thus, both uncontrolled inflammation and infection at wounds may block the action of growth factors using this pathway, and delay the healing (**Figure 5**).

Although not properly known, the JAK/STAT signaling is regulated by SOCS proteins, having an influence on the action of cytokines and growth factors, as well as on the cells involved in the wound repair process [52]. SOCS have been related to inflammatory diseases,

http://dx.doi.org/10.5772/intechopen.80978

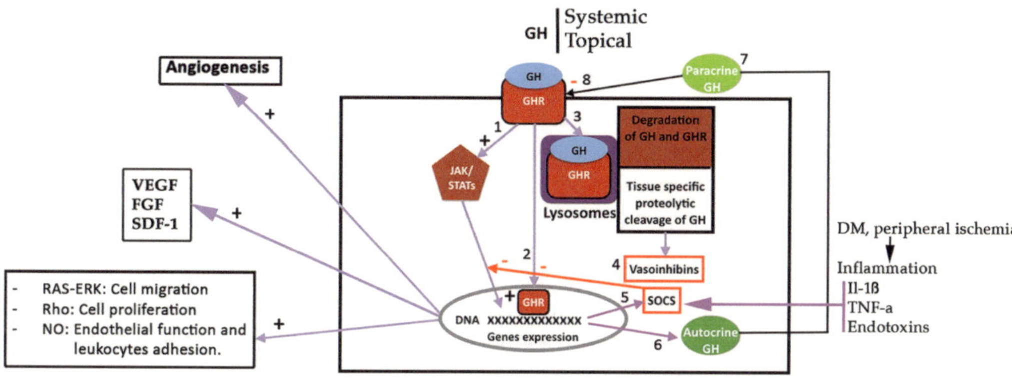

Figure 5. Activation of the GHR by GH, administered subcutaneously or secreted by the pituitary gland (systemic) or locally applied on the wound (topical). (1) After the interaction between GH and its receptor (GHR) a cascade of signaling pathways is initiated by JAK2 activation leading to the expression of a number of genes. (2) The GHR may be internalized together with GH and translocated to the nucleus, where it may also activate gene expression. (3) GH and GHR may suffer a lysosomal degradation after being internalized, but also, depending on the tissue, the hormone may suffer a specific proteolytic cleavage giving origin to vasoinhibins (4) which may block angiogenesis and arteriogenesis. (5) SOCS are expressed after GHR translocation to the nucleus of the cell, and they act by inhibiting GH signaling, directly or affecting the translocation of the GHR to the nucleus. (6, 7) Cells may express GH that acts in an autocrine (6) or paracrine (7) manner. This cellular production of the hormone may lead to an interaction with the membrane GHR (8) impeding the effects of endocrine, or exogenously administered hormone, or topically applied; these auto/paracrine GHs even may produce the desensitization of GHR, therefore impeding GH actions at this level. On the left of the figure, signals induced by GH on the expression of several genes leading to several positive effects, such as angiogenesis. On the right of the figure, it can be seen that some pathological situations, such as diabetes mellitus (DM) or peripheral ischemia lead to inflammation. In this situation, Il-1β, TNF-α or endotoxins, induce the expression or activation of SOCS which block GH signaling pathways. Blue arrows: stimulation; red arrows and squares, inhibition. +: activation; −: inhibition.

since in the absence of SOCS3, IL-6 acts decreasing tumor necrosis factor alpha (TNFα), by inhibiting the STAT3 signaling. It has to be highlighted that immune response, crucial in wound healing, is modulated by IL6 [59]. SOCS4 and SOCS5 have also been linked to EGF signaling, regulating its receptor (EGFR), and affecting its signaling capacity in senescent fibroblast cells [53].

The effects of the JAK/STAT pathway seem to be time-dependent: positive and protective in early phases, while negative and inhibitory in the later chronic phase [60].

Upregulation of the STAT genes and activation of the STAT proteins have been directly linked to wound healing in intestinal epithelial cells [61].

Further investigations into cellular and molecular mechanisms and signaling pathways involved in wound healing, and methods of activating senescent cells through various treatments will add possible benefits on this process in the future; therefore GH, the anti-aging factor for excellence, could be one of them.

2.2. GH, circadian rhythm disorders, and wound healing

All organisms have an adaptive mechanism, and several of their functions are synchronized to environmental factors and possess biological clocks that endogenously estimate the time. Consequently, functions such as the sleep-wake cycle and secretion of various hormones exhibit a rhythm with a characteristic period of ~24 hours (the so-called circadian rhythms). There is a relationship between feeding, the organs involved in food intake, metabolic networks, and circadian physiology. One of the most important endocrine axes involved in circadian rhythm is the axis Ghrelin-GH-IGF-1. The coordinating role of these hormones lies in regulating appetite, behavior, growth, and cell proliferation, with a clear influence in the metabolic regulation of nutrients and all those processes dependent of them, as it is wound healing. Some hormones have been implied in the regulation of circadian GH production, as cortisol, thyrotropin (TSH), and insulin, in addition to some important neurotransmitters [62].

Although GH is mainly released by the anterior pituitary gland, there is a peripheral GH production in practically all the organism, highly dependent on developmental stages, at the level of tissues as nervous system, or the immune, cardiovascular, gonadal, and musculoskeletal system. This peripheral GH plays an autocrine and paracrine role [63]. In humans, plasma GH shows a circadian pattern of secretion, different according to sex and age; during puberty, the hormone reaches its highest plasma values, but once puberty ends, the secretion of the hormone begins to decline until being practically undetectable in elder people [64].

The circadian pattern of GH is affected by nutritional status (caloric intake), age, stress, sex, physical exercise, and lack of sleep. Nutritional status is a key determinant in the regulation of GH secretion; thus, while fasting increases the frequency of GH secretion pulses, while IGF-1 levels decrease, in obesity the opposite occurs, at least during childhood [65]. During fasting, GHR are downregulated [66, 67]. Evidence for a circadian effect on the reduction of human GH gene expression has been demonstrated in response to excess caloric intake [68], and obesity has been associated to the suppression of circulating GH [69].

The highest pulse amplitude of GH secretion is observed during the REM phase of the sleep, while sleep deprivation leads to a strong inhibition of nocturnal GH secretion [70, 71].

Several studies have shown that prolonged sleep deprivation, with the subsequent stress, leads to a reduction in body mass, elevated energy metabolism, changes in circulating hormones, and loss of immune system integrity [72]. Stress mediators act on immune cells to modulate the production of key regulatory cytokines [73, 74]. Thus, circadian rhythm disorders affect the levels of IL-1, IL-2, IL-6, TNFα, natural killer cells, adrenocorticotropic hormone (ACTH), cortisol, GH, and melatonin, all of them playing a key role in wound healing [75–77]. Melatonin has potential effects on the immune system, as inhibition of pineal melatonin synthesis with propranolol or pinealectomy results in immunosuppression and negative effects on wound healing [78]. Yet another study found that melatonin improved wound healing when given at night, coinciding with its normal circadian period of secretion [79].

Notwithstanding all these data, some studies disagree with the concept that sleep exerts a predominant influence on GH release and its effects whatever the conditions be, as it seems to occur compensatory mechanisms promoting GH pulses during wakefulness [80].

Thus, GH influences on wound healing progression. Physiologic circadian rhythm, with higher levels of the hormone during the night, will make a faster healing of wounds during the night, and the alteration of this pattern by different factors might exert a deleterious effect on wound healing via GH and others hormones related to it, although compensatory mechanisms have been described in the long-term.

3. IGF-1 and wound healing

IGF-1 is considered as the main mediator of GH actions, and it has been considered as the "authentic" GH, at least for growing, although GH exerts many actions directly without the participation of IGF-1 [27].

IGF-1 is a polypeptide structural and functionally similar to insulin. It is produced in the liver and practically all extrahepatic tissues, and its production depends not only of GH, but also is strongly influenced by the nutritional status of the organism, at least in the liver. The local production of IGF-1 has been shown to regulate many physiological and pathophysiological states such as fetal development, atherosclerosis, and tissue repair. During tissue repair, IGF-1 is secreted by platelets, macrophages, and fibroblasts of the wound [5].

In wounds, IGF-1 increases protein production and cell proliferation and migration, which are crucial in the healing process [81, 82]. IGF-1 expression is enhanced in subcutaneous [5], and incisional [83] wounds, and in postburn injuries [84]. Some studies have shown that the administration of exogenous IGF-I enhanced protein synthesis in severely burned experimental animals [85].

Moreover, the levels of this growth factor are reduced in the wound environment of diabetic patients. Wound-related parameters as proteins, DNA, hydroxyproline, and macrophages have been shown to be decreased as a consequence of diabetes. After 14 days of treatment with IGF-1 in rats with diabetes produced by streptozotocin, it was observed that the total values of hydroxyproline, DNA, proteins, and macrophages increased by 48, 52, 31, and 40%, respectively [5]. These data support the fact that the suppression of IGF-1 and the macrophage function impairment within the wound environment by the diabetic state are responsible, at least in part, for the delay of wound healing in this disease.

In this context, the relationship between the IGF-1 receptor (IGF-1R) and the estrogen receptor (ER) is of interest. Locally administered IGF-1 promotes wound repair in an estrogen-deprived animal model, the ovariectomized (Ovx) mouse, mainly by dampening the local inflammatory response and promoting re-epithelialization. Using specific IGF-1R and ER antagonists it has been shown how IGF-1-mediated effects on re-epithelialization were directly mediated by IGF-1R [86]. In contrast, the anti-inflammatory effects of IGF-1 were predominantly mediated by ERs, in particular ERa (**Figure 6**). When ERa-null mice were used, IGF-1 could not promote healing and local inflammation increased [86]. These findings illustrate the great complexity of interactions between growth factors at the cutaneous level.

Recent data on the systemic administration of IGF-1 have shown an apparent lack of effect in wound healing. Therefore, perhaps only the IGF-1 produced locally by fibroblasts and macrophages contributes to the regulation of wound healing [46, 47], although it is also possible that the dose used and the type of administration do not have been the most appropriate in this case. If the systemic IGF-1 is ineffective in wound healing, topical administration of IGF-1 could be considered, as other growth factors such as EGF, TGFβ, or the own GH. In addition, IGF-1 systemic administration produces mild complications as hypoglycemia and hypotension. These limit its clinical usefulness.

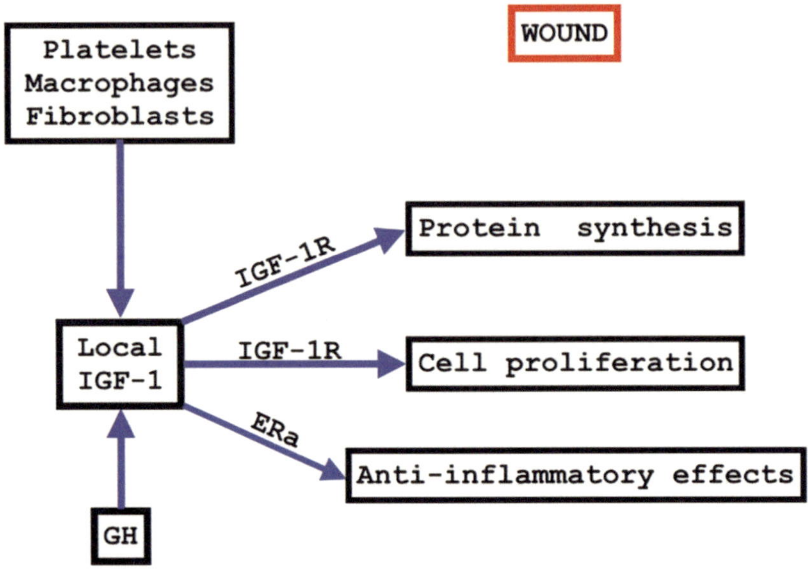

Figure 6. Local expression of IGF-1 in a wound. This expression may be induced by GH, but also IG-1 may proceed from platelets, macrophages, and fibroblasts. Local IGF-1 induces protein synthesis and cell proliferation by interacting with its receptor IGF-1R, and also has anti-inflammatory effects, although in this case IGF-1 seems to act via the estrogen receptor a (ERa).

4. Analogs of growth hormone-releasing hormone (GHRH) and wound healing

The complexity of GH regulation seems to be related to the multiple roles that GH plays in the human body, very far than those classically thought [27]. Interestingly, some of these roles are played in conjunction with GH-stimulating factors.

As described, growth hormone-releasing hormone (GHRH) is an important neuroendocrine peptide secreted by the hypothalamus, regulating the synthesis and release of GH [87]. Classically, it was thought that the role of GHRH simply was the regulation of the synthesis and secretion of GH [88, 89]. However, the detection of GHRH and its receptors, as well as the expression of GHRH gene in several extra-hypothalamic tissues, including placenta, ovary, testis, digestive tract, and tumors [90, 91], suggests that GHRH plays a wider role than simply acting on the regulation of pituitary GH secretion; in fact, it seems to be particularly involved in conditions aimed at tissue regeneration and repair. The presence of the peptide in peripheral tissues highlights the possibility that locally produced GHRH might act as an autocrine growth factor playing a role in cell proliferation. In addition to its own actions in various tissues, several GHRH agonists have been developed showing that the effects of this neuropeptide could include direct actions on wound healing. For example, a pioneer work demonstrated that the GHRH agonist JI-38 stimulates the proliferation and migration of mouse embryonic fibroblasts (MEF) [92]. The upregulation of GHRH receptor (GHRH-R) and its splicing variant 1 (SV1) in GHRH-R negative 3T3 fibroblasts has been shown to promote its proliferation when GHRH and its analogs are given [93, 94]. Despite it is logical to think that fibroblast stimulation by GHRH agonist could be mediated by GH/IGF-1. Some authors have found that using MR-409 and MR-502 GHRH agonists, there was a promotion of wound healing by stimulating the proliferation and survival of dermal fibroblast through phosphorylation of the ERK1/2 and AKT pathways, although neither GH nor IGF-1 was found to be significantly increased in fibroblasts after 4 hours exposure to these agonists. Moreover, none of the agonists showed an effect on the expression levels of either IGF-1 receptor (IGF1-R) or its phosphorylated isoform. Thus, these findings imply direct effects of GHRH and its agonists on extra-pituitary cells and tissues [95].

GHRH affects the proliferation of fibroblasts as well as their migration and the expression of smooth muscle actin α (α-SMA) [92], which is organized into stress fibers and exerts contractile forces on the extracellular matrix [96]. Therefore, it seems that GHRH can regulate, simultaneously, both the kinetic profile and the differentiation of fibroblasts in myofibroblasts (**Figure 7**).

The suppression of growth of fibroblasts in not healing-wound environment is partially due to the decreased sensitivity of resident cells and rapid degradation of growth factors used in different therapies by proteases released from inflammatory cells and bacteria [97, 98]. Therefore, it would be necessary to have a factor that exerted a strong mitogen action on the fibroblasts, while being resistant to proteolytic degradation. In this sense, unlike the natural GHRH [95], the above mentioned MR agonists seem to have an increased resistance to degradation by proteases, because many of the coded amino acids in the peptide chain have been replaced with synthetic non-natural and/or non-coded amino acids which are much less susceptible to such degradation [99]. Consequently, these analogs have demonstrated a greatly prolonged half-life in vivo, making them promising agents for use in wound healing, where an environment rich in proteases is often found. Even more, it was found that MR class agonists do not stimulate tumor growth or neoplastic transformation [95].

Another factor supporting the use of GHRH agonists has been found in human dermal microvascular endothelial cells (HDMEC), that seems to express both pituitary GHRH-R and its splicing variant 1 (SV1). HDMEC is responsible for angiogenesis, a critical event for granulation tissue formation [95].

The endogenous GHRH produced by fibroblasts regulates its own activity, and the role that GHRH signaling may play in physiological maintenance of wound healing could improve with some GHRH agonists.

The high concentration of glucose in diabetic patients inhibits the proliferation of fibroblasts and favors resistance to growth factors, decreasing wound healing. Interestingly, MR-409 enhances the survival of transplanted pancreatic islets and helps to lower blood glucose in diabetic SCID mice [100]; therefore, it would be interesting to investigate whether it might benefit diabetic wounds which are hard to cure, partially because of the special adverse bacterial environment. However, some other aspects of diabetic injuries should also be addressed; such is the case of the affectation of the neuropathic response, the true conductor in this process.

Despite these data, the precise physiologic and biochemical mechanism for GHRH accelerating wound healing remains unclear. Besides, the production of GHRH in dermal wounds still seems not to be clear. Moreover, given its short lifetime, it is unlikely that plasma GHRH

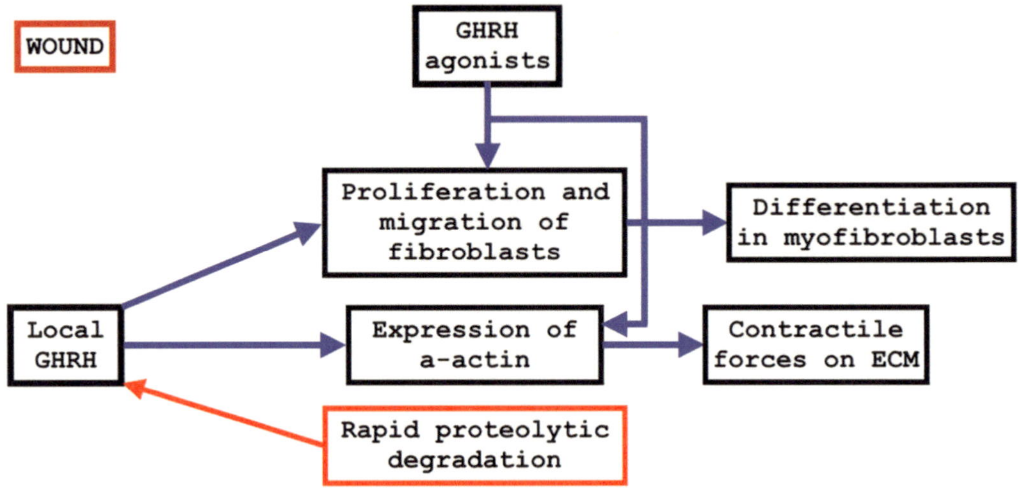

Figure 7. Possible effects of GHRH on wound healing. The possibility exists that GHRH is expressed in cells in a wound, since its short life in plasma does not explain its effects on wound healing. However, GHRH agonists do not suffer proteolytic degradation; therefore, they may mimic the effects of GHRH on the proliferation and migration of fibroblasts and its differentiation in myofibroblasts, as well as inducing the expression of smooth muscle a-actin which favors the appearance of contractile forces on the extracellular matrix (ECM). Blue arrows: induction or activation; red arrow: inhibition.

may reach adequate levels to contribute to wound healing. A possibility, not explored, is that some GHRH agonists produced in dermal wounds during healing might be responsible for the activity of GHRH on wound healing.

Whether this apparently novel function of GHRH is operational in a different kind of healing or it is indicative of the activity of a structurally related peptide(s), should be investigated more extensively to elucidate some of the basic aspects of skin biology and repair, as well as in view of its potential implications in therapeutic wound healing.

5. Wound healing in catabolic states: the role of growth hormone

The balance between anabolic and catabolic states and hormones may affect wound healing, since the overall protein compartment status has a great influence on this process [101]. Protein synthesis restores and maintains lean body mass, composed of muscle, skin, and the immune system, all of them having a role during wound repair. When anabolic activity decreases, as occurs during stress, aging, or chronic disease, there is a derivation of proteins to the energy compartment and, therefore, affects wound healing as a result of protein depletion in the wound to restore lost lean mass. Impaired immunity and healing during catabolic states are directly proportional to the degree of lean mass loss [102, 103]. Protein depletion appears to delay wound healing by prolonging the inflammatory phase (inhibits fibroplasia, synthesis of collagen, and proteoglycans), affects the proliferation phase (neoangiogenesis) and inhibits wound remodeling [104]. It has been shown that protein depletion models produce a decrease in tensile strength of wounds in animals, and rats fed with a protein-deficient diet showed a decrease in wound integrity and resistance as compared to control animals [105].

Burn injury induces acute and severe inflammation and a hypermetabolic state which are strongly correlated to the size of the burn [106]. The inflammatory process reaches a peak during the first week postburn and persists to a lesser extent throughout convalescence [107]. The hypermetabolic state begins 5 days after the burn, and may last up to 1 year after the injury, with energy requirements that reach 150–200% of the basal metabolic rate [108].

GH is one of the most important anabolic hormones and, like other anabolic hormones, has an anti-cortisol activity, lowering the catabolic response of this steroid, without altering its protective anti-inflammatory activity. Many studies have demonstrated the usefulness of anabolic hormones in existing wounds in catabolic states. However, it remains difficult to determine whether the benefit is due to the increase in the systemic anabolic state or to a direct effect on the anabolic state of the wound [109].

Starvation and intense exercise, both being catabolic states, are potent stimuli of GH, while acute or chronic injury or illness inhibits GH release, especially in the elderly [109]. GH leads to an increased influx of amino acids into the cell, decreasing the flow of these from the same. The increase in fatty metabolism that GH produces is also beneficial, since it preserves the amino acids for the synthesis of proteins, instead of being used as an energy resource.

Severe burns and injuries, people with HIV infection with wasting and elderly people, all of them catabolic states, are populations that could benefit from GH therapy. GH increases lean mass, muscle strength, and immune function in these states, but requires an intake of a high-protein, high-energy diet [109].

The skin is a target tissue for GH, and GHRs have been found on the surface of epidermal cells. Recent data indicate that IGF-1 and insulin also provide some of the anabolic effects of GH therapy in wounds [110, 111]. GH administered exogenously increases the thickness of the skin even in normal people [112]. It has been shown that GH can improve the re-epithelialization rate of sites where a skin graft has taken place in adults and children with severe burns or trauma [7, 10]. In addition, it has been seen, in experimental models, that GH also accelerates the healing by increasing wound collagen content, granulation tissue, and wound tensile strength, as well as the local production of IGF-1 by fibroblasts [109, 113].

A study conducted on burned children also supports the role of GH in catabolic states, since no differences were found in mortality, organ failure, or clinically significant morbidity between the groups, and the requirements for albumin supplementation were reduced by 65%, as well as episodes of hypocalcemia, an unexpected benefit of the hormone [114]. As it will be discussed at the end of the chapter, unlike it happens in children, it has been reported an increase of mortality in adult with burns when GH was used [115]. However, the authors of the study in pediatric population have been treating severely burned children with rhGH for more than 10 years, and they have reported that 0.2 mg/kg/day of rhGH in this catabolic state has some benefits, accelerating donor site wound healing by up to 30% and reducing a 25% the hospital stay and costs. They have also shown that GH increased protein synthesis by more than 25%. Another study has also found that GH causes significant serum elevations in other different parameters as total catecholamines, insulin, glucagon, or free fatty acids. GH therapy even showed a rise in blood flow of the leg [114].

In summary, the use of GH together with adequate nutrition and protein intake, at the appropriate doses, clearly improves anabolic activity and, as a consequence, positively impacts wound healing, even in patients with spinal cord injuries, as **Figure 8** shows. Although many data suggest that the effect of GH on wound healing can be direct, it is still unknown whether some other hormones could contribute to this positive effect.

5.1. Ghrelin, GH, and wound healing

Ghrelin (GH-releasing peptide or GHRP) is a small peptide found in the gastrointestinal tract in 1999 [116]. Although it is mainly secreted by the stomach, it is known that Ghrelin is also produced in other territories, such as the intestine or placenta, for example.

In addition to its known actions on the regulation of appetite and energy expenditure, it has also been discovered that this hormone plays a role in the control of inflammation and metabolism, as do leptin and adiponectin. In fact, all three hormones are interrelated in chronic disease states [117–119]. Interestingly, in a study that addressed the relationship between these hormones in burns, the authors came to the surprising conclusion that they acted in two different ways: one in normal physiological conditions or chronic disease states, and another after severe acute stresses such as burn injury [120]. This can be an adaptive mechanism that depends on the physiological situation or the type of the pathological condition.

Recently, it was demonstrated that Ghrelin improves hemodynamic and metabolic alterations and attenuates cancer, heart affectations, and cachexia induced by burns, and also again protects the damage induced by burns and facilitates the healing of wounds [121].

In relation to the hemodynamic role of this hormone, receptors for Ghrelin have been found in the aorta, the left cardiac ventricle, and the left cardiac atrium in rats. In healthy humans, the intravenous infusion of Ghrelin decreases blood pressure, increases the cardiac index, and produces a greater volume of the pulse [122].

Ghrelin also has an anti-inflammatory effect, by inhibiting the secretion of IL-6 and TNFα from monocytes and T5 cells [119, 123]. The protective role of Ghrelin appears to depend on the integrity of GH/IGF-1 axis, since in studies of inflammation with pancreatitis, protection against inflammation did not occur in hypophysectomized rats unless they received IGF-1 in parallel with Ghrelin. In these studies, when normal GH secretion was reached, the

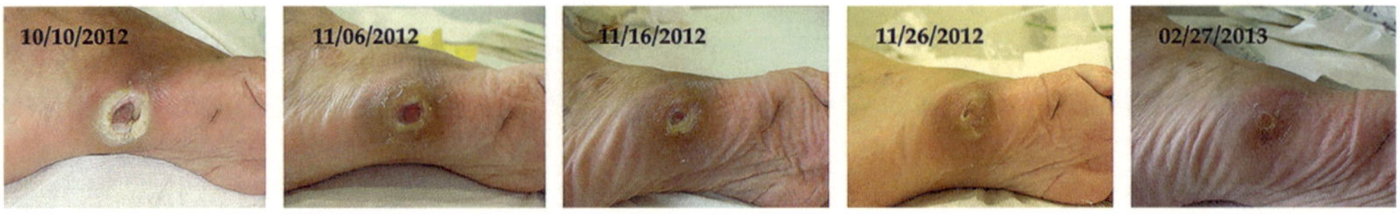

Figure 8. Evolution of a pressure ulcer in the foot of a quadriplegic patient (complete spinal cord injury, C5-C6) treated with GH applied topically (0.4 mg/day, 5 days/week), before the treatment (10/10/2012) and throughout it until the healing of the wound (02/27/2013).

inflammation was reduced in severity, with a more rapid regeneration of the pancreas, resulting in a reduction in the serum concentrations of interleukin 1-β pro-inflammatory (IL-1β) as well as the amylase and lipase activities. In addition, there was an increase in pancreatic blood flow, and DNA synthesis increased in this organ. This demonstrates that the possible role of Ghrelin during catabolic states needs an adequate functioning of the GH/IGF-1 axis [124]. This last statement has also been supported by models of colitis in which treatment with Ghrelin clearly improved the area of damage in the colonic mucosa in intact pituitary rats, but increased it in hypophysectomized animals. In addition, it was shown that rats with a normal production of GH-IGF-1 had improved blood flow in the colonic mucosa and increased mucosal cell proliferation while treated with Ghrelin, as well as reduced levels of IL1-1β and myeloperoxidase; just the opposite of what was found in hypophysectomized rats [125].

The therapeutic effect of Ghrelin on wound healing has also been evaluated using a rat model in which the administration of radiation was combined with the induction of a wound. The altered healing of a wound caused by radiation often occurs in clinical practice and the exact mechanisms by which this occurs are not yet clear. In this wound model, the administration of Ghrelin promoted the healing of skin wounds, and also reduced the average time of wound closure [126]. Ghrelin inhibited the induction of serum pro-inflammatory mediators, especially TNFα, and promoted wound healing in a dose-dependent manner [127]. After the isolation and analysis of the granulation tissues, a greater synthesis of DNA, hexosamine, nitrate, and nitrite, a high content of collagen and an enhanced neovascularization was observed after treatment with Ghrelin. The hormone also increased the expression of VEGF and TGFβ, responsible for wound healing as described. Again, when a GH 1a secretagogue receptor blocker (GHS-R1a) was administered, all of these therapeutic effects of Ghrelin were affected [126]. These results identify Ghrelin as a peptide that could be used for the affected wound healing induced by radiation, although it is necessary that there is a normal secretion of GH so that its effects occur. These effects of Ghrelin are shown in **Figure 9**.

5.2. Cellular senescence and wound healing: benefit of GH therapy

Cellular senescence is the consequence of DNA damage secondary to oxidative stress associated with aging or chronic morbid conditions such as diabetes. This seems to be an antitumor mechanism [128]. The number of senescent cells is low in young individuals, while it increases with age in all tissues, including the skin [129, 130].

At skin level, senescence has been reported in keratinocytes, melanocytes, endothelial cells, epithelial cells, T-lymphocytes, and even in stem cells [131–133].

This concept has emerged as a possible cause of general tissue dysfunction [134, 135], since, although senescent cells are unable to divide, they remain metabolically active. This high metabolic activity is associated with the release of a multitude of cytokines, chemokines, and pro-inflammatory growth factors, which leads to its denomination as the secretion phenotype associated with senescence (SASP) [136]. These factors would include interleukin (IL) 6 and IL-8, chemokines such as monocyte chemoattractant protein (MCPs), macrophage inflammatory proteins, and growth factors as VEGF, granulocyte/macrophage colony-stimulating factor (GMCSF), TGFβ, and proteinases such as matrix metalloproteinases [128, 137]. All these

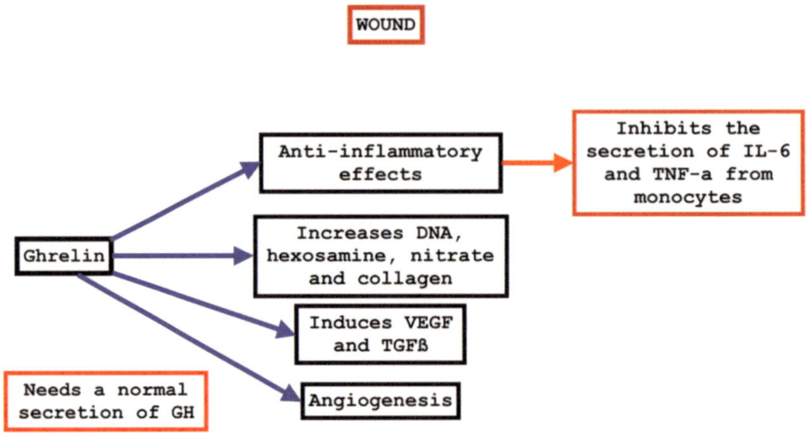

Figure 9. Ghrelin effects on a wound. While many positive effects appear at very different levels during wound healing, there is a need for a normal pituitary secretion of GH, so that these Ghrelin effects can occur. Therefore, it is not clear whether these effects depend on Ghrelin or on GH, although the possibility exists that GH could induce Ghrelin expression in the wound.

factors can act in an autocrine and paracrine way, also having effects on the surrounding cells and their environment. Therefore, the senescent cell itself could initiate a feedback mechanism by spreading this phenomenon to nearby cells [138].

Characteristically, the inflammation resulting from cellular senescence is sterile or is not associated with pathogens [137]. It has been suggested that chronic low-level inflammation that is often observed during aging in tissues without obvious infection is due to senescent cells and SASP [139]. In addition, a low number of senescent cells can have systemic effects, and it is already evident that the senescence process can be transmitted to normal cells by SASP in a paracrine or autocrine manner [128].

The basis of this senescence is mitochondrial dysfunction, which in turn causes oxidative stress, which has been implicated as a cause of aging [140].

Understanding this process would help develop different strategies that could mitigate chronic inflammation and, therefore, cellular senescence. These dysfunctional and destructive signs are also found in the wounds of diabetic or elderly patients, altering the normal healing process.

At this point, it is important to note that GH is a mitochondrial protector [141–143], therefore, playing a positive role in this process. GH restores the redox imbalance, improving the mitochondrial respiratory chain and the production of energy.

In situations of GH deficiency (GHD) there is an accelerated aging process. In mice with GHD, GH replacement therapy increases stress resistance by altering the functional capacity of the glutathione S-transferase system (GST) through the regulation of specific members of the GST family [144]. The hormone also affects the regulation of thioredoxins (TRX) and glutaredoxins (GRX), which are factors that regulate the post-translational modification of proteins and the redox balance, also influencing resistance to stress [144]. Patients with GHD show a decrease in their life expectancy with a twice higher risk of death from cardiovascular disease. In this regard, after 24 weeks of GH replacement therapy in the GREAT study, the hormone significantly lowered plasma diacron-reactive oxygen metabolites and improved endothelial function, as measured by reactive hyperemia index [145]. This indicates that GH can exert a protective role in redox balance in GHD, in which predominates a pro-oxidant environment, corrected by short-term GH administration [146]. Klotho, a GH-releasing factor that currently is gaining in interest, also lowers the oxidative stress, decreasing apoptosis and senescence of the vascular system in an atherogenic risk rat model [147]. The hormone also affects the regulation of TRX and GRX, which are factors that regulate the post-translational modification of proteins and the redox balance, also influencing resistance to stress [41]. As a consequence of the antioxidant action of GH, the hormone produces a benefit in the inflammatory state associated with senescence [22]. It has been reported that this protection against oxidative stress is mediated by GH induction of the RAS/ERK pathways [148].

However, the exact role of GH in the redox equilibrium has not been fully understood, since in some cases of oxidative stress, overproduction, or administration of GH in excess may enhance oxidation [149]. Thus, both the overproduction of GH and its deficiency are closely related to increased oxidative stress.

5.3. Contrary studies not supporting a GH role in wound healing

As described in the introduction, GH needs specific stimuli to exert its effects. In fact, there is a study carried out to determine the effect of rhGH on the rate of wound healing in normal individuals. In each subject was performed a split-thickness wound in one buttock and a full-thickness wound in the other. The full-thickness wound healed significantly more slowly in the group treated with rhGH compared to the control group treated with placebo, while no statistically significant difference was observed in the healing of the split-thickness wounds. This study concluded that rhGH may delay healing in normal patients with full-thickness wounds, although it could not be ruled out if the healing delay associated to rhGH group was due to the quality of the scab, thereby, appearing only as an alteration of the wound healing process [18].

In another trial, the serum levels of some hormones, GH, insulin, and cortisol were analyzed in normal and diabetic rats during wound healing. It was shown that the rate of wound healing in normal rats is faster than that of diabetics. The serum insulin concentrations were lower in the diabetic rats compared to the normal and control groups and showed a correlation with the wound healing process in diabetic rats. Serum cortisol concentrations decreased in the normal and diabetic groups during wound healing, but did not show a significant correlation with this process. Serum GH levels did not change significantly in any of the groups, nor did they show a significant correlation with the wound healing process [150]. As described above, a possible explanation for these findings is that the main effect of GH in this case could occur as a consequence of the local production of the hormone, something that was overlooked because it was not measured. A small wound on the back of the animal is not a stimulus strong enough to increase systemic GH, which seems to be related, as demonstrated, to more intense catabolic states.

A recent report from two prospective, randomized, double-blind, placebo-controlled Phase III trials conducted in Europe, which studied the effects of rhGH in critically ill burned adult patients, in an intensive care unit, revealed a significant increase in mortality among catabolic patients treated with rhGH (42 vs. 18%) [115]. GH, in fact, can increase cell adhesion molecules (CAM), since the serum of healthy patients treated with GH significantly increased the expression of VCAM-1 in cultured umbilical vein endothelial cells [151], and this could be the mechanism involved, but it must be taken into account that in these studies high doses of GH were used (10–20 times greater than the usual treatment dose), which would facilitate the appearance of side effects produced by the hormone. In contrast to these data, when the same study was carried out in burned children, no differences were found in mortality, but other beneficial effects were found.

6. Conclusion

Despite all data here presented, it is necessary to remember that the patient with a problem in the wound healing needs to be addressed in a holistic way. That is, "we do not treat a hole in the patient, but the whole patient". Normal wounds in healthy people are not a problem. However, a delaying wound always appears in a patient with a morbid condition, normally in an elderly patient or that with a catabolic state or a chronic disease as diabetes mellitus. Therefore, using only a topical wound treatment seems to be an unrealistic approach to healing. However, a total approach will be more beneficial to not only accelerate the healing process but also decrease the possibility of a new wound.

The knowledge of the molecular aspects related to wound repair and tissue regeneration, as well as the whole circumstances affecting also the patients is crucial to success dealing with this topic.

We cannot overlook the high amount of data regarding the role of GH and its secretagogues, not only in the healing process, but also improving the pro-oxidant state of the patients. GH therapy is a cheap and well known drug, and may increase many growth factors when is locally used in wounds. Maybe the combination of appropriate doses of systemic GH and topical application in the wound would be a good option. The combination of GH or its secretagogues and IGF-1 in a topical way, could be also a beneficious approach for wounds repair.

Acknowledgements

This chapter has been funded by the Carlos III Health Institute and the European Regional Development Fund (ISCIII-FEDER), Madrid, Spain, (grant number PI 13-00790). We thank the Foltra Medical Center for the transfer of some images for this chapter.

Diego Caicedo and Jesús Devesa participated in a similar way in the realization of this work.

Conflict of interest

The authors declare that no conflict of interest exists.

Author details

Diego Caicedo[1]* and Jesús Devesa[2]

*Address all correspondence to: diego.caicedo.valdes@sergas.es

1 Service of Vascular Surgery, University Hospital of Santiago de Compostela, Santiago de Compostela, Spain

2 Scientific Direction, Medical Center Foltra, Teo, Spain

References

[1] Eming SA, Krieg T, Davidson JM, Hall RP. Inflammation in wound repair: Molecular and cellular mechanisms. The Journal of Investigative Dermatology. 2007;**127**:514-525. DOI: 10.1038/sj.jid.5700701

[2] Gurtner GC, Werner S, Barrandon Y, Longaker MT. Wound repair and regeneration. Nature. 2008;**453**:314-321. DOI: 10.1038/nature07039

[3] Barrientos S, Brem H, Stojadinovic O, Tomic-Canic M. Clinical application of growth factors and cytokines in wound healing. Wound Repair and Regeneration. 2014;**22**:569-578. DOI: 10.1111/wrr.12205

[4] Eming SA, Martin P, Tomic-Canic M. Wound repair and regeneration: Mechanisms, signaling, and translation. Science Translational Medicine. 2014;**6**:265sr6. DOI: 10.1126/scitranslmed.3009337

[5] Bitar MS. Insulin-like growth factor-1 reverses diabetes-induced wound healing impairment in rats. Hormone and Metabolic Research. 1997;**29**:383-386. DOI: 10.1055/s-2007-979060

[6] Lee SW, Kim SH, Kim JY, Lee Y. The effect of growth hormone on fibroblast proliferation and keratinocyte migration. Journal of Plastic, Reconstructive and Aesthetic Surgery. 2010;**63**:e364-e369. DOI: 10.1016/j.bjps.2009.10.027

[7] Ghofrani A, Höller D, Schuhmann K, Saldern S, Messmer BJ. The influence of systemic growth hormone administration on the healing time of skin graft donor sites in a pig model. Plastic and Reconstructive Surgery. 1999;**104**:470-475

[8] Weiming Z, Ning L, Jieshou L. Effect of recombinant human growth hormone and enteral nutrition on short bowel syndrome. JPEN Journal of Parenteral and Enteral Nutrition. 2004;**28**:377-381. DOI: 10.1177/0148607104028006377

[9] Vara-Thorbeck R, Guerrero JA, Rosell J, Ruiz-Requena E, Capitán JM. Exogenous growth hormone: Effects on the catabolic response to surgically produced acute stress and on postoperative immune function. World Journal of Surgery. 1993;**17**:530-537; discussion 537-538

[10] Lal SO, Wolf SE, Herndon DN. Growth hormone, burns and tissue healing. Growth Hormone and IGF Research. 2000;**10**:539-543. DOI: 10.1016/S1096-6374(00)80008-8

[11] Herndon DN, Hawkins HK, Nguyen TT, Pierre E, Cox R, Barrow RE. Characterization of growth hormone enhanced donor site healing in patients with large cutaneous burns. Annals of Surgery. 1995;**221**:649-656; discussion 656-659

[12] Losada F, García-Luna PP, Gómez-Cía T, Garrido M, Pereira JL, Marín F, et al. Effects of human recombinant growth hormone on donor-site healing in burned adults. World Journal of Surgery. 2002;**26**:2-8. DOI: 10.1007/s00268-001-0170-9

[13] Rasmussen LH, Karlsmark T, Avnstorp C, Peters K, Jørgensen M, Jensen LT. Topical human growth hormone treatment of chronic leg ulcers. Phlebology. 1991;**6**:23-30. DOI: 10.1177/026835559100600105

[14] Rasmussen LH, Garbarsch C, Schuppan D, Moe D, Hørslev-Pedersen K, Gottrup F, et al. Influence of human growth hormone on granulation tissue formation, collagen deposition, and the aminoterminal propeptide of collagen type III in wound chambers in rats. Wound Repair and Regeneration. 1994;**2**:31-36. DOI: 10.1046/j.1524-475X.1994.20106.x

[15] Jørgensen PH, Oxlund H. Growth hormone increases the biomechanical strength and collagen deposition rate during the early phase of skin wound healing. Wound Repair and Regeneration. 1996;**4**:40-47. DOI: 10.1046/j.1524-475X.1996.40108.x

[16] Zaizen Y, Ford EG, Shimada H, Kosi M, Costin G, Atkinson JB. Growth hormone effects on wound healing in malnourished animals: A histological study. European Journal of Pediatric Surgery. 1995;**5**:226-230. DOI: 10.1055/s-2008-1066211

[17] Vakili H, Jin Y, Nagy JI, Cattini PA. Transgenic mice expressing the human growth hormone gene provide a model system to study human growth hormone synthesis and secretion in non-tumor-derived pituitary cells: Differential effects of dexamethasone and thyroid hormone. Molecular and Cellular Endocrinology. 2011;**345**:48-57. DOI: 10.1016/j.mce.2011.07.010

[18] Welsh KM, Lamit M, Morhenn VB. The effect of recombinant human growth hormone on wound healing in normal individuals. The Journal of Dermatologic Surgery and Oncology. 1991;**17**:942-945

[19] Thorey IS, Hinz B, Hoeflich A, Kaesler S, Bugnon P, Elmlinger M, et al. Transgenic mice reveal novel activities of growth hormone in wound repair, angiogenesis, and myofibroblast differentiation. The Journal of Biological Chemistry. 2004;**279**:26674-26684. DOI: 10.1074/jbc.M311467200

[20] Borrione P, Grasso L, Pautasso M, Parisi A, Quaranta F, Ciminelli E, et al. Impact of different concentrations of human recombinant growth hormone on T lymphocytes. International Journal of Immunopathology and Pharmacology. 2012;**25**:87-97. DOI: 10.1177/039463201202500111

[21] Caicedo D, Devesa P, Arce VM, Requena J, Devesa J. Chronic limb-threatening ischemia could benefit from growth hormone therapy for wound healing and limb salvage. Therapeutic Advances in Cardiovascular Disease. 2017;**12**:53-72. DOI: 10.1177/1753944717745494

[22] Caicedo D, Díaz O, Devesa P, Devesa J. Growth hormone (GH) and cardiovascular system. International Journal of Molecular Sciences. 2018;**19**:290. DOI: 10.3390/ijms19010290

[23] Luque RM, Gahete MD, Valentine RJ, Kineman RD. Examination of the direct effects of metabolic factors on somatotrope function in a non-human primate model, Papio anubis. Journal of Molecular Endocrinology. 2006;**37**:25-38. DOI: 10.1677/jme.1.02042

[24] Root AW, Root MJ. Clinical pharmacology of human growth hormone and its secretagogues. Current Drug Targets—Immune, Endocrine and Metabolic Disorders. 2002; **2**:27-52

[25] Jørgensen PH, Andreassen TT. A dose-response study of the effects of biosynthetic human growth hormone on formation and strength of granulation tissue. Endocrinology. 1987;**121**:1637-1641. DOI: 10.1210/endo-121-5-1637

[26] Messias de Lima CF, de Araújo Vieira LF, de Carvalho Wanderley LA, de Souza Ferro JN, Smaniotto S. Topical growth hormone accelerates wound healing in mice. Wounds: A Compendium of Clinical Research and Practice. 2017;**29**:387-392

[27] Devesa J, Almengló C, Devesa P. Multiple effects of growth hormone in the body: Is it really the hormone for growth? Clinical Medicine Insights: Endocrinology and Diabetes. 2016;**9**:47-71. DOI: 10.4137/CMED.S38201

[28] Fasshauer M, Klein J, Kralisch S, Klier M, Lossner U, Bluher M, et al. Monocyte chemoattractant protein 1 expression is stimulated by growth hormone and interleukin-6 in 3T3-L1 adipocytes. Biochemical and Biophysical Research Communications. 2004;**317**:598-604. DOI: 10.1016/j.bbrc.2004.03.090

[29] Meazza C, Pagani S, Travaglino P, Bozzola M. Effect of growth hormone (GH) on the immune system. Pediatric Endocrinology Reviews. 2004;**1**(Suppl 3):490-495

[30] Inoue T, Saito H, Tsuno N, Fukatsu K, Lin MT, Inaba T, et al. Effects of growth hormone and insulin-like growth factor I on opsonin receptor expression on local and systemic phagocytes in a lethal peritonitis model. Critical Care Medicine. 1998;**26**:338-343

[31] Napolitano LA, Schmidt D, Gotway MB, Ameli N, Filbert EL, Ng MM, et al. Growth hormone enhances thymic function in HIV-1-infected adults. The Journal of Clinical Investigation. 2008;**118**:1085-1098. DOI: 10.1172/JCI32830

[32] Singer AJ, Clark RA. Cutaneous wound healing. The New England Journal of Medicine. 1999;**341**:738-746. DOI: 10.1056/NEJM199909023411006

[33] Igarashi A, Okochi H, Bradham DM, Grotendorst GR. Regulation of connective tissue growth factor gene expression in human skin fibroblasts and during wound repair. Molecular Biology of the Cell. 1993;**4**:637-645

[34] Marchese C, Felici A, Visco V, Lucania G, Igarashi M, Picardo M, et al. Fibroblast growth factor 10 induces proliferation and differentiation of human primary cultured keratinocytes. The Journal of Investigative Dermatology. 2001;**116**:623-628. DOI: 10.1046/j.0022-202x.2001.01280.x

[35] Werner S, Smola H. Paracrine regulation of keratinocyte proliferation and differentiation. Trends in Cell Biology. 2001;**11**:143-146

[36] Trompezinski S, Berthier-Vergnes O, Denis A, Schmitt D, Viac J. Comparative expression of vascular endothelial growth factor family members, VEGF-B, -C and -D, by normal human keratinocytes and fibroblasts. Experimental Dermatology. 2004;**13**:98-105. DOI: 10.1111/j.0906-6705.2004.00137.x

[37] Rasmussen LH, Garbarsch C, Schuppan D, Moe D, Hørslev-Pedersen K, Gottrup F, et al. Dose response profiles of human growth hormone in subcutaneous wound chambers in rats. The European Journal of Surgery. 1995;**161**:157-162

[38] Messias de Lima CF, dos Santos Reis MD, da Silva Ramos FW, Ayres-Martins S, Smaniotto S. Growth hormone modulates in vitro endothelial cell migration and formation of capillary-like structures. Cell Biology International. 2017;**41**:577-584. DOI: 10.1002/cbin.10747

[39] Li J, Liu X, Tang H, Zhou X, Huang Y. Influence of some topical antibiotics and FGF2, EGF and rhGH on the biological characteristics of fibroblasts in vitro. Zhonghua Shao Shang Za Zhi. 2006;**22**:33-37

[40] Suk HK,Eun JH, Sang WL. The effect of topically applied recombinant human growth hormone on wound healing in pigs. Wounds. 2009;**21**:150-152

[41] Thum T, Hoeber S, Froese S, Klink I, Stichtenoth DO, Galuppo P, et al. Age-dependent impairment of endothelial progenitor cells is corrected by growth hormone mediated increase of insulin-like growth factor-1. Circulation Research. 2007;**100**:434-443. DOI: 10.1161/01.RES.0000257912.78915.af

[42] Clapp C, Thebault S, Jeziorski MC, Martínez De La Escalera G. Peptide hormone regulation of angiogenesis. Physiological Reviews. 2009;**89**:1177-1215. DOI: 10.1152/physrev.00024.2009

[43] Zheng H, Fu G, Dai T, Huang H. Migration of endothelial progenitor cells mediated by stromal cell-derived factor-1alpha/CXCR4 via PI3K/Akt/eNOS signal transduction pathway. Journal of Cardiovascular Pharmacology. 2007;**50**:274-280. DOI: 10.1097/FJC.0b013e318093ec8f

[44] Scott CD, Martin JL, Baxter RC. Production of insulin-like growth factor I and its binding protein by adult rat hepatocytes in primary culture. Endocrinology. 1985;**116**:1094-1101. DOI: 10.1210/endo-116-3-1094

[45] Pell JM, Bates PC. Differential actions of growth hormone and insulin-like growth factor-I on tissue protein metabolism in dwarf mice. Endocrinology. 1992;**130**:1942-1950. DOI: 10.1210/endo.130.4.1547721

[46] Robertson JG, Walton PE, Dunshea F, Dunaiski V, Ballard FJ, Belford DA. Growth hormone but not insulin-like growth factor-I improves wound strength in pigs. Wound Repair and Regeneration. 1997;**5**:168-174. DOI: 10.1046/j.1524-475X.1997.50209.x

[47] Dunaiski V, Belford DA. Contribution of circulating IGF-I to wound repair in GH-treated rats. Growth Hormone and IGF Research. 2002;**12**:381-387

[48] Steenfos HH, Jansson JO. Growth hormone stimulates granulation tissue formation and insulin-like growth factor-I gene expression in wound chambers in the rat. The Journal of Endocrinology. 1992;**132**:293-298

[49] Harrison DA. The Jak/STAT pathway. Cold Spring Harbor Perspectives in Biology. 2012;**4**:pii, a011205. DOI: 10.1101/cshperspect.a011205

[50] Abroun S, Saki N, Ahmadvand M, Asghari F, Salari F, Rahim F. STATs: An old story, yet mesmerizing. Cell Journal. 2015;**17**:395-411

[51] Soldevila G, García-Zepeda EA. The role of the Jak-Stat pathway in chemokine-mediated signaling in T lymphocytes. Signal Transduction. 2007;**7**:427-438. DOI: 10.1002/sita.200700144

[52] Hunckler J, de Mel A. A current affair: Electrotherapy in wound healing. Journal of Multidisciplinary Healthcare. 2017;**10**:179-194. DOI: 10.2147/JMDH.S127207

[53] Jere SW, Abrahamse H, Houreld NN. The JAK/STAT signaling pathway and photobiomodulation in chronic wound healing. Cytokine and Growth Factor Reviews. 2017;**38**:73-79. DOI: 10.1016/j.cytogfr.2017.10.001

[54] Pilecka I, Whatmore A, Hooft van Huijsduijnen R, Destenaves B, Clayton P. Growth hormone signalling: Sprouting links between pathways, human genetics and therapeutic options. Trends in Endocrinology and Metabolism. 2007;**18**:12-18. DOI: 10.1016/j.tem.2006.11.004

[55] Rowland JE, Lichanska AM, Kerr LM, White M, D'Aniello EM, Maher SL, et al. In vivo analysis of growth hormone receptor signaling domains and their associated transcripts. Molecular and Cellular Biology. 2005;**25**:66-77. DOI: 10.1128/MCB.25.1.66-77.2005

[56] Belacortu Y, Paricio N. Drosophila as a model of wound healing and tissue regeneration in vertebrates. Developmental Dynamics. 2011;**240**:2379-2404. DOI: 10.1002/dvdy.22753

[57] Feng Y, Sanders AJ, Morgan LD, Harding KG, Jiang WG. Potential roles of suppressor of cytokine signaling in wound healing. Regenerative Medicine. 2016;**11**:193-209. DOI: 10.2217/rme.16.4

[58] Croker BA, Kiu H, Nicholson SE. SOCS regulation of the JAK/STAT signalling pathway. Seminars in Cell and Developmental Biology. 2008;**19**:414-422

[59] McFarland-Mancini MM, Funk HM, Paluch AM, Zhou M, Giridhar PV, Mercer CA, et al. Differences in wound healing in mice with deficiency of IL-6 versus IL-6 receptor. Journal of Immunology. 2010;**184**:7219-7228. DOI: 10.4049/jimmunol.0901929

[60] Wang T, Yuan W, Liu Y, Zhang Y, Wang Z, Zhou X, et al. The role of the JAK-STAT pathway in neural stem cells, neural progenitor cells and reactive astrocytes after spinal cord injury. Biomedical Reports. 2015;**3**:141-146. DOI: 10.3892/br.2014.401

[61] Beigel F, Friedrich M, Probst C, Sotlar K, Göke B, Diegelmann J, et al. Oncostatin M mediates STAT3-dependent intestinal epithelial restitution via increased cell proliferation, decreased apoptosis and upregulation of SERPIN family members. PLoS One. 2014;**9**:e93498. DOI: 10.1371/journal.pone.0093498

[62] Giustina A, Veldhuis JD. Pathophysiology of the neuroregulation of growth hormone secretion in experimental animals and the human. Endocrine Reviews. 1998;**19**:717-797. DOI: 10.1210/edrv.19.6.0353

[63] Harvey S. Extrapituitary growth hormone. Endocrine. 2010;**38**:335-359. DOI: 10.1007/s12020-010-9403-8

[64] Goldenberg N, Barkan A. Factors regulating growth hormone secretion in humans. Endocrinology and Metabolism Clinics of North America. 2007;**36**:37-55. DOI: 10.1016/j.ecl.2006.11.003

[65] Ho KY, Veldhuis JD, Johnson ML, Furlanetto R, Evans WS, Alberti KG, et al. Fasting enhances growth hormone secretion and amplifies the complex rhythms of growth hormone secretion in man. The Journal of Clinical Investigation. 1988;**81**:968-975. DOI: 10.1172/JCI113450

[66] Harvey S, Scanes C, Daughaday WH. Growth hormone release: Integrative hypothalamic control. In: Growth Hormone. Boca Ratón, Florida: CRC Press; 1995. pp. 131-162. ISBN 0-8493-8697-7

[67] Clemmons DR, Underwood LE. Nutritional regulation of IGF-I and IGF binding proteins. Annual Review of Nutrition. 1991;**11**:393-412. DOI: 10.1146/annurev.nu.11.070191.002141

[68] Vakili H, Jin Y, Cattini PA. Evidence for a circadian effect on the reduction of human growth hormone gene expression in response to excess caloric intake. The Journal of Biological Chemistry. 2016;**291**:13823-13833. DOI: 10.1074/jbc.M116.722744

[69] Møller N, Jørgensen JOL. Effects of growth hormone on glucose, lipid, and protein metabolism in human subjects. Endocrine Reviews. 2009;**30**:152-177. DOI: 10.1210/er.2008-0027

[70] Van Cauter E, Plat L, Copinschi G. Interrelations between sleep and the somatotropic axis. Sleep. 1998;**21**:553-566

[71] Van Cauter E, Kerkhofs M, Caufriez A, Van Onderbergen A, Thorner MO, Copinschi G. A quantitative estimation of growth hormone secretion in normal man: Reproducibility and relation to sleep and time of day. The Journal of Clinical Endocrinology and Metabolism. 1992;**74**:1441-1450. DOI: 10.1210/jcem.74.6.1592892

[72] Everson CA, Bergmann BM, Rechtschaffen A. Sleep deprivation in the rat: III. Total sleep deprivation. Sleep. 1989;**12**:13-21

[73] Elenkov IJ, Chrousos GP. Stress hormones, proinflammatory and antiinflammatory cytokines, and autoimmunity. Annals of the New York Academy of Sciences. 2002;**966**:290-303

[74] Lorton D, Lubahn CL, Estus C, Millar BA, Carter JL, Wood CA, et al. Bidirectional communication between the brain and the immune system: Implications for physiological sleep and disorders with disrupted sleep. Neuroimmunomodulation. 2006;**13**:357-374. DOI: 10.1159/000104864

[75] Bjorvatn B, Pallesen S. A practical approach to circadian rhythm sleep disorders. Sleep Medicine Reviews. 2009;**13**:47-60. DOI: 10.1016/j.smrv.2008.04.009

[76] Dickstein JB, Moldofsky H. Sleep, cytokines and immune function. Sleep Medicine Reviews. 1999;**3**:219-228

[77] Moldofsky H, Lue FA, Davidson JR, Gorczynski R. Effects of sleep deprivation on human immune functions. The FASEB Journal. 1989;**3**:1972-1977

[78] Drobnik J, Dabrowski R. Melatonin suppresses the pinealectomy-induced elevation of collagen content in a wound. Cytobios. 1996;**85**:51-58

[79] Pugazhenthi K, Kapoor M, Clarkson AN, Hall I, Appleton I. Melatonin accelerates the process of wound repair in full-thickness incisional wounds. Journal of Pineal Research. 2008;**44**:387-396. DOI: 10.1111/j.1600-079X.2007.00541.x

[80] Brandenberger G, Weibel L. The 24-h growth hormone rhythm in men: Sleep and circadian influences questioned. Journal of Sleep Research. 2004;**13**:251-255. DOI: 10.1111/j.1365-2869.2004.00415.x

[81] Ando Y, Jensen PJ. Epidermal growth factor and insulin-like growth factor I enhance keratinocyte migration. The Journal of Investigative Dermatology. 1993;**100**:633-639

[82] Lee YR, Oshita Y, Tsuboi R, Ogawa H. Combination of insulin-like growth factor (IGF)-I and IGF-binding protein-1 promotes fibroblast-embedded collagen gel contraction. Endocrinology. 1996;**137**:5278-5283. DOI: 10.1210/endo.137.12.8940346

[83] Gartner MH, Benson JD, Caldwell MD. Insulin-like growth factors I and II expression in the healing wound. The Journal of Surgical Research. 1992;**52**:389-394

[84] Ghahary A, Shen YJ, Wang R, Scott PG, Tredget EE. Expression and localization of insulin-like growth factor-1 in normal and post-burn hypertrophic scar tissue in human. Molecular and Cellular Biochemistry. 1998;**183**:1-9

[85] Strock LL, Singh H, Abdullah A, Miller JA, Herndon DN. The effect of insulin-like growth factor I on postburn hypermetabolism. Surgery. 1990;**108**:161-164

[86] Emmerson E, Campbell L, Davies FCJ, Ross NL, Ashcroft GS, Krust A, et al. Insulin-like growth factor-1 promotes wound healing in estrogen-deprived mice: New insights into cutaneous IGF-1R/ERα cross talk. The Journal of Investigative Dermatology. 2012;**132**:2838-2848. DOI: 10.1038/jid.2012.228

[87] Kovács M, Schally AV, Varga JL, Zarándi M. Endocrine and antineoplastic actions of growth hormone-releasing hormone antagonists. Current Medicinal Chemistry. 2008;**15**:314-321

[88] Toogood AA, Shalet SM. Growth hormone replacement therapy in the elderly with hypothalamic-pituitary disease: A dose-finding study. The Journal of Clinical Endocrinology and Metabolism. 1999;**84**:131-136. DOI: 10.1210/jcem.84.1.5408

[89] Melmed S. In: Melmed S, editor. The Pituitary. 4th ed. Academic Press; 2017. ISBN 978-0-12-804169-7

[90] Meigan G, Sasaki A, Yoshinaga K. Immunoreactive growth hormone-releasing hormone in rat placenta. Endocrinology. 1988;**123**:1098-1102. DOI: 10.1210/endo-123-2-1098

[91] Bagnato A, Moretti C, Ohnishi J, Frajese G, Catt KJ. Expression of the growth hormone-releasing hormone gene and its peptide product in the rat ovary. Endocrinology. 1992;**130**:1097-1102. DOI: 10.1210/endo.130.3.1537276

[92] Dioufa N, Schally AV, Chatzistamou I, Moustou E, Block NL, Owens GK, et al. Acceleration of wound healing by growth hormone-releasing hormone and its agonists. Proceedings of the National Academy of Sciences of the United States of America. 2010; **107**:18611-18615. DOI: 10.1073/pnas.1013942107

[93] Kiaris H, Schally AV, Busto R, Halmos G, Artavanis-Tsakonas S, Varga JL. Expression of a splice variant of the receptor for GHRH in 3T3 fibroblasts activates cell proliferation responses to GHRH analogs. Proceedings of the National Academy of Sciences of the United States of America. 2002;**99**:196-200. DOI: 10.1073/pnas.012590999

[94] Barabutis N, Siejka A, Schally AV, Block NL, Cai R, Varga JL. Activation of mitogen-activated protein kinases by a splice variant of GHRH receptor. Journal of Molecular Endocrinology. 2010;**44**:127-134. DOI: 10.1677/JME-09-0121

[95] Cui T, Jimenez JJ, Block NL, Badiavas EV, Rodriguez-Menocal L, Granda AV, et al. Agonistic analogs of growth hormone releasing hormone (GHRH) promote wound healing by stimulating the proliferation and survival of human dermal fibroblasts through ERK and AKT pathways. Oncotarget. 2016;**7**:52661-52672. DOI: 10.18632/oncotarget.11024

[96] Serini G, Gabbiani G. Mechanisms of myofibroblast activity and phenotypic modulation. Experimental Cell Research. 1999;**250**:273-283. DOI: 10.1006/excr.1999.4543

[97] Yager DR, Chen SM, Ward SI, Olutoye OO, Diegelmann RF, Kelman Cohen I. Ability of chronic wound fluids to degrade peptide growth factors is associated with increased levels of elastase activity and diminished levels of proteinase inhibitors. Wound Repair and Regeneration. 1997;**5**:23-32. DOI: 10.1046/j.1524-475X.1997.50108.x

[98] Stanley AC, Park HY, Phillips TJ, Russakovsky V, Menzoian JO. Reduced growth of dermal fibroblasts from chronic venous ulcers can be stimulated with growth factors. Journal of Vascular Surgery. 1997;**26**:994-999.discussion 999-1001

[99] Cai R, Schally AV, Cui T, Szalontay L, Halmos G, Sha W, et al. Synthesis of new potent agonistic analogs of growth hormone-releasing hormone (GHRH) and evaluation of their endocrine and cardiac activities. Peptides. 2014;**52**:104-112. DOI: 10.1016/j.peptides.2013.12.010

[100] Zhang X, Cui T, He J, Wang H, Cai R, Popovics P, et al. Beneficial effects of growth hormone-releasing hormone agonists on rat INS-1 cells and on streptozotocin-induced NOD/SCID mice. Proceedings of the National Academy of Sciences of the United States of America. 2015;**112**:13651-13656. DOI: 10.1073/pnas.1518540112

[101] Ziegler TR, Gatzen C, Wilmore DW. Strategies for attenuating protein-catabolic responses in the critically ill. Annual Review of Medicine. 1994;**45**:459-480. DOI: 10.1146/annurev.med.45.1.459

[102] Roubenoff R, Kehayias JJ. The meaning and measurement of lean body mass. Nutrition Reviews. 1991;**49**:163-175

[103] Tierney R, Pierson N. Magnitude of body-cell-mass depletion death from wasting in A1DS13 and the timing. The American Journal of Clinical Nutrition. 1989;**50**:444-447

[104] Ruberg RL. Role of nutrition in wound healing. The Surgical Clinics of North America. 1984;**64**:705-714

[105] Peacock EE. Effect of dietary proline and hydroxyproline on tensile strength of healing wounds. Proceedings of the Society for Experimental Biology and Medicine. 1960;**105**:380-383

[106] Jeschke MG, Mlcak RP, Finnerty CC, Norbury WB, Gauglitz GG, Kulp GA, et al. Burn size determines the inflammatory and hypermetabolic response. Critical Care. 2007;**11**:R90. DOI: 10.1186/cc6102

[107] Finnerty CC, Herndon DN, Przkora R, Pereira CT, Oliveira HM, Queiroz DMM, et al. Cytokine expression profile over time in severely burned pediatric patients. Shock. 2006;**26**:13-19. DOI: 10.1097/01.shk.0000223120.26394.7d

[108] Herndon DN, Tompkins RG. Support of the metabolic response to burn injury. Lancet (London, England). 2004;**363**:1895-1902. DOI: 10.1016/S0140-6736(04)16360-5

[109] Demling RH. The role of anabolic hormones for wound healing in catabolic states. Journal of Burns and Wounds. 2005;**4**:46-59

[110] Lang CH, Frost RA. Role of growth hormone, insulin-like growth factor-I, and insulin-like growth factor binding proteins in the catabolic response to injury and infection. Current Opinion in Clinical Nutrition and Metabolic Care. 2002;**5**:271-279

[111] Ross RJ, Rodriguez-Arnao J, Bentham J, Coakley JH. The role of insulin, growth hormone and IGF-I as anabolic agents in the critically ill. Intensive Care Medicine. 1993;**19**(Suppl 2):S54-S57

[112] Mulligan K, Tai VW, Schambelan M. Use of growth hormone and other anabolic agents in AIDS wasting. JPEN Journal of Parenteral and Enteral Nutrition. 1999;**23**:S202-S209. DOI: 10.1177/014860719902300606

[113] Pierre EJ, Perez-Polo JR, Mitchell AT, Matin S, Foyt HL, Herndon DN. Insulin-like growth factor-I liposomal gene transfer and systemic growth hormone stimulate wound healing. The Journal of Burn Care and Rehabilitation. 1997;**18**:287-291

[114] Ramirez RJ, Wolf SE, Barrow RE, Herndon DN. Growth hormone treatment in pediatric burns: A safe therapeutic approach. Annals of Surgery. 1998;**228**:439-448

[115] Takala J, Ruokonen E, Webster NR, Nielsen MS, Zandstra DF, Vundelinckx G, et al. Increased mortality associated with growth hormone treatment in critically Ill adults. The New England Journal of Medicine. 1999;**341**:785-792. DOI: 10.1056/NEJM199909093411102

[116] Kojima M, Hosoda H, Date Y, Nakazato M, Matsuo H, Kangawa K. Ghrelin is a growth-hormone-releasing acylated peptide from stomach. Nature. 1999;**402**:656-660. DOI: 10.1038/45230

[117] Badman MK, Flier JS. The adipocyte as an active participant in energy balance and metabolism. Gastroenterology. 2007;**132**:2103-2115. DOI: 10.1053/j.gastro.2007.03.058

[118] Arvat E, Maccario M, Di Vito L, Broglio F, Benso A, Gottero C, et al. Endocrine activities of ghrelin, a natural growth hormone secretagogue (GHS), in humans: Comparison and interactions with hexarelin, a nonnatural peptidyl GHS, and GH-releasing hormone. The Journal of Clinical Endocrinology and Metabolism. 2001;**86**:1169-1174. DOI: 10.1210/jcem.86.3.7314

[119] Dixit VD, Taub DD. Ghrelin and immunity: A young player in an old field. Experimental Gerontology. 2005;**40**:900-910. DOI: 10.1016/j.exger.2005.09.003

[120] Levy R, Efrati O, Bujanover Y, Hashomer T. Leptin,ghrelin, and adiponectin in the metabolic adjustment to burn injury in children. Wounds. 2014;**26**(6):178-185

[121] Sehirli O, Sener E, Sener G, Cetinel S, Erzik C, Yeğen BC. Ghrelin improves burn-induced multiple organ injury by depressing neutrophil infiltration and the release of pro-inflammatory cytokines. Peptides. 2008;**29**:1231-1240. DOI: 10.1016/j.peptides.2008.02.012

[122] Nagaya N, Kojima M, Uematsu M, Yamagishi M, Hosoda H, Oya H, et al. Hemodynamic and hormonal effects of human ghrelin in healthy volunteers. American Journal of Physiology. Regulatory, Integrative and Comparative Physiology. 2001;**280**:R1483-R1487. DOI: 10.1152/ajpregu.2001.280.5.R1483

[123] Taub DD. Novel connections between the neuroendocrine and immune systems: The ghrelin immunoregulatory network. Vitamins and Hormones. 2008;**77**:325-346. DOI: 10.1016/S0083-6729(06)77014-5

[124] Ceranowicz D, Warzecha Z, Dembinski A, Ceranowicz P, Cieszkowski J, Kusnierz-Cabala B, et al. Role of hormonal axis, growth hormone—IGF-1, in the therapeutic effect of ghrelin in the course of cerulein-induced acute pancreatitis. Journal of Physiology and Pharmacology. 2010;**61**:599-606

[125] Ceranowicz P, Warzecha Z, Cieszkowski J, Ceranowicz D, Kuśnierz-Cabala B, Bonior J, et al. Essential role of growth hormone and IGF-1 in therapeutic effect of ghrelin in the course of acetic acid-induced colitis. International Journal of Molecular Sciences. 2017;**18**:pii, E1118. DOI: 10.3390/ijms18061118

[126] Liu C, Hao Y, Huang J, Li H, Yang Z, Zeng Y, et al. Ghrelin accelerates wound healing in combined radiation and wound injury in mice. Experimental Dermatology. 2017;**26**:186-193. DOI: 10.1111/exd.13224

[127] Liu C, Huang J, Li H, Yang Z, Zeng Y, Liu J, et al. Ghrelin accelerates wound healing through GHS-R1a-mediated MAPK-NF-κB/GR signaling pathways in combined radiation and burn injury in rats. Scientific Reports. 2016;**6**:27499. DOI: 10.1038/srep27499

[128] Campisi J, d'Adda di Fagagna F. Cellular senescence: When bad things happen to good cells. Nature Reviews. Molecular Cell Biology. 2007;**8**:729-740. DOI: 10.1038/nrm2233

[129] Tchkonia T, Morbeck DE, Von Zglinicki T, Van Deursen J, Lustgarten J, Scrable H, et al. Fat tissue, aging, and cellular senescence. Aging Cell. 2010;**9**:667-684. DOI: 10.1111/j.1474-9726.2010.00608.x

[130] Waaijer MEC, Parish WE, Strongitharm BH, van Heemst D, Slagboom PE, de Craen AJM, et al. The number of p16INK4a positive cells in human skin reflects biological age. Aging Cell. 2012;**11**:722-725. DOI: 10.1111/j.1474-9726.2012.00837.x

[131] Oh J, Lee YD, Wagers AJ. Stem cell aging: Mechanisms, regulators and therapeutic opportunities. Nature Medicine. 2014;**20**:870-880. DOI: 10.1038/nm.3651

[132] Bandyopadhyay D, Timchenko N, Suwa T, Hornsby PJ, Campisi J, Medrano EE. The human melanocyte: A model system to study the complexity of cellular aging and transformation in non-fibroblastic cells. Experimental Gerontology. 2001;**36**:1265-1275

[133] Rheinwald JG, Green H. Serial cultivation of strains of human epidermal keratinocytes: The formation of keratinizing colonies from single cells. Cell. 1975;**6**:331-343

[134] Kirkland JL, Tchkonia T. Clinical strategies and animal models for developing senolytic agents. Experimental Gerontology. 2015;**68**:19-25. DOI: 10.1016/j.exger.2014.10.012

[135] Muñoz-Espín D, Serrano M. Cellular senescence: From physiology to pathology. Nature Reviews. Molecular Cell Biology. 2014;**15**:482-496. DOI: 10.1038/nrm3823

[136] Kuilman T, Peeper DS. Senescence-messaging secretome: SMS-ing cellular stress. Nature Reviews. Cancer. 2009;**9**:81-94. DOI: 10.1038/nrc2560

[137] López-Otín C, Blasco MA, Partridge L, Serrano M, Kroemer G. The hallmarks of aging. Cell. 2013;**153**:1194-1217. DOI: 10.1016/j.cell.2013.05.039

[138] Nelson G, Wordsworth J, Wang C, Jurk D, Lawless C, Martin-Ruiz C, et al. A senescent cell bystander effect: Senescence-induced senescence. Aging Cell. 2012;**11**:345-349. DOI: 10.1111/j.1474-9726.2012.00795.x

[139] Franceschi C, Capri M, Monti D, Giunta S, Olivieri F, Sevini F, et al. Inflammaging and anti-inflammaging: A systemic perspective on aging and longevity emerged from studies in humans. Mechanisms of Ageing and Development. 2007;**128**:92-105. DOI: 10.1016/j.mad.2006.11.016

[140] Passos JF, Nelson G, Wang C, Richter T, Simillion C, Proctor CJ, et al. Feedback between p21 and reactive oxygen production is necessary for cell senescence. Molecular Systems Biology. 2010;**6**:347. DOI: 10.1038/msb.2010.5

[141] Ardail D, Debon A, Perret-Vivancos C, Biol-N'Garagba M-C, Krantic S, Lobie PE, et al. Growth hormone internalization in mitochondria decreases respiratory chain activity. Neuroendocrinology. 2010;**91**:16-26. DOI: 10.1159/000268289

[142] Nylander E, Grönbladh A, Zelleroth S, Diwakarla S, Nyberg F, Hallberg M. Growth hormone is protective against acute methadone-induced toxicity by modulating the NMDA receptor complex. Neuroscience. 2016;**339**:538-547. DOI: 10.1016/j.neuroscience.2016.10.019

[143] Keane J, Tajouri L, Gray B. The effect of growth hormone administration on the regulation of mitochondrial apoptosis in-vivo. International Journal of Molecular Sciences. 2015;**16**:12753-12772. DOI: 10.3390/ijms160612753

[144] Rojanathammanee L, Rakoczy S, Brown-Borg HM. Growth hormone alters the glutathione S-transferase and mitochondrial thioredoxin systems in long-living Ames dwarf mice. The Journals of Gerontology. Series A, Biological Sciences and Medical Sciences. 2014;**69**:1199-1211. DOI: 10.1093/gerona/glt178

[145] Suzuki K, Yanagi K, Shimizu M, Wakamatsu S, Niitani T, Hosonuma S, et al. Effect of growth hormone replacement therapy on plasma diacron-reactive oxygen metabolites and endothelial function in Japanese patients: The GREAT clinical study. Endocrine Journal. 2017;**65**:101-111. DOI: 10.1507/endocrj.EJ17-0330

[146] Scacchi M, Valassi E, Pincelli AI, Fatti LM, Pecori Giraldi F, Ascoli P, et al. Increased lipid peroxidation in adult GH-deficient patients: Effects of short-term GH administration. Journal of Endocrinological Investigation. 2006;**29**:899-904. DOI: 10.1007/BF03349194

[147] Ikushima M, Rakugi H, Ishikawa K, Maekawa Y, Yamamoto K, Ohta J, et al. Anti-apoptotic and anti-senescence effects of Klotho on vascular endothelial cells. Biochemical and Biophysical Research Communications. 2006;**339**:827-832. DOI: 10.1016/j.bbrc.2005.11.094

[148] Gu Y, Zou Y, Aikawa R, Hayashi D, Kudoh S, Yamauchi T, et al. Growth hormone signalling and apoptosis in neonatal rat cardiomyocytes. Molecular and Cellular Biochemistry. 2001;**223**:35-46. DOI: 10.1023/A:1017941625858

[149] Kokoszko A, Lewiński A, Karbownik-Lewińska M. The role of growth hormone and insulin-like growth factor I in oxidative processes. Endokrynologia Polska. 2008; **59**:496-501

[150] Zadeh ZA, Kesmati M, Galehdari H, Rezai A, Seyednezhad SM, Torabi M. Evaluation of the relationship between serum levels of insulin, cortisol and growth hormones with wound healing in normal and diabetic rats. Physiology and Pharmacology. 2014;**18**:92-100

[151] Hansen TK, Fisker S, Dall R, Ledet T, Jørgensen JOL, Rasmussen LM. Growth hormone increases vascular cell adhesion molecule 1 expression: In vivo and in vitro evidence. The Journal of Clinical Endocrinology and Metabolism. 2004;**89**:909-916. DOI: 10.1210/jc.2003-030223

Chapter 9

Autologous Platelet-Rich Plasma and Mesenchymal Stem Cells for the Treatment of Chronic Wounds

Peter A. Everts

Additional information is available at the end of the chapter

http://dx.doi.org/10.5772/intechopen.80502

Abstract

Emerging autologous cellular therapies, utilizing platelet-rich plasma and mesenchymal stem cell applications, have the potential to play an adjunctive role in a standardized wound care treatment plan in patients suffering from chronic and recalcitrant wounds. The use of platelet-rich plasma growth is based on the fact that platelet growth factors can support the three phases of wound healing and then ultimately contribute to full wound closure. Mesenchymal stem cell-based therapies are also an attractive approach for the treatment of these difficult-to-heal wounds. This field of regenerative medicine focuses primarily on stem cells, which are specialized cells with the ability to self-renew and differentiate into multiple cell types. Mesenchymal stem cells can be isolated from bone marrow and adipose tissue via minimally manipulative and cell-processing techniques, at point of care. Both platelet-rich plasma and mesenchymal stem cell applications have the potential to become an effective and ideal autologous biological cell-based therapy, which can be applied to chronic wounds to effectively change the wound bed microenvironment to enable and accelerate wound closure.

Keywords: chronic wounds, microenvironment, wound healing, clinical platelet-rich plasma, platelet-rich plasma gel, mesenchymal stem cells, bone marrow concentrate, adipose tissue

1. Introduction

In the Western world, approximately 1–2% of the population will develop a chronic wound during their lifetime. These numbers will increase worldwide as a result of the aging population, increase in diabetes and obesity, and cardiovascular disease as well [1–3]. In particular, chronic leg wounds represent the largest fraction, with venous and diabetic foot ulcers (DFUs) accounting for 70–90% of these ulcers [4]. Concomitantly, the costs of wound care services are rising, with the market of wound care products surpassing $15 billion annually.

There is an unmet need to stimulate the healing of acute and chronic wounds to a level that is not possible with the current standard care measures and therapy approaches.

An area of medicine that holds promise for the treatment of recalcitrant and difficult-to-heal wounds is regenerative medicine. Therefore, it is critical to use more effective and efficient treatment options from patient and cost perspectives. The use of autologous biologics, such as platelet-rich plasma (PRP)- and mesenchymal stem cell (MSC)-based therapies, holds substantial promise to enhance tissue regeneration and repair in many different diseases and could therefore also be potentially effective in chronic wound care management strategies.

This review aimed to describe the scientific rationale and clinical experiences of two different autologous biological therapies to support the healing of chronic and recalcitrant wounds. First is the use of clinical PRP, prepared at point of care using a dual spin buffy coat device, and second is the local application of MSCs, derived from either bone marrow concentrate or adipose tissue.

2. Skin layers

The skin consists of three layers. The epidermis is the most outer layer, consisting of multilayered epithelium extending from the basement membrane, which separates the dermis from the air. The basement membrane contains progenitor stem cells, which undergo continuous self-renewal and differentiate into keratinocytes. The keratinocytes migrate towards the surface of the skin where they normally undergo terminal differentiation and maturation [5]. The dermis is the thickest layer, just below the epidermis. The dermis is a connective tissue, composed of the extracellular matrix (ECM), fibroblasts, vascular endothelial cells, and skin appendages such as sweat glands and hair follicles [6]. Fibroblasts are cells that secrete molecules including collagen and elastin, which provide mechanical strength and elasticity to the skin. The third layer is the hypodermis, which is underneath the dermis and composed of adipose tissue, providing insulation and cushioning between the skin and bone, muscle, tendon, and other skeletal structures [6]. A skin defect is repaired through cutaneous wound healing processes to recover loss of integrity, facilitate tensile strength, and provide a barrier for the skin [7]. Normal cutaneous wound repair is a multifaceted process.

3. Normal wound healing and cellular mechanisms

Wound healing is a well-orchestrated and complex series of events involving cell-cell and cell-matrix interactions, with platelet growth factors (PGFs), their dedicated receptors, and stem cells serving as messengers to regulate the various processes involved. The "wound healing" process as a whole has to be considered from the point of view of the type of lesion, which will in turn dictate the degree of healing that can be obtained. A partial thickness skin abrasion heals almost entirely by epithelialization, whereas deep pressure chronic ulcers rely mainly on matrix synthesis, angiogenesis, fibroplasia, and wound contraction.

3.1. Platelet clot and degranulation

With wounds and also after surgical incisions, repair begins with platelet clot formation, activation of the coagulation cascade, and subsequent platelet degranulation, releasing PGFs. After tissue damage, specific growth factors, including platelet-derived growth factor (PDGF) and fibroblast growth factor (FGF), are already being produced by the injured tissue cells [8]. Once a platelet plug is in place, platelets will get trapped in the fibrin mesh and start to degranulate, releasing PGFs, among other molecular components. Different growth factors have different characteristics and thus biological activities. Chemotactic and mitogenic capabilities have been demonstrated with regard to inflammatory cells (i.e., neutrophils, monocytes, and macrophages) [9]. At wound sites, PDGF subunits AB and transforming growth factor-β (TGF-β) are the most important growth factors initiating the wound healing process.

3.2. Inflammatory cell mechanisms

During the first 2 days of wound healing, an inflammatory process is initiated by the migration of inflammatory cells (neutrophils, macrophages, and T-lymphocytes) to the wound site to accomplish phagocytosis with the removal of bacteria, cellular debris, and damaged tissue. After the early inflammatory phase subsides, the predominant macrophage population assumes a wound healing phenotype that is characterized by the production of numerous growth factors and cytokines, including PDGF, transforming growth factor β1 (TGF-β1), insulin-like growth factor 1 (IGF-1), and vascular endothelial growth factor-a (VEGF-a), which promote cell proliferation and blood vessel development [10, 11]. Activated macrophages can be classified into different phenotypes. M1-type, with antimicrobial and antitumor properties, is activated upon wound formation by inflammatory signals from interferon-y (IFN-y) and tumor necrosis factor-α (TNF-α) or when pathogen-associated molecular patterns or endogenous danger signals are recognized. Their main role is host-defense mechanisms in the early healing process, releasing IL-12, promoting pro-inflammatory Th1 immune responses [12]. Conversely, the M2 macrophage phenotype downregulates inflammation and initiates tissue repair by releasing anti-inflammatory cytokines, such as IL-10 [13, 14]. Apoptotic wound neutrophils are ingested by these M2 macrophages, which release cytokines to promote macrophage recruitment and synthesize mediators critical to remodeling and angiogenesis, including TGF-β, VEGF, and epidermal growth factor (EGF) [15, 16].

3.3. Proliferative cell activity

Angiogenesis and fibroplasia are the next phases of wound healing, the proliferative phase. New blood vessel formation and the migration of fibroblasts, which deposit new ECM, are facilitated by EGF, keratinocyte growth factors (KGFs), and TGF-α [17, 18]. Keratinocytes migrate from the wound edges between the dermis facilitated by the production of collagenase and other proteases in the epidermis. Fibroblasts migrate, proliferate, and produce ECM in the wound bed, resulting in early granulation and tissue formation [19]. This process leads to an early increase in wound breaking strength, which is an important wound healing parameter of surgical wounds.

3.4. Epithelialization

The final phase of wound closure is epithelialization, characterized by the exit of inflammatory cells, a decrease in growth factor release, an increase in the ratio of collagen deposition to fibroblasts, and the cross-linking and organization of collagen molecules. Remodeling takes place over a much longer period of time in which the newly formed tissue is reorganized for higher tensile strength [17]. Hence, the normal wound healing process constitutes a delicate balance of cells secreting and regulating the many cytokines, chemokines, proteins, and growth factors.

4. Chronic wound healing characteristics

A vast majority of chronic wounds begin as minor traumatic injuries, such as penetrating injuries, insect bites, or even simple scratches of dry skin. Normally, these wounds heal within a few days/weeks. However, aging and underlying pathologies, such as diabetes-induced and nondiabetic neuropathies, can lead to the development of poor or non-healing wounds [20]. Furthermore, arterial and venous vascular pathologies with hyperglycemia could further complicate the wound healing process. Chronic wounds are chronically inflamed and can be characterized by dysfunctional cellular events and aberrant cytokine and growth factor activities, leading to failure of normal wound closure with the potential for infections [19, 21]. Wound infections trigger extensive recruitment of inflammatory cells, particularly resulting in high concentrations of neutrophils, serine elastase, and inflammatory macrophages, while cell extravasation is facilitated by disproportionate expression of vascular cell adhesion molecules and interstitial cell adhesion molecules by resident endothelial cells. The accumulated inflammatory cells in the wound bed lead to protease activity, with elevated levels of matrix metalloproteases (MMP) 2, 8, and 9, successively prolonging inflammation [22]. Moreover, tissue inhibitor of MMP 1 is decreased in non-healing wounds, thereby increasing collagenolytic activity. Furthermore, neutrophils also produce various reactive oxygen species (ROS), inducing considerable oxidative stress and thus damaging structural elements of the ECM and wound biochemical microenvironment [23]. Nonetheless, together with proinflammatory cytokines, an abnormally prolonged inflammatory phase will result in wound chronicity, which might lead to premature cell senescence [24]. Tissue hypoxia and repeated wound infections will continue to promote MMP enzyme activity, resulting in decreased growth factor functions, and fibrin deficits will transpire. It has been demonstrated that a chronically inflamed wound microenvironment subjects proteins and cytokines to degradation and sequestration, in particular the growth factors PDGF, EGF, and TGF-β [25, 26]. In addition, Cooper et al. demonstrated that a number of growth factors were markedly reduced in wound fluids from chronic wounds as compared to acute wounds [27]. Moreover, FGF and TGF-β concentrations were significantly downregulated in chronic wounds. Decreased growth factor levels and upregulation of proinflammatory cytokines and chemokines will worsen normal progression of wound healing and consequently the potential for full wound closure. In chronic wounds, the microenvironment must be modified to be an active and effective intervention, eliminating the factors that impede healing.

http://dx.doi.org/10.5772/intechopen.80502

To succeed in the reparative phase of wound healing, chronic wound care treatment strategies should have a dual approach. This includes the treatment of any underlying systemic disease and wound-microenvironmental tissue therapy. Evidence-based principles for local and systemic wound care management exist in the literature but are not further discussed in this chapter [28, 29]. In these traditional wound care treatment options, the application of autologous cellular biologics, such as platelet-rich plasma (PRP) growth factor therapy and MSC applications, is not anticipated, but discussed in detail here below.

5. Platelets in platelet-rich plasma therapy

PRP therapies have been used for a variety of indications, for more than 30 years. More than 10,000 references are currently in PubMed, using the search term platelet-rich plasma. These countless applications have given rise to considerable interest in the potential of autologous PRP in numerous regenerative medicine indications. In the last decade, numerous studies and reviews have been published on PRP therapies as a biological, adjunctive, therapy option in the management of chronic wounds.

5.1. Platelets and their intracellular content

Platelets are formed from megakaryocytes and are synthesized in bone marrow by pinching off from their progenitor cell. Thereafter, platelets are released into the peripheral circulation. Platelets are small, anucleate, discoid blood cells (1–3 μm), with an in vivo half-life of 7 days. The average platelet count in adults ranges from 150 to 350 × 10^6/mL of circulating blood. Platelets have a ring of contractile microtubules (cytoskeleton) around their periphery, containing actin and myosin. Inside platelets, there are a number of intracellular structures, including α-granules comprising PGFs and angiogenesis regulators and dense granules containing ADP, ATP, serotonin, histamine, calcium, and mitochondria. Other complex platelet biological components include adhesins and coagulation and immunological molecules. These molecules serve a multitude of functions, first within the clotting cascade and finally as initiators of tissue-healing processes. Platelets are equipped with an extensively invaginated membrane with an intricate canalicular system, which is in constant contact with the extracellular fluid [30]. Normally, platelets are in a resting state, non-thrombogenic. They require a 'trigger' before they become a potent and an active player in hemostasis and an accelerator of the wound healing cascade, depending upon the microenvironmental effectors.

5.2. Platelet-rich plasma gel, growth factors, and platelet receptors

When PRP is indicated to treat recalcitrant wounds, in the vast majority of these applications, PRP is delivered as a topical semiviscous coagulum so that concentrated platelets and various cytokines can adhere to the surface of the wound bed. For platelets to stick to a prepared wound bed, the PRP sample needs to be activated, thereby changing from a resting, inactive state to an active form. The platelet discoid shape changes, with the development of pseudopodia (**Figure 1**). This change in platelet shape and configuration is facilitated by the

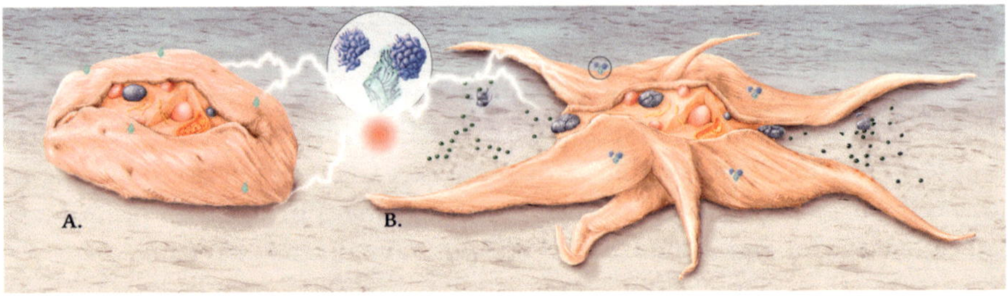

Figure 1. Graphic illustration of non-activated and an activated platelet. (A) A normal, discoid, resting platelet in a non-activated state, with platelet glycoprotein surface receptors on the outside of the platelet. (B) Following activation, the platelet shape is changed, with the development of pseudopods and the release of platelet granules and other intracellular storage vesicles via the opened canalicular system into the local microenvironmental milieu.

addition of platelet agonists (e.g., autologous or bovine thrombin, calcium, tissue factor, or other platelet-activating proteins) to a volume of PRP. Platelet activation and aggregation then leads to the creation of the semiviscous coagulum, that is, platelet clot, referred to in the literature as platelet-rich plasma gel (PRP-G). In this constitution, PRP-G can then be exogenously applied to soft tissues and chronic wounds.

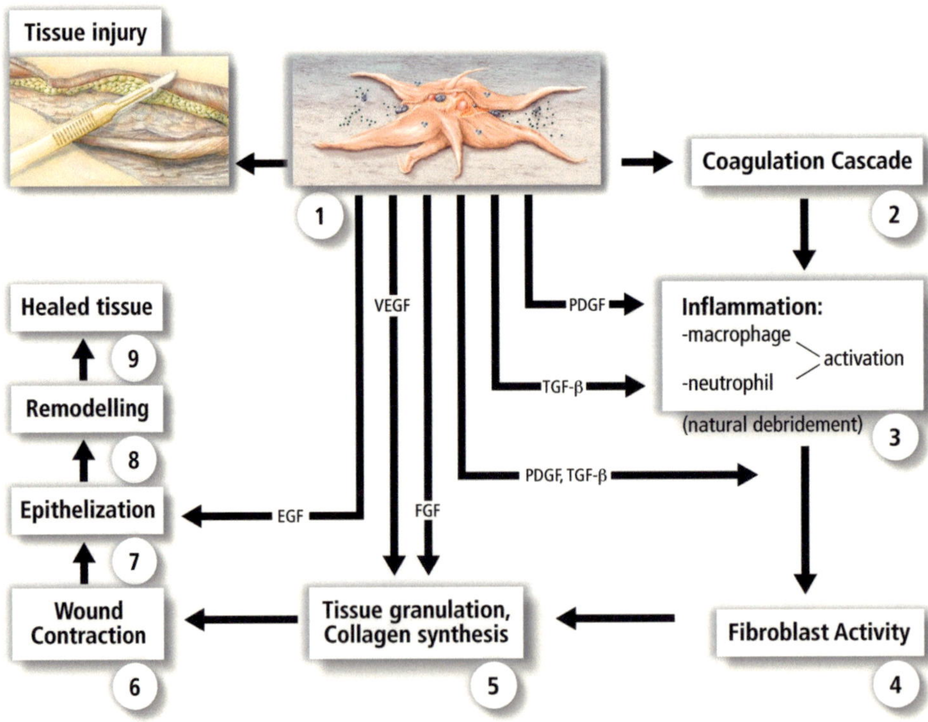

Figure 2. Schematic illustration of the activities of platelet growth factors during the different stages of the wound healing cascade. The numbers indicate the sequence of the phased stages of the wound healing process in which platelet growth factors have pivotal roles (EGF, epidermal growth factor; FGF, fibroblast growth factor; PDGF, platelet derived growth factor; TGF-β, transforming growth factor beta; VEGF, vascular endothelial growth factor).

http://dx.doi.org/10.5772/intechopen.80502

Following a PRP-G application on a debrided wound bed, fibrinolysis occurs over time and the platelets start to disintegrate, subsequently releasing their PGFs and other plasma proteins. This is the onset of PGF-mediated stimulation of cell proliferation, promotion of cell differentiation and chemotaxis, and induction of migration of various (stem) cells to the wound area [31, 32]. The rational for applying PRP-G to wound bed tissues is the delivery of a diversity of concentrated platelet-derived growth factors and other biological mediators (e.g., adhesive proteins, fibrinogen, fibronectin, vitronectin, and thrombospondin-1) to mimic, and accelerate, physiologic wound healing cascades and regenerative tissue repair processes (**Figure 2**) [33].

After disintegration of the topical semiviscous coagulum, PGFs and other platelet molecules accumulate in the ECM and the released growth factors interact and bind with a specific platelet tyrosine kinase receptor (TKR), present on the outer surface of cell membranes (ligand-receptor interaction). TKRs are membrane spanning proteins that extend into the cytoplasm of the cell. After growth factors interact with their specific cell membrane TKR, activation of (inactive) messenger proteins in the cytoplasm occurs. The activated TKR cytoplasmic tail now serves as a binding site for the messenger proteins. An activated protein is generated through a signaling cascade, capable of entering the cell nucleus, where it triggers the genes responsible for controlling cell division. Subsequently, transcription of mRNA is induced, producing a biological response that initiates cascades that induce tissue repair and regeneration (**Figure 3**) [34, 35].

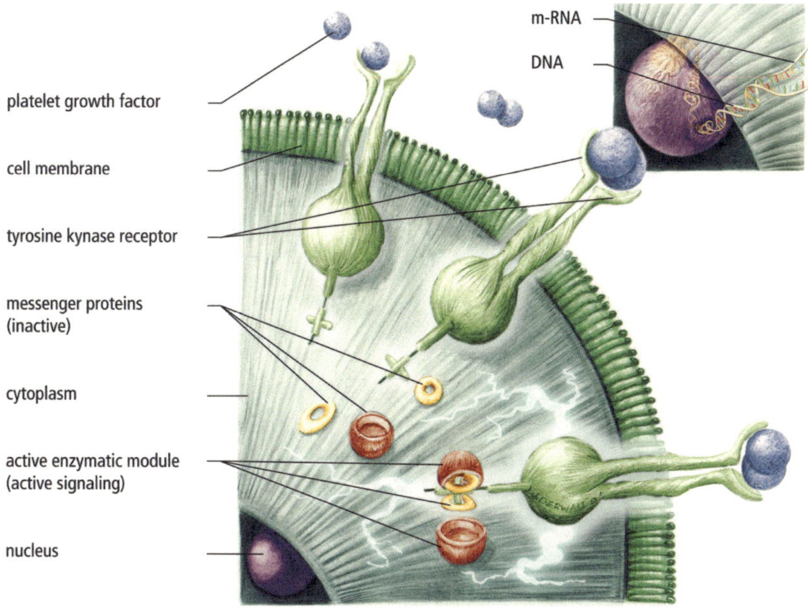

Figure 3. Illustrative representation of the mechanisms involved in platelet growth factor binding to their receptor. Specific platelet growth factors find their dedicated cell membrane tyrosine kinase receptor on the outside cell membrane. Following coupling, active enzymatic intracellular signaling occurs, with transmission to the cell nucleus via messenger ribonucleic acid.

Platelet growth factor	Growth factor sources	Biological activities
Platelet-derived growth factor, PDGF(a-b)	Platelets, osteoblasts, endothelial cells, macrophages, monocytes, smooth muscle cells	Mitogenic for mesenchymal cells and osteoblasts; stimulates chemotaxis and mitogenesis in fibroblast/glial/smooth muscle cells; regulates collagenase secretion and collagen synthesis; stimulates macrophage and neutrophil chemotaxis
Transforming growth factor, TGF(α-β)	Platelets, extracellular matrix of bone, cartilage matrix, macrophages/monocytes, and neutrophils	Stimulates undifferentiated mesenchymal cell proliferation; regulates endothelial, fibroblastic, and osteoblastic mitogenesis; regulates collagen synthesis and collagenase secretion; regulates mitogenic effects of other growth factors; stimulates endothelial chemotaxis and angiogenesis; inhibits macrophage and lymphocyte proliferation
Vascular endothelial growth factor, VEGF	Platelets, endothelial cells	Increases angiogenesis and vessel permeability; stimulates mitogenesis for endothelial cells
Epidermal growth factor, EGF	Platelets, macrophages, monocytes	Stimulates endothelial chemotaxis/angiogenesis; regulates collagenase secretion; stimulates epithelial/mesenchymal mitogenesis
Fibroblast growth factor, FGF(a-b)	Platelets, macrophages, mesenchymal cells, chondrocytes, osteoblasts	Promotes growth and differentiation of chondrocytes and osteoblasts; mitogenic for mesenchymal cells, chondrocytes, and osteoblasts
Connective tissue growth factor, CTGF	Platelets through endocytosis from extracellular environment in bone marrow	Promotes angiogenesis, cartilage regeneration, fibrosis, and platelet adhesion
Insulin-like growth factor-1, IGF-1	Plasma, epithelial cells, endothelial cells, fibroblasts, osteoblasts, bone matrix	Chemotactic for fibroblasts and stimulates protein synthesis. Enhances bone formation by proliferation and differentiation of osteoblasts
Interleukin-8, IL-8	Platelets, macrophage, epithelial cells	Stimulates mitosis of epidermal cells and supports angiogenesis

Adapted from Everts [130].

Table 1. Comprehensive description of the most known platelet α-granule components as they appear in PRP.

A synopsis of the most well-known PRP growth factors is provided in **Table 1**, along with a description of the growth factor sources and their individual specific functions [36–47]. Besides the numerous activities of their growth factors, platelets also contribute to many adjunctive and supportive activities (**Table 2**) via paracrine, autocrine, and endocrine modes of actions [35, 37]. Because of these unique modes of action, PGFs are capable of exerting effects on multiple cell types, showing a series of morphometric and mitogenic functions. The morphometric growth factors, involved in bone growth, can turn undifferentiated multipotent MSCs into immature and mature osteoprogenitor cells through the presence of the so-called bone morphogenetic proteins (BMPs) [48]. Most PGFs have mitogenic actions that increase the population of healing cells and degranulate by mitogenesis.

http://dx.doi.org/10.5772/intechopen.80502

Proteins-chemokines-cytokines	Biological activities
Adhesive proteins	Cell contact interactions
	Extracellular matrix composition
Proteases and anti-proteases	Angiogenesis
	Vascular remodeling
	Cellular regulation
	Cellular behavior
Mitogenic factors	Increases angiogenesis
	Cell proliferation
	Chemotaxis
Chemokines and cytokines	Cellular interaction
	Vascular remodeling
	Bone formation
Membrane glycoproteins	Platelet aggregation
	Platelet adhesion
	Inflammation
	Platelet and leukocyte interaction
Granules	Capillary permeability
	Vascular local regulation

Table 2. Non-platelet growth factor-related adjunctive effects of PRP therapy.

6. PRP device technology and cellular formulations of clinical PRP

PRP treatment protocols have evolved immensely over the past 20 years. Through laboratory, experimental, and clinical research, followed by more recent meta-analyses, physicians, medical practitioners, and scientists have gained a better understanding of platelets in PRP cellular physiology. The platelet secretome consists of all the proteins that are released upon platelet activation, which can be measured through proteomic-based techniques [49]. This proteomic profiling has increased our current understanding of the functional importance of the platelet granule contents [50], especially with regard to the biological cellular functions of the multifaceted platelet secretome and other plasma constituents, affecting PRP treatment outcomes.

6.1. Autologous blood predonation and PRP processing devices

The starting point for any PRP preparation is whole blood. At point of care, a fresh unit of autologous blood is drawn via a phlebotomy, following standard operating procedures.

The median cubital vein is often used as this is an easily accessible and superficial vein, enabling the introduction of 18- to 21-gauge butterfly systems. Blood is collected in a syringe containing an anticoagulant to prevent clotting. The blood predonation volume depends on the PRP device of choice to prepare PRP and the volume needed for specific single, or multiple, wound care treatments in the same patient. Directly after blood collection, the PRP centrifugation process should be initiated in order to produce a sample of PRP.

Currently, physicians can choose from more than 30 PRP processing systems. However, a lack of consensus on standardizing PRP has contributed to the variation in PRP devices, which produce dissimilar platelet concentrations and cellular compositions [51, 52].

Optimal blood separation is best safeguarded by so-called double-spin PRP centrifuges with dedicated disposable platelet concentration devices. These double-spin PRP devices create a layered buffy coat stratum based on different centrifugal forces and specific gravities and densities of the individual blood components (**Figure 4**). Single-spin devices, or plasma-PRP

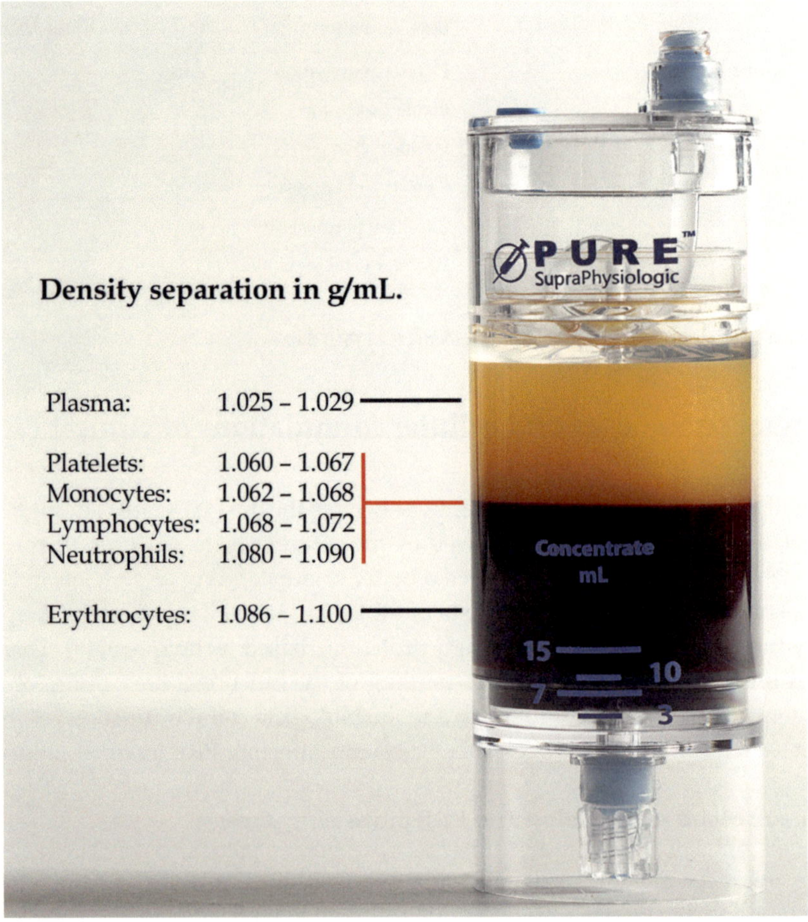
Density separation in g/mL.
Plasma: 1.025 - 1.029
Platelets: 1.060 - 1.067
Monocytes: 1.062 - 1.068
Lymphocytes: 1.068 - 1.072
Neutrophils: 1.080 - 1.090
Erythrocytes: 1.086 - 1.100
PURE™
SupraPhysiologic
Concentrate
mL
15
10
7
3

Figure 4. Cellular density separation of whole blood by centrifugation. After the first centrifugation procedure, the whole blood components are separated in the PRP device from the plasma as a result of the different densities in two basic layers. The top layer is the platelet plasma suspension, consisting of plasma and the multicomponent buffy coat layer, containing platelets, monocytes, lymphocytes, and neutrophils. The second layer consists of erythrocyte pack. The range of the specific cell densities varies between individuals.

http://dx.doi.org/10.5772/intechopen.80502

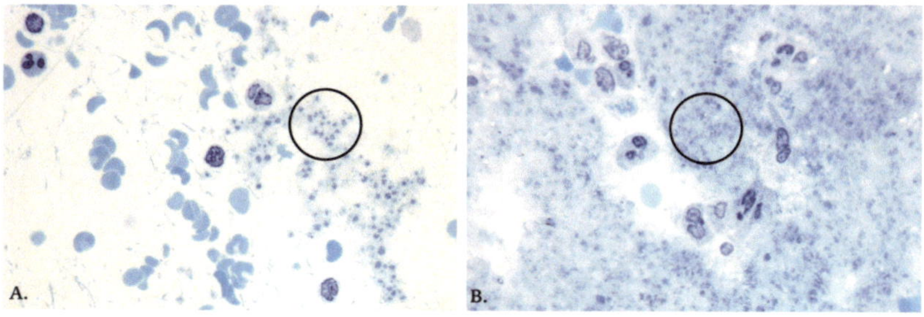

Figure 5. Whole blood and PRP smears with non-activated platelet. (A) Peripheral blood smear of whole blood inside the circle, platelets are visible (platelet count of the smear is 276,000/μL), next to white blood cells, erythrocytes, and fibrin. (B) Platelet-rich plasma smear. A high density of platelets inside the circle, with minimal leukocytes and erythrocytes (platelet count of 2,208,000/μL, prepared with the EmCyte System).

devices, prepare a product from the acellular plasma layer, excluding erythrocytes and leukocytes, while collecting as many platelets as possible from the plasma layer [53]. These differences in cellular compositions, and thus PRP characteristics, have recently been recognized in the literature [54]. Marques et al. found that inferior treatment outcomes following PRP applications correlated directly with poor quality and inconsistent PRP products [55]. Therefore, PRP devices should be versatile and compliant to enable the production of different PRP formulations, while maintaining supraphysiologic platelet numbers (**Figure 5**). More specifically, the final cellular PRP treatment sample should be tailored to serve treatment protocols contingent to wound bed condition, wound size and depth, and undermining tissue.

6.2. Definition of clinical-PRP and platelet dose

PRP can be characterized as a complex composition of autologous multicellular components in a small volume of plasma, with a substantial supraphysiologic concentration of platelets compared to baseline values, with minimal red blood cell contamination.

Clinical PRP (C-PRP) contains a clinical dose of concentrated platelets in a treatment sample. Marx demonstrated enhancement of bone and soft tissue healing with a minimum platelet count of 1×10^9/mL [56]. Furthermore, Giusti et al. revealed in an experimental study that 1.5×10^9 platelets/mL are needed for inducing a functional angiogenic response, via endothelial cell activity, in tissue repair mechanisms [57]. Therefore, to significantly induce an angiogenic response in circulatory compromised chronic wounds, C-PRP should contain at least 7.5 billion deliverable platelets in a 5-mL treatment sample. These platelets should then be able to release their entire content after (tissue) activation has occurred, as visualized in **Figure 6** by electron microscopic imaging. Furthermore, this platelet dose will correspondingly induce cell proliferation and cell migration. Ultimately, an increase in wound bed microcirculation would contribute to ECM remodeling and wound epithelialization [58]. Consequently, C-PRP containing a platelet dose of 1.5×10^9 platelets/mL has the ability to stimulate (neo)angiogenesis and elicit the healing of chronic wounds.

6.3. Leukocytes in C-PRP

Leukocytes have a great impact on the intrinsic biology of chronic wounds because of their immune and host-defense mechanisms. Therefore, the presence of leukocytes in

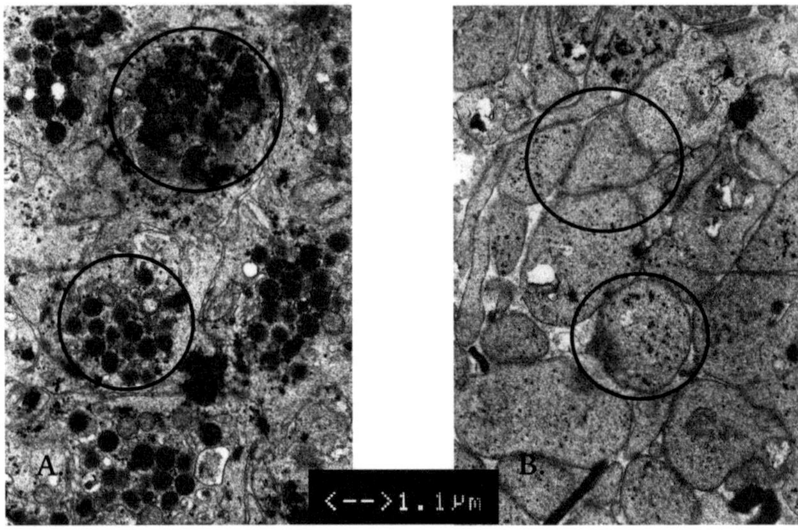

Figure 6. (A) Electron microscopic image of a single platelet in the circles. The internal platelet α and dense granules (black and gray structures, respectively) and lysosomes are visible with intact cellular membranes. (B) Electron microscopic image of activated platelets in the circles. The platelet membranes are ruptured, and their granular content is no longer visible. The platelet growth factors and other vesicles have been released to the extracellular matrix.

re-establishing wound healing attempts in chronic non-healing wounds can be turntables in the wound healing process [59].

The eventual presence of leukocytes in PRP specimen depends on the operating and design principles of PRP devices. Most ideally, PRP processing devices should be able to produce different PRP cellular formulations, including leukocyte composition and concentration. PRP formulations should be based on a disease-specific pathology, medical condition, and tissue types.

Leukocytes develop from multipotential hemopoietic stem cells in the bone marrow and mature along several differentiation pathways. Via common myeloid progenitor cells and myeloblasts, they become differentiated granular (neutrophils, eosinophils, basophils) and a-granular cells (lymphocytes and monocytes) [60]. However, during PRP preparation, the cell membranes of eosinophils and basophils are destroyed following the centrifugation procedure. Interactive wound healing processes involve mediators, extracellular matrix components, resident cells, including platelets, and infiltrating leukocytes. They participate in the classical pathway of wound healing: hematoma, inflammation, tissue formation, and ultimately tissue remodeling.

In PRP, lymphocytes are more concentrated than other leukocytes. They produce insulin-like growth factors, and they may contribute to tissue remodeling [61].

Monocytes are non-inflammatory white blood cells and are the precursors to macrophages. Macrophages are important cells of the immune system that, similar to neutrophils, are formed to fight infection or engulf accumulating damaged or dead cells. Unlike neutrophils, monocytes do not lead to a prolonged inflammatory condition but play important roles in tissue healing.

M1 macrophages are responsible for producing several inflammatory cytokines that support host defense through pathogen clearance, necrotic tissue clearance, and reactive oxygen species. Furthermore, the M1 phenotype produces growth factors such as VEGF and FGF. M2 macrophages have anti-inflammatory capacities and generate precursors for collagen and fibroblast stimulating factor, thus supporting their role in extracellular matrix deposition. Generally, the plasticity of monocytes is dependent on the microenvironment in which they are present. Monocytes and macrophages release additional pro-regenerative growth factors that lead to neovascularization, proliferation of myogenic precursor cells, and stimulation of the activity of satellite cells, playing key roles in wound repair and inflammatory control [21, 62].

Neutrophils have a clear function in healing cascades since they form a dense barrier against invading pathogens and counteract infections [63]. Their presence in PRP can be desirable in wound care treatment to functionally destroy and clear bacteria from the wound bed, in certain types of open surgical procedures to prevent wound infections, or within specific treatment protocols that require higher levels and longer periods of inflammation [64]. However, when PRP samples containing very high neutrophil concentrations are used, for example, in non-infected and granulating wound beds, this neutrophil-rich PRP poses a potential risk of progressive and persistent microenvironmental inflammation via the secretion of proteases and toxic oxygen metabolites. PRP products containing elevated levels of proinflammatory neutrophils facilitate a strong leukocytic chemotaxis to induce a phagocytic response, not contributing to wound epithelialization [65, 66].

6.4. Erythrocytes in C-PRP and effects of eryptosis on the wound microenvironment

Detrimental consequences of erythrocytes or red blood cells (RBCs) on tissues have been studied by several groups. In a study by Hooiveld and coworkers, chondrocytes and synoviocytes were exposed to RBCs causing tissue degeneration and destruction, including apoptosis [67]. In another study, it was postulated that erythrocytes inhibit fibroblast proliferation in a collagen scaffold. These findings indicate potential negative effects on the healing of soft tissue cellular structures when using PRP that contains high concentrations of erythrocytes [68]. Indeed, the use of PRP containing RBCs should be avoided in wound healing strategies to prevent wound breakdown.

Another rare phenomenon occurs when a PRP preparation including RBCs is applied to tissues. Under normal physiological circumstances, erythrocytes are removed from the circulatory system by the process of senescence after approximately 120 days. In tissues treated with PRP-containing erythrocytes, natural mechanisms of erythrocyte elimination are no longer valid, and erythrocytes undergo eryptosis before they reach their full lifespan [69]. Typical features of eryptosis are similar compared to apoptosis: membrane blebbing and cell shrinkage, resulting in the release of platelet activating factor (PAF). PAF plays a role in control mechanisms of inflammation and stimulating ceramide release and intracellular stress response, while eryptotic RBCs bind to endothelial cells and impede microcirculation [70]. Therefore, the application of PRP containing RBCs in the chronic wound microenvironment finally leads to tissue inflammation and an intracellular stress response, causing oxidative destruction in the wound vasculature.

7. PRP preparation protocol to produce PurePRP®SP

In this paragraph, a detailed and specific PRP preparation procedure is described to produce Pure Platelet-Rich Plasma-Supra Physiologic (PurePRP®SP, EmCyte Corporation, Fort Myers, FL, USA). This autologous cellular platform technology is able to generate C-PRP with high concentrations of platelets; there are protocol options to produce neutrophil-poor or -rich PRP, with minimal erythrocyte contamination (**Figure 7**). Furthermore, this platform technology enables clinicians to also concentrate bone marrow aspirate to retrieve, among other cells, concentrated mesenchymal cells [71]. Additionally, the same technology is capable of creating concentrated and viable adipose tissue complex. Both bone marrow and adipose biological tissue types will be discussed in another paragraph to emphasize the ability to use viable MSCs for wound care treatment.

7.1. PRP preparation and procedural therapy application steps

At point of care, 54 mL of fresh whole blood is predonated in a 60-mL syringe preloaded with 6 mL of 3.8% sodium citrate (anticoagulant). The PurePRP®SP device is loaded from the top and placed in a centrifuge with pre-programmed settings. Following a first centrifugation of 1.5 min, the whole blood is sequestered in a Platelet-Poor Plasma Suspension (PPS) containing a buffy coat layer and RBCs. Using a syringe, the PPS is aspirated until a band of RBCs, which holds mature platelets, is captured with the PPS. This volume is then transferred to the bottom part of the same device, the concentration chamber, and placed in the centrifuge for a 5-min second spin. During this period, a final cell PPS separation is achieved, with the concentrated platelets pelleted at the bottom of the chamber. Excessive platelet-poor plasma (PPP) is removed, leaving a PurePRP®SP volume, generally between 3 and 7 mL. This PPP

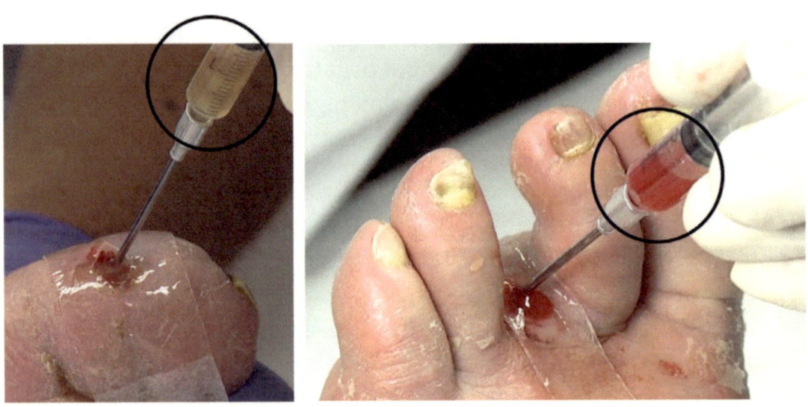

A B

Figure 7. (A) Typical aspect of a neutrophil-poor PurePRP®SP sample, with a more yellow coloring. This PRP is intended to treat a wound that does not require proinflammatory PRP stimulation. (B) Typical aspect of a neutrophil-rich PurePRP®SP sample. This formulation is defined as a full buffy coat PRP, containing a significant concentration of platelets, neutrophils, monocytes, and lymphocytes. The red color in this preparation is due to the erythrocytes present in the PRP, as the collected neutrophils are on top of the red cells when they are from the platelet-plasma suspension (PurePRP®SP, pure platelet-rich plasma supraphysiologic; PRP, platelet-rich plasma).

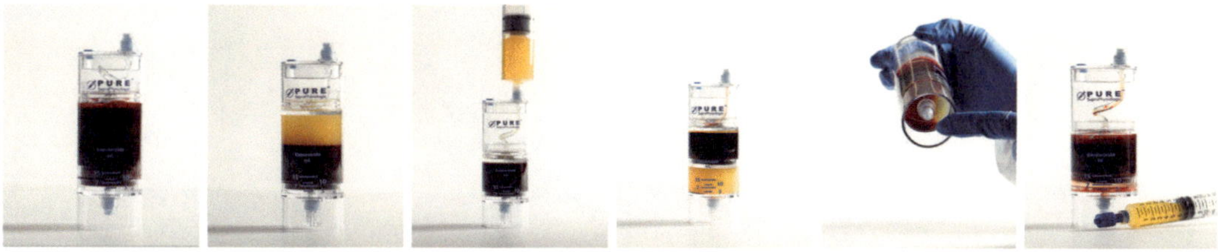
A B C D E F

Figure 8. PurePRP®SP preparation procedure. (A) The PRP device is loaded with anticoagulated whole blood. (B) After first spin, the PPS is created following gravity centrifugal separation. (C) The PPS evacuated from the top chamber and meticulously injected in bottom part of the PRP device for the second spin procedure. (D) After the second spin, the PPS is further refined in a PPP fraction and concentrated platelets. (E) PPP has been softly removed with a syringe, leaving a desired volume behind to gently resuspend the supraphysiologic platelet concentrate, which is attached to the bottom of the second chamber of the device. (F) The platelets are aspirated in a small volume of plasma and the PurePRP®SP product is collected in a syringe prior to application (PPS, platelet plasma suspension; PRP, platelet-rich plasma; PPP, platelet poor plasma; PurePRP®SP is a registered trademark of EmCyte corporation, Fort Myers FL, USA).

volume is used to resuspend the platelets from the bottom of the device back into the PPP by gentle swirling of the device. When the bottom part is clear, all platelets are resuspended in the plasma and the PurePRP®SP is then withdrawn with a 12-mL syringe (**Figure 8**).

Depending on the biological wound treatment strategies, different PRP application techniques can be used. Before starting any PRP procedure, a meticulous sharp wound debridement should be done. Microfracturing the wound bed, with removal of cellular/plasma debris or dead tissue, allows PGFs to function more effectively while being resistant to rapid degradation by proteolytic wound activities.

The application of PRP, or PRP-G, can be done using different techniques. First, PRP can be injected intralesionally, including the wound edges [72]. This technique delivers the platelets directly into the deeper tissue structures. The objective of this technique is to stimulate tissue regeneration faster in more stagnant wounds and wound edges or to prepare the wound bed for a final reconstructive procedure [73]. Second, PRP mixed with bovine or autologous thrombin creates a PRP-G coagulum, where this topical "primary" biological wound dressing covers and sticks to the wound bed. The PRP-G can be applied to a wound bed via a single syringe technique or delivered using a double syringe spray device to ultimately generate a solid graft (**Figure 9**). Lastly, wounds with undermining can be filled with PRP-G using a single syringe and blunt needle approach. Furthermore, the same technique using a sharp needle is suitable for injecting the wound perimeter with adipose tissue, with or without PRP (**Figure 10**).

After PRP has been applied to the wound bed, wound undermining areas, and wound edges, platelets will slowly start to lyse, releasing their PGFs, cytokines, and other proteins; inducing cell signaling processes; and initiating regeneration and tissue healing [74].

The literature is not clear on the number of PRP treatments needed to treat a wound and the associated outcomes. Several studies indicate multiple treatments over a period of time. Everts et al. performed initially two treatments weekly for 2 weeks. Thereafter, the procedure was bi-weekly, until final wound closure was expected. In the same study, the PRP procedure was followed by using a naturally derived porcine intestinal submucosa matrix graft to support building the

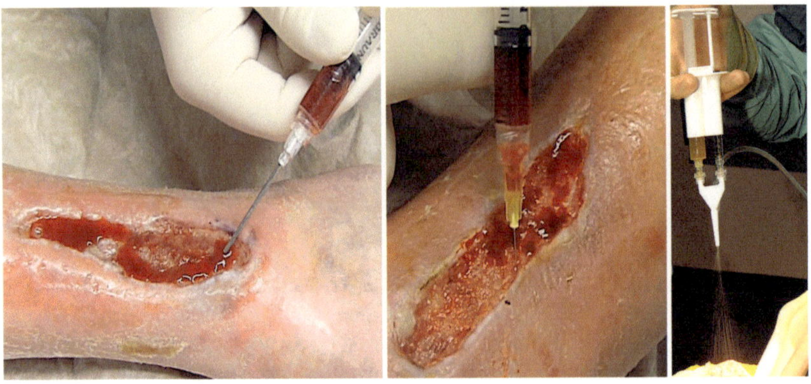

A B C

Figure 9. PRP application techniques. (A) A semiviscous PRP-G coagulum is topically placed on a wound bed via a single syringe technique. PRP and thrombin are mixed in the same syringe and delivered via a blunt needle covering the entire wound bed. (B) Intralesional injection of PRP with a 30-gauge needle in the wound bed and/or wound edges. (C) Spray application using an aerosol delivery technique, with PRP and autologous thrombin in separate syringes. The content mixes at the tip of the spray catheter, where after PRP-G is formed at the tissue site (PRP-G, platelet-rich plasma gel; PRP, platelet-rich plasma).

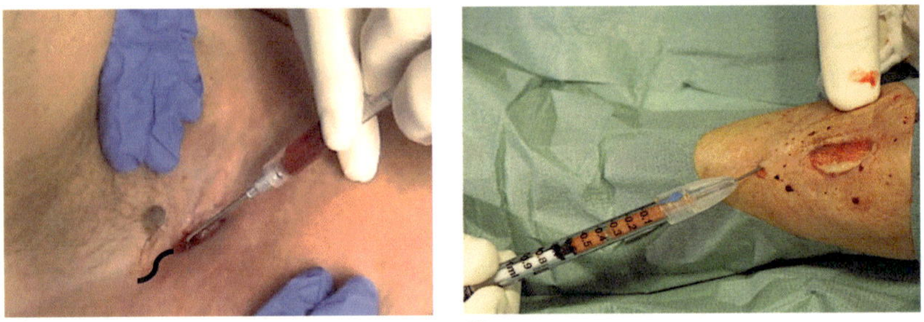

A B

Figure 10. (A) Filling an undermining of a wound with PRP-G, using a single syringe technique in which both PRP and thrombin have been mixed to a semiviscous coagulum (the black line indicates the direction of the undermining). (B) The wound perimeter of the chronic wound is injected with a mixture of PRP and concentrated adipose tissue to deliver PGFs and adipose tissue constituents like MSCs (PRP-G, platelet-rich plasma gel; PRP, platelet-rich plasma; PGFs, platelet growth factors; MSCs, mesenchymal cells).

ECM and limited permeability to keep the lysing platelet fluids in place (OASIS® Wound Matrix, Cook Biotech, Inc., West Lafayette, IN, USA), followed by a hydrocolloid secondary dressing (DuoDERM® Extra Thin Dressing, ConvaTec, Greensboro, NC, USA) [73]. Others have used, for example, a non-absorbent sterile transparent sheet (Tegaderm™, 3M Medical Inc.) or a knitted cellulose acetate non-adherent dressing impregnated with a petrolatum emulsion (Adaptic, Systagenix Wound Management Limited, North Yorkshire, UK) [75].

Recent review articles do not provide clear information on post-PRP treatment protocols [76, 77]. This author's experiences with PRP wound care treatments included no dressing changes for 5 days post-treatment. Thereafter, minimal wound cleaning and no sharp debridement are standard wound care activities, until the next PRP application. During all patient visits, the wounds were assessed according to the TIME wound grading system [78], which was designed for tissue evaluation, infectious condition, and moisture evaluation, and the condition of the wound edges was checked at every visit to monitor progress and regression of wound healing.

8. Overview of some of the most relevant studies using autologous PRP to treat chronic wounds

The characteristics of biological PRP and PRP-G suggest that they might be a beneficial tool in the surgical armamentarium. PRP-G has been successfully used in maxillofacial surgery, orthopedics, cosmetic surgery, and dental implantology. Furthermore, several randomized controlled clinical trials studied the effect of PRP-G in wound rehabilitation and tissue engineering. Eleven studies were identified involving the use of different PRP formulations in venous and diabetic leg ulcers between 2007 and 2018 [79–89]. A summary of all the studies is shown in **Table 3**. A general comment from these studies is that some of them were underpowered [79, 81]. The PRP interventions were highly variable with regard to platelet dosing, formulations, the total number of PRP applications, and the interval between applications. PRP-G was produced using bovine thrombin and/or $CaCl_2$ or calcium gluconate to initiate a platelet coagulum. The presence of leukocytes in PRPs and the platelet dose relative to peripheral blood were hardly described. The frequency of application varied between twice weekly and weekly. Time to wound healing or wound size reduction was the most common outcome measurement. Six trials involved predominantly diabetic patients [81–83, 87, 88], while mixed ulcer etiology was included in the other studies. Outcome results favored experimental treatments with PRP, in all studies presented. Furthermore, Carter et al. conducted a review in 2011, analyzing published prospective and retrospective studies and meta-analyzed the use of PRP and PRP-G in wound healing in acute and chronic conditions [90]. Their paper included 24 studies, from which 3 studies were systematic reviews and 9 studies were included in the meta-analysis. The systematic review and meta-analysis stated that PRP applications in cutaneous wounds exposed complete and partial wound healing when compared to control wound care. Furthermore, the presence of infection was reduced in acute wounds treated with PRP. Martinez-Zapata and co-workers presented their results from a systematic review, including10 randomized controlled trials (RCTs) in chronic wounds in their meta-analysis [91]. Three of these RCTs involved DFU and three studies involved venous leg ulcers. Their results indicated that autologous PRP can enhance DFU healing when compared with standard care.

A condensed summary review by Everts et al. revealed the efficacy and safety of PRP-G treatments when used by different institutions [92]. Picard et al. published a literature review, comprising 12 studies, to summarize evidence-based data regarding the treatment of diabetic chronic wounds with PRP. In 87.5% of controlled studies, they found a significant benefit for the use of PRP therapy to treat chronic diabetic wounds, which remained unhealed after standard wound care treatment [93]. However, more studies remain necessary to produce strong evidence eliminating poor design and high bias [90, 91].

Year; author [reference]	Study design	N patients in study; indication	Duration of wound	Outcomes
2007; Kakagi [77]	RCT	51; foot tissue defects	>3 months	Ulcer reduction in treatment group
2010; Jeong [77]	RCT	100; DFU	>4 weeks	Complete wound healing
2011; Saad Setta [79]	RCT	24; non-healing DFU	>8 weeks	PRP treated group healed significantly faster
2015; Karimi [80]	RCT	50; DFU	No limit	PRP significantly reduced wound surface and depth in 3 weeks
2015; Li [81]	RCT	117; DFU	>2 weeks	PRP significant better healing than standard care
2016; Pravin [82]	RCT	31; 22 VLU and DFU; 9 others	>8 weeks	Leukocyte free PRP healed better, 86% ulcer healing
2017; Moneib [83]	RCT	40; venous ulcers	>6 months	Significant ulcer reduction
2017; Obolensky [84]	CT	100; non-healing, mixed etiology	>6 weeks	Earlier epithelialization; shorter hospitalization; less total costs
2017; Babaei [85]	PT	150; DFU	>3 weeks	Full closure after 8.8 weeks
2017; Milek [86]	CT	100; DFU	>6 months	Full wound closure treatment group controls only small wounds
2018; Etugov [87]	PT	23; VLU	>4 weeks	Significant ulcer size reduction compared to control

RCT, randomized controlled trial; CT, controlled trial; PT, prospective trial; DFU, diabetic foot ulcer; VLU, venous leg ulcer; PRP, platelet-rich plasma.

Table 3. Overview of some of the most relevant studies using autologous PRP technology to treat chronic wounds.

Presently, more studies are ongoing to clarify optimized PRP protocols to improve its angiogenic and regenerative properties to be implemented as a standard practice of care in advanced wound care treatment plans.

9. Comprehensive background on stem cells

In any regenerative tissue microenvironment, there are essentially stem cells, growth factors, and a biological scaffold to provide the necessary biological milieu for cell-tissue regeneration and cell renewal. MSCs originating from either bone marrow or adipose tissue are now extensively being used in a variety of patients who have an indication for minimally invasive, regenerative medicine therapies to enhance tissue repair and regeneration. Traditionally, bone marrow aspirate (BMA) has been utilized as a source of bone marrow-derived mesenchymal stem cells (BM-MSC), hematopoietic stem cells (HSCs), progenitor cells, and platelets. Lately, MSCs derived from adipose tissue have emerged in a variety of regenerative treatment protocols. However, in chronic wound care strategies, autologous, non-cultured, MSC therapies are rarely used. However, Hocking reported from preclinical and clinical trials that MSC therapy has the potential to effectively treat wounds with delayed healing, resulting in accelerated wound closure [94]. A stem cell is, by definition, the one cell capable of duplicating itself (self-renewal) and resuming its undifferentiated status, while also originating progeny that can differentiate into one or more final products that are physiologically defined by their specific functions. Stem cells can be classified on the basis of their origin and their potential to proliferate and differentiate. According to Wagers and Weissman, the classification of stem cells is based on their plasticity and potential for differentiation [95]: totipotent, able to give rise to all embryonic and extraembryonic cell types; pluripotent, able to give rise to all cell types of the embryo proper; multipotent, able to give rise to a subset of cell lineages; oligopotent, able to give rise to a restricted subset of cell lineages; and unipotent, able to contribute only one mature cell type. Adult stem cells have a multipotent lineage and are able to transdifferentiate into various progenies, forming cells of multipotent lineages, such as HSCs and MSCs [95]. HSCs are pluripotent cells that further differentiate via hematopoiesis into distinct progenitor cells which mature into blood cells of myeloid lineages (monocyte, granulocyte, erythrocyte, and megakaryocyte/platelets) and lymphoid cells (B, T and NK cells) [96].

10. Mesenchymal stem cells

MSCs are multipotent adult stem cells and can be obtained from various adult tissues, including bone marrow stroma, adipose tissue, and other tissue types. According to the International Society of Cellular Therapy, MSCs are defined as those cells that are able to adhere to plastic and express a number of cell surface markers (including CD73, CD90, and CD105) while undergoing multilineage differentiation. Furthermore, MSCs should have the ability for self-renewal [97]. MSCs can also be identified as specialized populations of mural cells/pericytes. They provide a niche for HSCs and have the ability to differentiate into various mesodermal lineages. Under appropriate conditions and an optimal microenvironment, MSCs can differentiate into mesodermal lineage cells such as osteoblasts, endothelial cells, adipose tissue, and smooth muscle cells [4]. These capabilities have led to the use of MSC as a potential strategy for treating various diseases since they promote biological processes, such as angiogenesis and cell proliferation and differentiation [98]. Furthermore, they synthesize mediators (cytokines and trophic factors) that participate in tissue repair processes, immune modulation, and the regulation of inflammatory processes. [99]. The trophic effects are facilitated by the MSC secretion of reparative cytokines and growth factors, including TGF-β, VEGF, and EGF, to contribute to local tissue repair [100]. Caplan also suggested that the modulation of inflammation is instigated by the suppression of inflammatory T-cell proliferation and inhibition of monocyte and myeloid cell maturation [101]. Based on above characteristics, one can see that MSCs are able to establish a regenerative microenvironment at the site of release, which could improve the recruitment, activation, and differentiation of endogenous stem cells with the potential for repair in wound healing. Currently, clinical research is investigating MSCs as a therapy to treat difficult-to-heal wounds.

10.1. Bone marrow mesenchymal stem cells

BM-MSCs from adult bone marrow tissue were first isolated by Pittenger et al. [102]. Since then, BM-MSCs are frequently used successfully as a biological product, like PRP, in regenerative

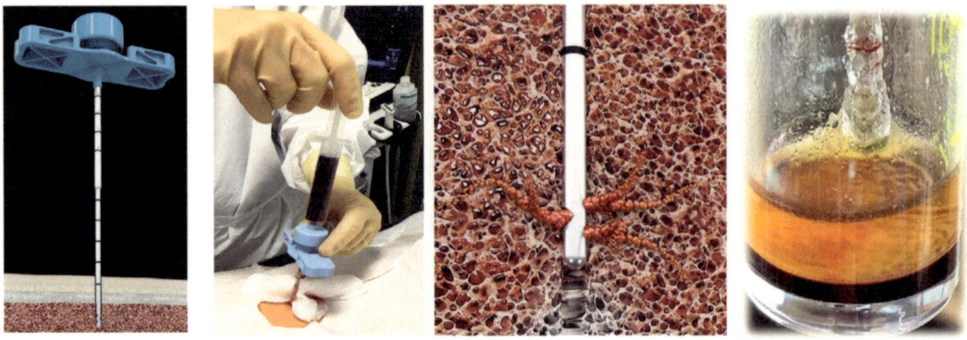

Figure 11. Aspire bone marrow aspiration from the posterior superior iliac spine area. (A) The introducer and aspiration needle are placed through the skin, sub cutaneous layer, and cortical bone into the marrow cavity. (B) The BMA device is placed in the PSIS. Bone marrow is meticulously aspirated via suction vacuum applied to a syringe, through the aspirator needle. (C) Bone marrow cells, including purified mesenchymal stem cell, hematopoietic stem cells, total nucleated cells, platelets, and progenitor cells, are collected through the fenestrated aspirator needle with a blunt tip from the cancellous bone. (D) The final BMC sample is produced following a 2-step proprietary centrifugation protocol. Inside the blue circle, concentrated bone marrow cells are visible, on the top of the erythrocyte layer (BMA, bone marrow aspirate; PSIS, posterior superior iliac spine; BMC, bone marrow concentrate; Aspire™ bone marrow aspiration system is trademark of EmCyte Corporation, Fort Myers FL, USA).

medicine therapies to treat a variety of musculoskeletal disorders, such as chondral defects, osteoarthritis, and rotator cuff lesions [103, 104]. BM-MSCs are relatively easy to acquire via a BMA procedure. Bone marrow can be harvested from a variety of anatomic sites during a surgical procedure in the operating room, or an office setting, with minimal morbidity. A variety of donor locations are available, including the anterior or posterior iliac crest, calcaneus, tibia, distal femur, and proximal humerus. The iliac crest is used frequently and known to be a rich source of BM-MSCs (**Figure 11**). BM-MSCs are transplanted autologously, therefore avoiding any ethical issues. Furthermore, the relatively simple preparation and separation and high genetic stability of BM-MSCs allow for their easy use in vitro and as an injectate. Imperative for an effective BM-MSC injection is the quality of the initial bone marrow aspiration procedure with regard to minimizing trauma to cellular content of the bone marrow niche, such as platelets, progenitor cells, and leukocytes, while maximizing cellular yields and minimizing peripheral blood infiltration [105].

Furthermore, the collected bone marrow cells should be viable, with no presence of disintegrated erythrocytes (hemolysis), as this would have a profound negative effect on tissue regeneration [106]. The author believes that a BMA sample should always be preceded by a 2-step centrifugation procedure to concentrate the sample to a bone marrow concentrate (BMC). This will concentrate the indispensable cellular content, such as MSCs (measured by CFU-f), HSCs, total nucleated cells, and platelets, above the baseline counts of these cells. Nonetheless, the centrifugation procedure will decrease hemolytic parameters as well as RBC levels. The effects of concentrating BMA with regard to some of the most important constituents and factors are shown in **Table 4**. Erythrocytes should also be avoided in a BMC specimen, for the same reasons as discussed in the above paragraph on C-PRP and effects

Laboratory parameters	BMA	BMC	Concentrating effect
TNC (−nRBCs) × 10^6/mL	28	142.8	5.1 × BL
Platelets × 10^6/mL	96	614	6.4 × BL
CD34+ cells × 10^5/mL	1.68	9.2	5.5 × BL
CFU-f (MSCs) × 10^3/mL	1.05	5.59	5.3 × BL
Hematocrit %	40.7	6.8	−83% × BL
Hemolysis %	6.3	1.8	−73% × BL
Cell viability %	95.9	97.3	+ 0.6% × BL

BMA, bone marrow aspirate; BMC, bone marrow concentrate; × BL, effects times baseline values; TNC, total nucleated cells; −nRBCs, minus red blood cells; CD34+, stem cell marker/expression on hematopoietic progenitor cells found in bone marrow; CFU-f, fibroblast colony-forming units: assay for bone marrow mesenchymal stem cell analysis; MSCs, mesenchymal stem cells.

Table 4. Effects of bone marrow aspirate concentration on cell counts, hematocrit, and the elimination of hemolytic red cells.

of eryptosis on the wound, as this will cause profound inflammation and compromise the microcirculation [69].

10.2. Adipose mesenchymal stem cells

Similar to BM-MSCs, adipose-derived mesenchymal stem cell (AD-MSC) has been used in regenerative medicine applications. AD-MSCs can be isolated following an adipose tissue (mini) liposuction procedure of subcutaneous fat tissue, mostly from the abdomen.

Various preparation techniques, including centrifugation, exist to collect, wash, and rinse adipose tissue to generate a concentrated adipose tissue concentrate (ATC). Adipocytes constitute almost 90% of adipose tissue volume and nearly 65% of the total cell number [107]. When enzymatically digested, adipose tissue yields a heterogeneous population of many cell types (pre-adipocytes, fibroblasts, vascular smooth muscle cells, endothelial cells, resident monocytes/macrophages, and lymphocytes), which upon isolation are termed the stromal vascular fraction (SVF) [108]. AD-MSCs have a multilineage cell differentiation potential, that is, they are capable of differentiating into adipogenic, chondrogenic, myogenic, osteogenic, and neurogenic cells [109]. Thus, AD-MSCs might be indicated in clinical applications for the repair of damaged tissues, as well as for angiogenic therapy to improve neovascularization [110].

The popularity of AD-MSCs in regenerative medicine treatment protocols and recently in a biological wound care treatment protocol as well is due to an abundance of MSCs, with a high proliferation capacity and differentiation potential, when compared to MSCs derived from bone marrow [111, 112]. Furthermore, Yun et al. described AD-MSC-mediated effects on the reduction of proinflammatory cytokines, chemokines, cellular apoptosis, and collagenases [113]. Moreover, AD-MSCs have been shown to be immune-privileged [114].

11. MSCs in cutaneous wound healing

Currently, cell-base therapy is an attractive approach for the treatment of recalcitrant chronic wounds. MSCs from adipose and bone marrow tissues are being investigated as a therapeutic strategy for a distinct group of pathological conditions, including chronic hard-to-heal wounds [115]. The orchestrated process of wound healing entails cellular and hormonal physiological processes of inflammation, epithelialization, proliferation, collagen matrix formation, and particular neoangiogenesis, regulated by various growth factors such as TGF-β, VEGF, PDGF, granulocyte macrophage colony-stimulating factor, the interleukin family, EGF, FGF, and TNF-α [116, 117]. However, the activity of these cytokines in chronic wounds is often reduced due to a prolonged inflammatory state, decreasing the neoangiogenic potential.

BM-MSCs and AD-MSCs have been studied as potential solutions for these major issues. Both types of MSCs have been shown to be effective in augmenting wound healing by modulating the immune response and secreting paracrine factors which promote therapeutic (neo) angiogenesis and thereby providing biological ingredients for wound tissue regeneration, and they are ultimately capable of inducing full wound closure (**Figure 11**; [118–121]).

Optimal wound bed preparation encompasses not only debridement and proper management of the bacterial load but also correction of the wound matrix and reconditioning of phenotypically altered resident cells which are present in chronic wounds. Based on their characteristics and biological activity, MSCs are capable of interacting with resident wound cells to transform resident cells to functional matrix building cells [122]. This might be of particular importance for the dermal rebuilding process to stimulate keratinocytes to accomplish epithelialization.

Given their higher isolation yield, ease of harvesting, and abundance of adipose tissue, some groups believe that AD-MSCs might be more clinically attractive. Not only because of their angiogenic capability, but they may also function in situ as pericytes providing vascular stability and they might communicate with endothelial cells in response to environmental stimuli [123, 124]. However, experienced clinicians may dispute the cited potential risk for complications with BMA, as they feel comfortable in performing BMA procedures in medical-office settings using local anesthetics and imaging to perform the aspiration. Shapiro and coworkers performed a prospective, single-blind, placebo-controlled trial on 25 patients with bilateral knee osteoarthritis and reported that the BMA, production, and use of BMC is a safe procedure [125].

11.1. Critical limb ischemia

BM-MSCs are frequently being studied in patients with critical limb ischemia, who also might suffer from chronic wounds and who are not eligible for the revascularization procedure due to several comorbidities, namely high operative risk, multiple failures of revascularization, and high rate of restenosis. These patients are suitable for biological cell-based therapy with MSCs. In particular, BM-MSCs protocols are newly emerging therapies to treat CLI in this subset of patients, promoting the regeneration of impaired endothelium and neoangiogenesis in ischemic tissues [126, 127]. The effects of several types of bone marrow cell therapy (e.g., bone marrow-derived mononuclear cells, CD34+ bone marrow cells, and mesenchymal stromal cells) have been studied in CLI patients. The outcomes of several cell-based therapy trials demonstrated that the rate of major amputation was significantly decreased [128]. It can be concluded that MSC application can be considered a promising target for future biological therapies in CLI patients [129].

12. Conclusions

Regenerative medicine technologies offer solutions to a number of compelling clinical problems that have not been able to adequately result in a solution through the use of drugs, surgery, or permanent replacement devices.

The purpose of this chapter was to review multiple aspects of both PRP and MSC biocellular therapies as part of a wound care treatment plan to support in the healing of chronic and recalcitrant wounds.

Numerous significant aspects that are still not well understood or standardized have been discussed, as well as the rationale for cell-based therapies. For platelet-rich plasma preparations, specific formulations, platelet dosing, processing, and the differences between systems were discussed. With regard to bone marrow and adipose tissue, as cell sources for obtaining high quality mesenchymal cells, some technicalities were provided.

Among both tissue-based cellular therapies, bone marrow mesenchymal cells have been the most frequently employed and reported on. In this review, evidence is shown on results from several clinical studies in which autologous biologics have been applied in patients with chronic wounds. The outcomes of these studies suggested that the application of biocellular products can reverse the microenvironment in chronic wounds, achieving the ultimate goal: full wound epithelialization in the shortest possible time. Furthermore, it was revealed that these treatments are safely executed without adverse effects for patients.

Conflict of interest

The author served also as Chief Scientific Officer of EmCyte Corporation.

Author details

Peter A. Everts

Address all correspondence to: peter@gulfcoastbiologics.com

Gulf Coast Biologics, Fort Myers, FL, USA

References

[1] Gottrup F. A specialized wound-healing center concept: Importance of a multidisciplinary department structure and surgical treatment facilities in the treatment of chronic wounds. American Journal of Surgery. 2004;**187**:38S-43S

[2] Edwards H, Finlayson K, Courtney M, Graves N, Gibb M, Parker C. Health service pathways for patients with chronic leg ulcers: Identifying effective pathways for facilitation of evidence based wound care. BMC Health Services Research. 2014;**13**:86

[3] Hostetler SG, Xiang H, Gupta S, Sen C, Gordillo JM. Discharge patterns of injury-related hospitalizations with an acute wound in the United States. Wounds. 2006;**18**:340-351

[4] Otero-Vin M, Falanga V. Mesenchymal stem cells in chronic wounds: The spectrum from basic to advanced therapy. Advances in Wound Care. 2016;**5**:149-163

[5] Gurtner G, Werner S, Barrandon Y, Longaker M. Wound repair and regeneration. Nature. 2008;**453**:314-321

[6] Harvey C. Wound healing. Orthopaedic Nursing. 2005;**24**:143-157

[7] Singer A, Thode H Jr, McClain S. Development of a histomorphologic scale to quantify cutaneous scars after burns. Academic Emergency Medicine. 2000;**7**:1083-1088

[8] McNeil PL. Cell wounding and healing. American Scientist. 1991;**79**:222-235

[9] Cromack DT, Pierce GF, Mustoe TA. TGF-b and PDGF medicated tissue repair: Identifying mechanisms of action using impaired and normal models of wound healing. In: Barbul A, Caldwell M, Eaglstein W, Hunt T, Marshall D, Pines E, Skower G, editors. Clinical and Experimental Approaches to Dermal and Epidermal Repair: Normal and Chronic Wounds. New York: Wiley; 1991. pp. 359-373

[10] Chujo S, Shirasaki F, Kondo-Miyazaki M, Ikawa Y, Takehara K. Role of connective tissue growth factor and its interaction with basic fibroblast growth factor and macrophage chemoattractant protein-1 in skin fibrosis. Journal of Cellular Physiology. 2009;**220**:189-195

[11] Wynn T, Vannella K. Macrophages in tissue repair, regeneration, and fibrosis. Immunity. 2016;**15**:450-462

[12] Sindrilaru A, Scharffetter-Kochanek K. Disclosure of the culprits: Macrophages-versatile regulators of wound healing. Advances in Wound Care. 2013;**2**:357-368

[13] Rodero MP, Khosrotehrani K. Skin wound healing modulation by macrophages. International Journal of Clinical and Experimental Pathology. 2010;**3**:643-653

[14] Mahdavian Delavary B, van der Veer WM, van Egmond M, Niessen FB, Beelen RH. Macrophages in skin injury and repair. Immunobiology. 2011;**216**:753-762

[15] Polverini PJ, Cotran P, Gimbrone MA Jr, Unanue ER. Activated macrophages induce vascular proliferation. Nature. 1997;**269**:804-806

[16] Snyder R, Lantis J, Kirsner R, et al. Macrophages: A review of their role in wound healing and their therapeutic use. Wound Repair and Regeneration. 2016;**24**:613-629

[17] Diegelmann R, Evans M. Wound healing: An overview of acute, fibrotic and delayed healing. Frontiers in Bioscience. 2004;**9**:283-289

[18] Shah JM, Omar E, Pai DR, Sood S. Cellular events and biomarkers of wound healing. Indian Journal of Plastic Surgery. 2012;**45**:220-228

[19] Agren M, Eaglstein W, Ferguson M, et al. Causes and effects of the chronic inflammation in venous leg ulcers. Acta Dermato-venereologica. Supplementum. 2000;**210**:3-17

[20] Shai A, Halevy S. Direct triggers for ulceration in patients with venous insufficiency. International Journal of Dermatology. 2005;**44**:1006-1009

[21] Leibovich S, Ross R. The role of the macrophage in wound repair. A study with hydrocortisone and antimacrophage serum. The American Journal of Pathology. 1975;**78**:71-100

[22] Mendez M, Stanley A, Park H, et al. Fibroblasts cultured from venous ulcers display cellular characteristics of senescence. Journal of Vascular Surgery. 1998;**28**:876-883

[23] Pradhan Nabzdyk L, Kuchibhotla S, Guthrie P, et al. Expression of neuropeptides and cytokines in a rabbit model of diabetic neuroischemic wound healing. Journal of Vascular Surgery. 2013;**58**:766-775

[24] Ben-Porath I, Weinberg RA. The signals and pathways activating cellular senescence. The International Journal of Biochemistry & Cell Biology. 2005;**37**:961-976

[25] Mast BA, Schultz GS. Interactions of cytokines, growth factors, and proteases in acute and chronic wounds. Wound Repair and Regeneration. 1996;**4**:411-420

[26] Robson MC. The role of growth factors in the healing of chronic wounds. Wound Repair and Regeneration. 1997;**5**:12-17

[27] Cooper DM, Yu EZ, Hennessey P, Ko F, Robson MC. Determination of endogenous cytokines in chronic wounds. Annals of Surgery. 1994;**219**:688-691

[28] Palfreyman S. Evidence-based decisions for local and systemic wound care. The British Journal of Surgery. 2012;**99**:1172-1183

[29] Flanagan M. Principles of wound management. In: Flanagan M, editor. Wound Healing and Skin Integrity. Vol. 2013. Oxford: Wiley-Blackwell. pp. 66-86

[30] Zucker-Franklin C. Megakaryocytes and platelets. In: Zucker-Franklin D, Greaves MF, Grossi CE, Marmont AM, editors. Atlas of Blood Cells. Philadelphia, PA: Lea & Febiger; 1998. pp. 621-634

[31] Giannoble WV. Periodontal tissue engineering by growth factors. Bone. 1996;**S19**:S23-S37

[32] Giannoble WV, Hernandez RA, Finkelman RA, et al. Comparative effects of platelet-derived growth factor-BB and insulin-like growth factor I, individually and in combination,

on periodontal regeneration in *Macaca fascicularis*. Journal of Periodontal Research. 1996;**31**: 301-312

[33] Rožman P, Semenič D, Maja Smrke D. The role of platelet gel in regenerative medicine. In: Wislet-Gendebien, editor. Advances in Regenerative Medicine. Rijeka: InTech; 2011. ISBN: 978-953-307-732-1. Available from: http://www.intechopen.com/books/advances-in-regenerative-medicine/the-role-ofplatelet-gel-in-regenerative-medicine

[34] Antoniades H, Williams L. Human platelet-derived growth factor: Structure and functions. Federation Proceedings. 1983;**81**:2396-2400

[35] Trippel S, Coutts R, Einhorn T, Mundy G, Rosenfeld R. Growth factors as therapeutic agents. The Journal of Bone and Joint Surgery. American Volume. 1996;**78**:1272-1286

[36] Pierce G, Mustoe T, Altrock B, Deuel T, Thomason A. Role of platelet-derived growth factor in wound healing. Journal of Cellular Biochemistry. 1991;**45**:319-326

[37] Bames G, Kostenuik P, Gerstenfeld L, Einhorn T. Growth factor regulation of fracture repair. Journal of Bone and Mineral Research. 1999;**14**:1805-1815

[38] Rosier RN, O'Keefe RJ, Hicks DG. The potential role of transforming growth factor beta in fracture healing. Clinical Orthopaedics. 1998;(355 Suppl):S294-S300

[39] Wang J. Basic fibroblastic growth factor for stimulation of bone formation in osteoinductive or conductive implants. Acta Orthopaedica Scandinavica. 1996;**269**:1-33

[40] Friesel R, Maciag T. Molecular mechanisms of angiogenesis: Fibroblast growth factor signal transduction. The FASEB Journal. 1995;**9**:919-925

[41] Canalis E, McCarthy T, Centrella M. Effects of platelet-derived growth factor on bone formation in vitro. Journal of Cellular Physiology. 1989;**140**:530-537

[42] Steenfos HH. Growth factors and wound healing. Scandinavian Journal of Plastic and Reconstructive Surgery and Hand Surgery. 1994;**28**:95-105

[43] Martin P, Hopkinson-Woolley J, McClusky J. Growth factors and cutaneous wound repair. Progress in Growth Factor Research. 1992;**4**:25-44

[44] Rhee J, Black M, Schubert U, et al. The functional role of blood platelet components in angiogenesis. Thrombosis and Haemostasis. 2004;**92**:394-402

[45] Hom DB, Maisel RH. Angiogenic growth factors: Their effects and potential in soft tissue wound healing. The Annals of Otology, Rhinology, and Laryngology. 1992;**101**:349-354

[46] Kubota S, Kawata K, Yanagita T, Doi H, Kitoh T, Takigawa M. Abundant retention and release of connective tissue growth factor (CTGF/CCN2) by platelets. Journal of Biochemistry. 2004;**136**:279-282

[47] Cicha I, Garlichs C, Daniel W, Goppelt-Struebe M. Activated human platelets release connective tissue growth factor. Thrombosis and Haemostasis. 2004;**91**:755-760

[48] Hock J, Canalis E. Platelet-derived growth factor enhances bone cell replication, but not differentiated function of osteoblasts. Endocrinology. 1994;**134**:301-312

[49] Senzel L, Gnatenko D, Bahou W. The platelet proteome. Current Opinion in Hematology. 2009;**16**(5):329-333

[50] McRedmond J. Proteomics of platelet granules, organelles and releasate. In: Garcia A, Senys A, editors. Platelet Proteomics: Principles, Analysis, and Applications. Hoboken, NJ: John Wiley& Sons; 2011. pp. 139-157

[51] Mazzucco L, Balbo V, Cattana E, et al. Not every PRP-gel is born equal. Evaluation of growth factor availability for tissues through four PRP-gel preparations: Fibrinet, RegenPRP-Kit, Plateltex and one manual procedure. Vox Sanguinis. 2009;**97**:110-118

[52] Everts P, Hoffmann J, Weibrich G, et al. Differences in platelet growth factor release and leucocyte kinetics during autologous platelet gel formation. Transfusion Medicine. 2006;**16**:363-368

[53] Fitzpatrick J, Bulsara M, McCrory P, Richardson M, Zheng M. Analysis of platelet-rich plasma extraction variations in platelet and blood components between 4 common commercial kits. Orthopaedic Journal of Sports Medicine. 2017;**5**:1-8

[54] Magalon J, Chateau A, Bertrand B, et al. DEPA classification: A proposal for standardizing PRP use and a retrospective application of available devices. BMJ Open Sport & Exercise Medicine. 2016;**2**:1-6

[55] Marques L, Stessuk T, Camargo I, et al. Platelet-rich plasma (PRP): Methodological aspects and clinical applications. Platelets. 2015;**26**:101-113

[56] Marx R. Platelet-rich plasma (PRP): What is PRP and what is not PRP? Implant Dentistry. 2001;**10**:225-228

[57] Giusti I, Rughetti A, D'Ascenzo S. Identification of an optimal concentration of platelet gel for promoting angiogenesis in human endothelial cells. Transfusion. 2009;**49**:771-778

[58] Lokmic Z, Mitchell G. Engineering the microcirculation. Tissue Engineering Part B. 2008;**14**:87-103

[59] Bielecki T, Dohan Ehrenfest D, Everts P, Wiczkowski A. The role of leukocytes from L-PRP/L-PRF in wound healing and immune defense: New perspectives. Current Pharmaceutical Biotechnology. 2012;**13**:1153-1162

[60] Eaves C. Hematopoietic stem cells: Concepts, definitions, and the new reality. Blood. 2015;**125**:2605-2613

[61] Gordon J, Ley S, Melamed M, et al. Immortalized B lymphocytes produce B-cell growth factor. Nature. 1984;**310**:145-147

[62] Das A, Sinha M, Datta S, et al. Monocyte and macrophage plasticity in tissue repair and regeneration. American Journal of Pathology. 2015;**185**:2596-2606

[63] Cook-Mills J, Deem T. Active participation of endothelial cells in inflammation. Journal of Leukocyte Biology. 2005;**77**:487-495

[64] Kovtun A, Bergdolt S, Wiegner R, et al. The crucial role of neutrophil granulocytes in bone fracture healing. European Cells & Materials. 2016;**32**:152-162

[65] Fitzpatrick J, Bulsara M, Zheng M. The effectiveness of platelet-rich plasma in the treatment of tendinopathy. A meta-analysis of randomized controlled clinical trials. American Journal of Sports Medicine. 2016;**45**(1):226-233

[66] Everts P, Delawi D, Brown Mahoney C, et al. Platelet leukocyte gel facilitates bone substitute growth and autologous bone growth in a goat model. Journal of Biomedical Materials Research. Part A. 2010;**92**:746-753

[67] Hooiveld M, Roosendaal G, Wenting M, et al. Short-term exposure of cartilage to blood results in chondrocyte apoptosis. American Journal of Pathology. 2003;**162**:943-951

[68] Harrison S, Vavken P, Murray M. Erythrocytes inhibit ligament fibroblast proliferation in a collagen scaffold. Journal of Orthopaedic Research. 2011;**29**:1361-1366

[69] Pretorius E, du Plooy J, Bester J. A comprehensive review on eryptosis. Cellular Physiology and Biochemistry. 2016;**39**:1977-2000

[70] Repsold L, Joubert A. Eryptosis: An Erythrocyte's suicidal type of cell death. BioMed Research International. 2018. DOI: 10.1155/2018/9405617

[71] Dragoo J, DeBaun M. Stem cell yield after bone marrow concentration. In: Proceedings of the AOSSM July 2017; Orthopaedic Journal of Sports Medicine

[72] Dionyssiou D, Demiri E, Foroglou P. The effectiveness of intralesional injection of platelet-rich plasma in accelerating the healing of chronic ulcers. An experimental and clinical study. International Wound Journal. 2012;**10**:397-406

[73] Everts P, Warbout M, de Veth D, et al. Use of epidermal skin grafts in chronic wounds: A case series. International Wound Journal. 2017;**14**:1213-1218

[74] Everts P, Knape J, Weibrich G, et al. Platelet rich plasma and platelet gel: A review. The Journal of Extra-Corporeal Technology. 2006;**38**:174-187

[75] Pinto N, Ubilla M, Zamora Y, et al. Leucocyte- and platelet-rich fibrin (L-PRF) as a regenerative medicine strategy for the treatment of refractory leg ulcers: A prospective cohort study. Platelets. 2018;**29**:468-475

[76] Burgos-Alonso N, Lobato I, Hernández I, et al. Adjuvant biological therapies in chronic leg ulcers. International Journal of Molecular Sciences. 2017;**18**:2561. DOI: 10.3390/ijms18122561

[77] Chicharro-Alcántara D, Rubio-Zaragoza M, Damiá-Giménez E. Platelet rich plasma: New insights for cutaneous wound healing management. Journal of Functional Biomaterials. 2018;**9**:10. DOI: 10.3390/jfb9010010

[78] Schultz G, Barillo D, Mozingo D, Chin G. Wound bed preparation and a brief history of TIME. International Wound Journal. 2004;**1**(1):19-32

[79] Kakagia D, Kazakos K, Xarchas K, et al. Synergistic action of protease-modulating matrix and autologous growth factors in healing of diabetic foot ulcers. A prospective randomized trial. Journal of Diabetes and its Complications. 2007;**21**:387-391

[80] Jeong S, Han S, Kim W. Treatment of diabetic foot ulcers using a blood bank platelet concentrate. Plastic and Reconstructive surgery. 2010;**125**:944-952

[81] Saad Setta H, Elshahat A, Elsherbiny K, et al. Platelet-rich plasma versus platelet-poor plasma in the management of chronic diabetic foot ulcers: A comparative study. International Wound Journal. 2011;**8**:307-312

[82] Karimi R, Afshar M, Salimian M, et al. The effect of platelet rich plasma dressing on healing diabetic foot ulcers. Nursing and Midwifery Studies. 2016;**5**:e30314. DOI: 10.117795/nmsjournal30314

[83] Li L, Chen D, Wang C, et al. Autologous platelet-rich gel for treatment of diabetic chronic refractory cutaneous ulcers: A prospective, randomized clinical trial. Wound Repair and Regeneration. 2015;**23**:495-505

[84] Pravin A, Sridhar V, Srinivasan B. Autologous platelet rich plasma (PRP) versus leucocyte-platelet rich fibrin (L-PRF) in chronic non-healing leg ulcers—A randomized, open labelled, comparative study. Journal of Evolution of Medical and Dental Sciences. 2016;**5**:7460-7462

[85] Moneib H, Youssef S, Aly D, et al. Autologous platelet-rich plasma versus conventional therapy for the treatment of chronic venous leg ulcers: A comparative study. Journal of Cosmetic Dermatology. 2018;**17**:495-501

[86] Obolenskiy V, Ermolova D, Laberko L. Clinical and economic effectiveness of the use of platelet-rich plasma in the treatment of chronic wounds. Wound Medicine. 2017;**19**:27-32

[87] Babaei V, Afradi H, Gohardani H, et al. Management of chronic diabetic foot ulcers using platelet-rich plasma. Journal of Wound Care. 2017;**26**:784-787

[88] Miłek T, Baranowski K, Zydlewski P, et al. Role of plasma growth factor in the healing of chronic ulcers of the lower legs and foot due to ischaemia in diabetic patients. Advances in Dermatology and Allergology. 2017;**6**:601-606

[89] Etugov D, Mateeva V, Mateev G. Autologous platelet-rich plasma for treatment of venous leg ulcers: A prospective controlled study. Journal of Biological Regulators and Homeostatic Agents. 2018;**32**:593-597

[90] Carter M, Fylling C, Parnell L. Use of platelet rich plasma gel on wound healing: A systematic review and meta-analysis. Eplasty. 2011;**11**:e38

[91] Martinez-Zapata M, Marti-Carvajal A, Sola I, et al. Autologous platelet-rich plasma for treating chronic wounds. Cochrane Database of Systematic Reviews. 2016;**25**(5). DOI: 10.1002/14651858.CD006899.pub3

[92] Everts P, Hoogbergen M, Weber T, et al. Is the use of autologous platelet-rich plasma gels in gynecologic, cardiac, and general, reconstructive surgery beneficial? Current Pharmaceutical Biotechnology. 2012;**3**:1163-1172

[93] Picard F, Hersant B, Bosc R, Meningaud J-P. The growing evidence for the use of platelet-rich plasma on diabetic chronic wounds: A review and a proposal for a new standard care. Wound Repair and Regeneration. 2015;**23**:638-643

[94] Hocking A. Mesenchymal stem cell therapy for cutaneous wounds. Advances in Wound Care. 2012;**4**:166-171

[95] Wagers A, Weissman I. Plasticity of adult stem cells. Cell. 2004;**116**:639-648

[96] Maclean A, Lo Celso C, Stumpf M. Concise review: Stem cell population biology: Insights from hematopoiesis. Stem Cells. 2017;**35**:80-88

[97] Ikebe C, Suzuki K. Mesenchymal stem cells for regenerative therapy: Optimization of cell preparation protocols. BioMed Research International. 2014:951512. DOI: 115/2014/951512

[98] Meirelles L d S, Fontes A, Covas D, Caplan A. Mechanisms involved in the therapeutic properties of mesenchymal stem cells. Cytokine & Growth Factor Reviews. 2009;**20**:419-427

[99] Bashir J, Sherman A, Lee H, et al. Mesenchymal stem cell therapies in the treatment of musculoskeletal diseases. PMR. 2014;**6**:61-69

[100] Caplan A, Correa D. The MSC: An injury drugstore. Cell Stem Cell. 2011;**9**:11-15

[101] Caplan A. Why are MSCs therapeutic? New data: New insight. The Journal of Pathology. 2009;**217**:318-324

[102] Pittenger M, Mackay A, Beck S, et al. Multilineage potential of adult human mesenchymal stem cells. Science. 1999;**284**:143-147

[103] Orozco L, Munar A, Soler R, et al. Treatment of knee osteoarthritis with autologous mesenchymal stem cells: Two-year follow-up results. Transplantation. 2014;**97**:e66-e68

[104] Hernigou P, Flouzat Lachaniette C, Delambre J, et al. Biologic augmentation of rotator cuff repair with mesenchymal stem cells during arthroscopy improves healing and prevents further tears: A case-controlled study. International Orthopaedics. 2014;**38**:1811-1818

[105] Oh M, Nor J. The perivascular niche and self-renewal of stem cells. Frontiers in Physiology. 2015;**6**:article 367. DOI: 10.3389/fphys.2015.00367

[106] Schaer D, Buehler P, Alayash A, Belcher J, Vercellotti G. Hemolysis and free hemoglobin revisited: Exploring hemoglobin and hemin scavengers as a novel class of therapeutic proteins. Blood. 2013;**121**:1276-1284

[107] Kokai L, Marra K, Rubin J. Adipose stem cells: Biology and clinical applications for tissue repair and regeneration. Translational Research. 2014;**163**:399-408

[108] Mizuno H, Tobita M, Uysal A. Concise review: Adipose-derived stem cells as a novel tool for future regenerative medicine. Stem Cell. 2012;**30**:804-810

[109] Wagner W, Wein F, Seckinger A, et al. Comparative characteristics of mesenchymal stem cells from human bone marrow, adipose tissue, and umbilical cord blood. Experimental Hematology. 2005;**33**:1402-1416

[110] Miranville A, Heeschen C, Sengenès C, et al. Improvement of postnatal neovascularization by human adipose tissue derived stem cells. Circulation. 2004;**110**:349-355

[111] Baer P. Adipose-derived mesenchymal stromal/stem cells: An update on their phenotype in vivo and in vitro. World Journal of Stem Cells. 2014;**6**:256-265

[112] Dmitrieva R, Minullina I, Bilibina A, et al. Bone marrow and subcutaneous adipose tissue-derived mesenchymal stem cells: Differences and similarities. Cell Cycle. 2012;**11**:377-383

[113] Yun S, Ku S, Kwon Y. Journal of Orthopaedic Surgery and Research. 2016;**11**:9. DOI: 10.1186/s13018-016-0342-9

[114] Gonzalez-Rey E, Gonzalez M, Varela N, et al. Human adipose-derived mesenchymal stem cells reduce inflammatory and T cell responses and induce regulatory T cells in vitro in rheumatoid arthritis. Annals of the Rheumatic Diseases. 2010;**69**:241-248

[115] Yang M, Sheng L, Zhang T, Li Q. Stem cell therapy for lower extremity diabetic ulcers: Where do we stand? BioMed Research International. 2013:462179. DOI: 10.1155/2013/462179

[116] Robson MC. Growth factors as wound healing agents. Current Opinion in Biotechnology. 1991;**2**:863-867

[117] Goldman R. Growth factors and chronic wound healing: Past, present, and future. Advances in Skin & Wound Care. 2004;**17**:24-35

[118] Lawall H, Bramlage P, Amann B. Stem cell and progenitor cell therapy in peripheral artery disease. Thrombosis and Haemostasis. 2010;**103**:696-709

[119] Badiavas E, Falanga V. Treatment of chronic wounds with bone marrow-derived cells. Archives of Dermatology. 2003;**139**:510-516

[120] Na Y, Ban J, Lee M, Im W, Kim M. Wound healing potential of adipose tissue stem cell extract. Biochemical and Biophysical Research Communications. 2017;**5**:30-34

[121] Kuo Y, Wang C, Cheng JT, Kao G, Chiang YG. Adipose-derived stem cells accelerate diabetic wound healing through the induction of autocrine and paracrine effects. Cell Transplantation. 2016;**25**:71-81

[122] Falanga V, Sablonski M. A bilayered living skin construct (APLIGRAF) accelerates complete closure of hard-to heal venous ulcers. Wound Repair and Regeneration. 1999;**7**:201-207

[123] Hassan W, Greiser U, Wang G. Role of adipose-derived stem cells in wound healing. Wound Repair and Regeneration. 2014;**22**:313-325

[124] Cherubino M, Rubin P, Miljkovic N, et al. Adipose-derived stem cells for wound healing applications. Annals of Plastic Surgery. 2011;**66**:210-215

[125] Shapiro S, Kazmerchak S, Heckman M, et al. A prospective, single-blind, placebo-controlled trial of bone marrow aspirate concentrate for knee osteoarthritis. The American Journal of Sports Medicine. 2017;**45**:82-90

[126] Uccioli L, Meloni M, Izzo V, Giurato L, Merolla S, et al. Critical limb ischemia: Current challenges and future prospects. Vascular Health and Risk Management. 2018;**14**:63-74

[127] Teraa M, Sprengers R, van der Graaf Y, et al. Autologous bone marrow-derived cell therapy in patients with critical limb ischemia: A meta-analysis of randomized controlled clinical trials. Annals of Surgery. 2013;**258**:922-929

[128] Ko S, Bandyk D. Therapeutic angiogenesis for critical limb ischemia. Seminars in Vascular Surgery. 2014;**27**:23-31

[129] Pignon B, Sevestre M, Kanagaratnam L, et al. Autologous bone marrow mononuclear cell implantation and its impact on the outcome of patients with critical limb ischemia. Results of a randomized, double blind, placebo-controlled trial. Circulation Journal. 2017;**81**:1713-1720

[130] Everts PAM. Autologous platelet-leukocyte enriched gel. Basics and efficacy [thesis]. Utrecht: Utrecht University; 2007

The Wound Healing Responses and Corneal Biomechanics after Keratorefractive Surgery

Wenjing Wu and Yan Wang

Additional information is available at the end of the chapter

http://dx.doi.org/10.5772/intechopen.81886

Abstract

Corneal biomechanics have been concerned recently since it is not only found to play an important role in the wound healing process after corneal refractive surgeries, but also essential to improve the predictability and safety of refractive procedures. Corneal biomechanics and wound healing responses are linked in time and space and may also cause complications of keratectasia, haze formation, and regression. This review focuses on wound healing and biomechanics of the corneal refractive procedures. Identifying corneal wound healing from the biomechanical point of view is mandatory to improve the outcomes and reduce the complications.

Keywords: wound healing, refractive surgery, corneal biomechanics

1. Introduction

Over the past 30 years, corneal refractive surgery has successfully corrected the refractive error for millions of patients. The spread of laser corneal refractive surgery is increasing the interest in the study of the safety and predictability. Many studies showed that the wound healing process influences the predictability and safety. Corneal wound healing is a major contributor to the success of refractive surgeries. Biological differences in wound healing responses are thought to be a major factor limiting the predictability of refractive surgery [1]. In some cases, mechanical instability or an abnormal wound healing process can lead to serious complications such as keratectasia or severe haze.

Hence, it is important to investigate and understand the corneal biomechanics and wound healing process for a better vision after corneal refractive surgery.

2. The wound healing responses and corneal biomechanics after keratorefractive surgery

2.1. Corneal refractive surgery

Corneal refractive surgery changes the corneal curvature to correct the refractive error. The most common laser refractive procedures performed today are small incision lenticule extraction surgery (SMILE) [2, 3], femtosecond laser in situ keratomileusis (FS-LASIK), and surface ablation procedures, i.e., photorefractive keratectomy (PRK), laser epithelial keratomileusis (LASEK), and epi-LASIK [4]. With the development of the femtosecond laser, the SMILE surgery and FS-LASIK have become the most commonly used procedures in China for myopic subjects.

2.2. Corneal structure and biomechanics

The cornea is a highly specialized transparent avascular tissue and is composed of five layers. They are epithelium, stroma, Descemet's membrane, and endothelium. Stroma is the main part of the cornea, and any factor that changes the corneal structure may obviously influence the biomechanical properties of the cornea [5, 6].

2.2.1. Epithelium, Bowman's membrane, and biomechanics

The epithelium's contribution to corneal biomechanics was significantly lower than that of the stroma with respect to the stiffness. Bowman's membrane tissue is a transparent sheet of approximately 12 μm. It is acellular and is composed of densely packed collagen fibrils that are in random direction. The fibrils are continuous with those in the stroma, which is believed to stabilize the corneal curvature [5].

2.2.2. Corneal stroma and biomechanics

The stroma constitutes nearly 90% of the corneal thickness. And its biomechanical properties are influenced by the collagen fibers and extracellular matrix (ECM), which further determine the corneal strength, shape, and transparency [7, 8].

The stroma is a fibrous layer of lamellae made up of connective tissue. Interlamellar branching is more extensive in the anterior stroma than in the posterior stroma. The density of the collagen lamellae is higher, and their arrangement and directionality are more complicated anteriorly than posteriorly. The collagen lamellae in the corneal stroma are organized into a complex, highly intertwined three-dimensional meshwork of transversely oriented fibers, which contributes to the corneal shape and stromal stiffness. Another critical component for corneal stromal biomechanics is the ECM. The ECM is mostly composed of proteoglycans (PGs), which comprise a core protein and are located in the spaces among the collagen fibers in the corneal stroma. PGs play a critical role in collagen fibril assembly and spacing, and their mechanical importance may be greater than currently recognized [9].

2.2.3. *Descemet's membrane and biomechanics*

Descemet's membrane is approximately 10-nm thick and considered as a secretion of endothelial cells. The membrane is comprised of type IV collagen fibers. It is highly elastic and represents a barrier against punctures. Descemet's membrane serves as an endothelial basement membrane. Bowman's layer and Descemet's membrane accounted for 20% of the bending rigidity of the cornea through the Finite element evaluation [5].

2.2.4. *Endothelium and biomechanics*

The endothelium is composed of one layer of cells, which adhere to the Descemet's membrane. The endothelium cells cannot regenerate after damage or aging, but can spread and enlarge to maintain the cornea clear and transparent, and further prevent the cornea from becoming hydrated. The corneal endothelium may indirectly affect the corneal stiffness by regulating corneal hydration. The loss of corneal endothelial cells will result in increased water absorption by the corneal stroma [8, 9].

2.3. Corneal biomechanics and corneal wound healing after refractive surgeries

It is noteworthy that the corneal biomechanics and wound healing responses are linked in time and space. Specifically, the corneal biomechanics involves the stromal healing responses; the better stromal healing process will contribute to better corneal biomechanics after surgery and more stable visual results.

2.3.1. *Epithelial wound healing*

Epithelial wound healing involves three main steps: sliding, proliferation, and stratification of epithelial cells. Specifically, the epithelium cells migrate to the wound surface; then the cells increase and divide; lastly the cells cover the wound area and multiple layers of the epithelium are regenerated [9].

Some studies suggest that many cytokines are involved in the healing process including the epithelial growth factor (EGF), hepatocyte growth factor (HGF), keratinocyte growth factor (KGF), and transforming growth factor β (TGF-β). [9] These changes permit cells to migrate, establishing dynamic adhesion with other epithelial cells and extracellular matrix components. In the epithelial cells surrounding the wound edge, there is an increased expression of CD44. After the migration of epithelial cells, the phase of proliferation begins.

2.3.2. *Corneal epithelial and stromal interactions*

When the basal membrane is damaged, cytokines, neuropeptides, growth factors, chemokines, and matrix metalloproteinases can diffuse into the stroma and interact with keratocytes. These factors could stimulate the transformation of the keratocytes into myofibroblast cells [9]. One recent study [10] used the exosomes extracted from the epithelial cells, and cultured these exosomes with fibroblast cells; they found that the stroma cells transformed into myofibroblast cells with higher expression of TGF-β, CD63, and PDGF-B. This study indicates that the epithelial cells are very important for stromal wound healing, and they may use exosomes to transmit the wound healing signals in order to regulate the process [10].

After the epithelial and stromal damage, soluble mediators could be secreted through the epithelium and move to the stroma area. These molecules, like TGF-β and TSP-1, could stimulate the wound healing process and make keratocytes transform into myofibroblasts. The myofibroblasts lay down the ECM and generate alpha-smooth muscle actin (α-SMA) to close the wound. However, abnormal wound healing synthesizes excessive α-SMA, exerts traction forces across the ECM, and causes unorganized tissue architecture, haze, and regression after corneal refractive surgery [11, 12]. Only when the EBM is appropriately re-established, proper stromal levels of TGF-β and PDGF cause myofibroblast apoptosis, keratocyte repopulation, clearing of the abnormal ECM, and restoring of corneal transparency [13]. A delay in the regeneration of the EBM, due to damage, dystrophy, or elevated levels of MMP-2 and MMP-9, causes TGF-β and PDGF to continue entering the corneal stroma.

2.3.3. Stromal wound healing and corneal biomechanics

The wound healing of the stroma is end when the collagen fibrils fully connected the wound edge. Activated cells migrate to the wound area. The keratocytes are changed through the reorganization of the cytoskeleton and the development of stress fibers and focal adhesion structures. Genes that encode fibronectin, metalloproteinases, and integrins are activated. The early matrix consists of fibronectin [14], which was conducive to cell migration and proliferation. Then the matrix is converted to a collagen and proteoglycan matrix that increases the tissue tensile strength and resilience. Growth factors increased stiffness and enhanced mechanical load through enhanced collagen fiber formation and cross-linking. The geometry of the collagen network will determine the mechanical properties of the wound. The collagen fiber diameter increases with time during the wound healing process and is related to tensile strength. Interweaving of collagen bundles between neighboring lamellae provides an important structural foundation for shear resistance and transfer of tensile loads between lamellae.

The transformation of keratocytes into myofibroblasts is curial in the wound healing process. These cells are characterized by the expression of α-smooth muscle actin, stress fibers, and focal adhesion complexes. The microfilament bundles of myofibroblasts form stress fibers, and they contract and remodel the adjacent ECM. Myofibroblasts extend from the anterior stroma to the posterior stroma in a progressive manner. These cells develop fibrotic tissue for repair. Besides that, deposition of the ECM is beneficial for the matrix stiffening and global cellular stress. However, excess myofibroblasts cause the deposition of disorganized collagen and glycosaminoglycan [15]. The underlying mechanism for the interaction between myofibroblast cells and matrix is the focal adhesions. They play the role of a mechanotransduction system, transmitting the force generated by stress fibers to the surrounding ECM and also transducing the extracellular mechanical signals into the intracellular signaling. Further investigations are needed to find whether we could regulate the mechanotransduction system to influence the corneal wound healing process.

2.4. Complications relevant to the corneal wound healing and biomechanics after laser refractive surgery

Corneal wound healing is important for the predictability and safety of corneal refractive surgery. The refractive outcome and its stability over time are strongly influenced by the corneal biomechanics and wound healing process. And the abnormal healing process or biomechanical instability could cause some complications after corneal refractive surgery.

2.4.1. Regression

Refractive regression is defined as a gradual loss of the attempted correction that limits prediction. Many studies showed loss of surgical outcome and the main cause seems to be the regression. The regression is mainly due to epithelial hyperplasia and stromal remodeling, two processes related to corneal wound healing. Refractive regression is a major challenge for myopia, especially for high levels of correction. Apoptosis, keratocyte proliferation, and myofibroblast cellular density have proved to be more intense following treatment for high myopia compared to treatments for mild myopia. Myofibroblasts are important effectors of regression. The changes of corneal biomechanics also induce the changes of the corneal shape and cause regression.

2.4.1.1. Keratectasia

Corneal ectasia is a rare complication induced by the corneal refractive surgery. It may occur due to an insufficient residual stromal thickness or unidentified subclinical keratoconus. Many advanced examinations have been used clinically to exclude the potential subclinical keratoconus. Moreover, surgeons have also used many ways to preserve as thicker corneal thickness as possible. However, it is still difficult to avoid the onset of keratectasia. It may be because the corneal stiffness or biomechanics is different among individuals [16]. And the postoperative stromal tensile strength is different for each procedure. This indicates that the risk evaluations for ectasia should take the residual stromal bed thickness and corneal biomechanical properties into account. Moreover, biomechanical changes can manifest clinically as changes of the corneal shape and increased sensitivity to shape changes. The role of biomechanics is therefore important to consider in routine refractive procedures and in special cases where the biomechanical status of the cornea is abnormal.

2.4.2. Haze

Corneal haze refers to the cornea opacity. It is commonly seen in surface ablation surgeries. Haze can potentially form in the interface between the LASIK flap and the stromal bed or directly underneath the newly formed epithelium overlying the stromal tissue after PRK surgery [17]. In modern refractive surgery, haze tends to be mild and resolves very quickly. In extremely rare instances, haze can cause decreased visual acuity and increased glare.

Abnormal regulation of the wound healing process can result in the formation of stromal haze with decreased corneal crystalline expression, increased light scattering, and production of a disorganized extracellular matrix. Myofibroblasts are major contributors to corneal opacity with reduced expression of crystallin, greater secretion of type III collagen, and spread morphology. Over a period of time ranging from several weeks to several months, the myofibroblasts tend to gradually disappear through a series of remodeling processes. This process may be closely related to the expression of matrix metalloproteinases. These proteins are a family of proteolysis enzymes, which could degrade abnormal collagen fibrils. The cytokines, growth factors, and inflammatory mediators could also regulate the synthesis of metalloproteinase [18–20].

3. Conclusions

Laser refractive surgeries are effective for the correction of refractive errors. A better understanding of corneal wound healing from the biomechanical point of view is mandatory if refractive surgery is ever to achieve more predictable and safer refractive results.

Author details

Wenjing Wu and Yan Wang*

*Address all correspondence to: wangyan7143@vip.sina.com

Tianjin Eye Hospital, Tianjin Eye Institute, Tianjin Key Laboratory of Ophthalmology and Visual Science, Nankai University, Tianjin, China

References

[1] Azar DT, Chang JH, Han KY. Wound healing after keratorefractive surgery: Review of biological and optical considerations. Cornea. 2012;**31**(Suppl 1):S9-S19. DOI: 10.1097/ICO.0b013e31826ab0a7

[2] Sekundo W, Kunert KS, Blum M. Small incision corneal refractive surgery using the small incision lenticuleextraction (SMILE) procedure for the correction of myopia and myopic astigmatism: Results of a 6 month prospective study. The British Journal of Ophthalmology. 2011;**95**(3):335-339. DOI: 10.1136/bjo.2009.174284

[3] Shah R, Shah S, Sengupta S. Results of small incision lenticule extraction: All-in-one femtosecond laser refractive surgery. Journal of Cataract and Refractive Surgery. 2011;**37**(1):127-137. DOI: 10.1016/j.jcrs.2010.07.033

[4] Murueta-Goyena A, Cañadas P. Visual outcomes and management after corneal refractive surgery: A review. Journal of Optometry. 2018;**11**(2):121-129. DOI: 10.1016/j.optom.2017.09.002

[5] Ma J, Wang Y, Wei P, Jhanji V. Biomechanics and structure of the cornea: Implications and association with corneal disorders. Survey of Ophthalmology. 2018;**63**(6):851-861. DOI: 10.1016/j.survophthal.2018.05.004

[6] Roberts CJ. Importance of accurately assessing biomechanics of the cornea. Current Opinion in Ophthalmology. 2016;**27**(4):285-291. DOI: 10.1097/ICU.0000000000000282

[7] Roberts CJ, Dupps WJ Jr. Biomechanics of corneal ectasia and biomechanical treatments. Journal of Cataract and Refractive Surgery. 2014;**40**(6):991-998. DOI: 10.1016/j.jcrs.2014.04.013

[8] Spadea L, Giammaria D, Trabucco P. Corneal wound healing after laser vision correction. The British Journal of Ophthalmology. 2016;**100**(1):28-33. DOI: 10.1136/bjophthalmol-2015-306770

[9] Baldwin HC, Marshall J. Growth factors in corneal wound healing following refractive surgery: A review. Acta Ophthalmologica Scandinavica. 2002;**80**(3):238-247. Review

[10] Han KY, Tran JA, Chang JH, Azar DT, Zieske JD. Potential role of corneal epithelial cell-derived exosomes in corneal wound healing and neovascularization. Scientific Reports. 2017;**7**:40548

[11] Kling S, Hafezi F. Corneal biomechanics—A review. Ophthalmic & Physiological Optics. 2017;**37**(3):240-252. DOI: 10.1111/opo.12345

[12] Shu DY, Lovicu FJ. Myofibroblast transdifferentiation: The dark force in ocular wound healing and fibrosis. Progress in Retinal and Eye Research. 2017;**60**:44-65. DOI: 10.1016/j.preteyeres.2017.08.001

[13] Kivanany PB, Grose KC, Petroll WM. Temporal and spatial analysis of stromal cell and extracellular matrix patterning following lamellar keratectomy. Experimental Eye Research. 2016;**153**:56-64. DOI: 10.1016/j.exer.2016.10.009

[14] Raghunathan VK, Thomasy SM, Strøm P, Yañez-Soto B, Garland SP, Sermeno J, et al. Tissue and cellular biomechanics during corneal wound injury and repair. Acta Biomaterialia. 2017;**58**:291-301. DOI: 10.1016/j.actbio.2017.05.051

[15] Ljubimov AV, Saghizadeh M. Progress in corneal wound healing. Progress in Retinal and Eye Research. 2015;**49**:17-45. DOI: 10.1016/j.preteyeres.2015.07.002

[16] Moshirfar MD, Desautels JD, Walker BS, Murri MC, Birdsong OC, Hoopes PSr. Optical regression following corneal laser refractive surgery: Epithelial and stromal responses. Medical Hypothesis, Discovery and Innovation in Ophthalmology. 2018;**7**(1):1-9

[17] Anitua E, Muruzabal F, Alcalde I, Merayo-Lloves J, Orive G. Plasma rich in growth factors (PRGF-Endoret) stimulates corneal wound healing and reduces haze formation after PRK surgery. Experimental Eye Research. 2013;**115**:153-161. DOI: 10.1016/j.exer.2013.07.007

[18] Daniels JT, Schultz GS, Blalock TD, Garrett Q, Grotendorst GR, Dean NM, et al. Mediation of transforming growth factor-beta(1)-stimulated matrix contraction by fibroblasts: A role

for connective tissue growth factor in contractile scarring. The American Journal of Pathology. 2003;**163**(5):2043-2052

[19] Torricelli AA, Santhanam A, Wu J, Singh V, Wilson SE. The corneal fibrosis response to epithelial-stromal injury. Experimental Eye Research. 2016;**142**:110-118. DOI: 10.1016/j.exer.2014.09.012

[20] Wilson SE. Corneal myofibroblast biology and pathobiology: Generation, persistence, and transparency. Experimental Eye Research. 2012;**99**:78-88. DOI: 10.1016/j.exer.2012.03.018

Chapter 11

Open Abdomen: The Surgeons' Challenge

José Santivañez Palomino, Arturo Vergara and
Manuel Cadena

Additional information is available at the end of the chapter

http://dx.doi.org/10.5772/intechopen.81428

Abstract

An open abdomen is defined as purposely foregoing fascial closure of the abdomen after the cavity is opened. Management of complex abdominal problems with the open abdomen and temporary abdominal closure techniques has become a common and valuable tool in surgery. Several challenging clinical situations can necessitate leaving the abdominal cavity open after surgery, resulting in an open abdomen. The indications for open abdomen are as follows: Damage control for life-threatening intraabdominal bleeding, severe acute pancreatitis, severe abdominal sepsis, and prevention and treatment of the abdominal compartment syndrome. Damage control surgery is based on a rapid control of bleeding and focuses on reversing physiologic exhaustion in a critically ill or injured patient. In severe abdominal sepsis, the intervention should be abbreviated due to suboptimal local conditions for healing and global susceptibility to spiraling organ failure. Abdominal compartment syndrome (ACS) is commonly encountered and the only solution is decreasing the pressure by decompressive laparotomy. Open abdomen is associated with significant complications, including wound infection, fluid and protein loss, a catabolic state, loss of abdominal wall domain, and development of enteroatmospheric fistula; however, if the indications are clear, it can become a most valuable resource in treating these conditions.

Keywords: open abdomen, laparostoma, damage control, abdominal compartment syndrome, abdominal sepsis

1. General aspects

The open abdomen is the most challenging of the wounds that a surgeon faces, that is because of the metabolic, physiological, and dynamic implications that this condition entails. An open abdomen is defined as a purposely foregoing fascial closure of the abdomen after the cavity has been opened [1]. Throughout the years, management of complex abdominal problems dealing with an open abdomen and techniques that handle the temporary closure of the abdominal wall have become common and valuable tools for the surgeon [2]. Several challenging clinical situations force the surgeon in leaving the abdominal cavity open after surgery, resulting in an open abdomen or laparostoma [3].

There are several indications for open abdomen, some of which are severe acute pancreatitis [4], damage control for life-threatening intra-abdominal bleeding (with a need for a "second look"), severe abdominal sepsis, and finally, prevention and treatment of an abdominal compartment syndrome [2]. In our recent experience, we have found that peritoneal failure, as the result of the imbalance between the mechanisms of defense of the guest and the peritoneal injury, is the clear indication of the need for the open abdomen.

2. Damage control

Damage control surgery is based on a rapid control of bleeding and focuses on reversing physiologic exhaustion in a critically ill or injured patient [5]. Initially, it was introduced in the field as a temporizing measure used to salvage trauma patients very near death. Through time, damage control surgery has evolved to become the *preferred method for those general surgical patients whose physiological derangements do not allow the completion of an intended operation* [6].

About 10–15% of all laparotomies performed specifically for a trauma patient are managed with damage control techniques [7]. *Persistent hypotension, acidosis* ($pH < 7.2$), *hypothermia* ($T < 34°C$), *and coagulopathy are strong predictors of the need to use damage control and open abdomen in trauma patients* [8]. However, damage control should not be an afterthought; it should be considered early in the decision process before the patient reaches a point of no return (before reaching the triad of death). Therefore before the surgery begins, there are many factors that should be considered: the available resources, the nature of the injuries, the experience of the surgeon, the clinical condition of the patient, and any comorbid conditions the patient might have [2].

During the damage control laparotomy, the primary goal of the trauma surgeon should be control of active hemorrhage (vascular shunting or ligation, direct packing, resection, etc.), followed by a strict control of contamination, and lastly temporary abdominal closure [6].

Despite the advancement of supportive care and the development of new sophisticated commercial devices for temporary abdominal closure, an open abdomen is still highly associated with serious postoperatively complications such as nutritional problems dealing with fluid and protein loss, loss of abdominal domain secondary to fascial retraction, frozen abdomen, and enteroatmospheric fistulas [4].

Following a damage control surgery, the abdomen should never be closed because of the high risk of intra-abdominal hypertension. The second stage within damage control procedures involves the stabilization of the physiological parameters in the intensive care unit, followed by the final stage of definitive surgical care in the operating room; this usually occurs within 24–48 h of the initial operation (preferably following the reversal of the lethal triad) [9].

2.1. Key points

- Open abdomen has become the preferred surgical method for patients whose physiological derangements do not allow the completion of an intended operation.
- Persistent hypotension, acidosis (pH < 7.2), hypothermia (T < 34°C), and coagulopathy are strong predictors of the need for damage control and open abdomen in trauma patients.
- Control of active hemorrhage must be the primary goal of the trauma surgeon during damage control laparotomy.
- Open abdomen is still associated with serious complications.
- The abdomen should never be closed because of the high risk of intra-abdominal hypertension.

3. Severe abdominal sepsis

The role of an open abdomen in the management of severe secondary peritonitis has been a controversial issue throughout time [2]. In severe secondary peritonitis, some patients may experience disease progression from severe sepsis and septic shock to progressive organ dysfunction, hypotension, myocardial depression, and coagulopathy, where a staged approach might be required [10].

If the patient is not in a condition where he can undergo definitive repair and/or abdominal wall closure (such as instability, elevated requirements of inotropics, etc.), *the intervention should be cut short* because of the suboptimal local conditions for healing [11]. In addition, *peritonitis and intra-abdominal sepsis can influence the intra-abdominal pressure* because of bowel distension, ascites, or parietal muscle contraction [12].

When facing the inability to completely control contamination in a single operation, it is recommended to postpone definitive intervention or anastomosis [13]. Extensive visceral edema and decreased abdominal wall compliance may increase the risk of developing abdominal compartment syndrome; therefore, primary fascial closure should not be attempted and the abdomen should be left open [12]. *Following the first* 24–48 h *after the initial surgery, the patient should be taken back to the operating room* for reoperation, lavage, drainage, source control, and if its feasible [13] the closure of the abdominal wall.

The CIAOW study reports that patients with abdominal sepsis have been shown to have worse outcomes after an open abdomen, with an increased incidence of fistula formation, intra-abdominal abscesses, and a higher-delayed primary closure rate [14, 15]. However, there is no definitive data or strong recommendation regarding the use of open abdomen in the face of severe peritonitis. Therefore, *when using an open abdomen approach under these circumstances, caution and individualization of patients should be the priority* [8].

3.1. Key points

- The role of an open abdomen in the management of severe secondary peritonitis has been a controversial issue.
- If the patient is not in a condition to undergo a definitive repair, the intervention should be cut short (hemodynamic instability, elevated requirements of inotropics, or insulated multi-organic failure).
- Peritonitis and intra-abdominal sepsis can influence the intra-abdominal hypertension.
- Following 24–48 h after the initial surgery, the patient should be taken back to the operating room.
- Caution and individualization of patients should be exercised when using open abdomen in severe abdominal sepsis.

4. Abdominal compartment syndrome

Intra-abdominal hypertension and abdominal compartment syndrome are commonly encountered among surgical and nonsurgical critically ill patients. Intra-abdominal hypertension is defined as a sustained pathologic increase in intra-abdominal pressure greater than or equal to 12 mm Hg. Abdominal compartment syndrome is defined as a sustained increase in intra-abdominal tension ≥20 mm Hg that is associated with new organ dysfunction or failure [2, 16].

$$\text{Abdominal perfusion pressure (APP)} = \text{mean arterial pressure (MAP)} - \text{intra-abdominal pressure (IAP)} \quad (1)$$

Intra-abdominal hypertension can lead to tissue hypoperfusion, especially of the abdominal viscera, as well as organ dysfunction. Uncontrolled intra-abdominal hypertension that exceeds 25 mm Hg can cause abdominal compartment syndrome, which is a potentially lethal complication. It is characterized by cardiorespiratory and renal dysfunction, as well as bacterial and toxin intestinal translocation and intracranial hypertension [17].

Abdominal compartment syndrome develops as a result of alterations in perfusion related to intra-abdominal hypertension. It can be classified as primary if it is the result of a pathophysiologic process within the abdominopelvic cavity. It can be caused by bleeding, acute accumulation of ascites, a rapidly growing tumor or another type of mass, retroperitoneal edema, even the packing of visceral injuries, etc. Secondary abdominal compartment syndrome refers to the development of abdominal compartment syndrome in the absence of a primary abdomino-pelvic process [4].

The organ dysfunction that can be seen with abdominal compartment syndrome is usually recognized by the changes in lung and renal function. As abdominal compartment syndrome develops, the pulmonary dynamics change, tidal volumes decrease or, if mechanical ventilation is being used, an increase in peak pressure can be observed with similar tidal volumes. Renal dysfunction can be seen when there is a decrease in urine output caused by decreased renal perfusion as the renal vein is compressed due to the increased abdominal pressure. Other organs can display changes after abdominal compartment syndrome including but not limited to the heart and brain [1]. Intra-abdominal hypertension and abdominal compartment syndrome can also generate changes in other intra-abdominal organs [18].

All patients in the intensive care unit should have measurements of their intra-abdominal pressure because the real incidence of abdominal compartment syndrome in the intensive care unit remains sub-diagnosed, and in some cases it is still unknown. When abdominal compartment syndrome is suspected, bladder pressures should be measured. This is accomplished by instilling a small amount of sterile saline into the bladder and attaching a Foley tube to a pressure transducer [1]; according to the findings, the following steps will be decided and a treatment will be administered (**Table 1**).

Management of this condition requires a multidisciplinary approach by the surgeon and the intensive care unit team, taking in account a specific staged process [4] (**Figure 1**).

There are four main principles when it comes to the management of intra-abdominal hypertension: first of all, serial monitoring of intra-abdominal pressure should be taken every 4–6 h; optimization of systemic perfusion and organ function in the patient with an increased intra-abdominal pressure; medical procedures to reduce intra-abdominal pressure that are institution of specific such as sedation, analgesia, or neuromuscular blockade, and prompt surgical decompressive laparotomy for refractory intra-abdominal hypertension [2] (**Figure 2**).

Medical interventions include sedation to improve abdominal wall compliance, as well as the placing of a nasogastric tube for gastric drainage, removing intraperitoneal fluid collections if they are present, limiting intravenous fluids if possible, diuresis, and also allowing hypercarbia by reducing tidal volumes. *Although all these interventions are promising, the only solution for ACS is decreasing the pressure by performing a decompressive laparotomy* [1, 2, 16, 19].

Intra-abdominal pressure (IAP)
Normal → 5–7 mm Hg
Intra-abdominal hypertension grade I → 12–15 mm Hg
Intra-abdominal hypertension grade II → 16–20 mm Hg
Intra-abdominal hypertension grade III → 21–25 mm Hg
Intra-abdominal hypertension grade IV → > 25 mm Hg

Table 1. Final 2013 consensus definitions of the World Society of the Abdominal Compartment Syndrome [19].

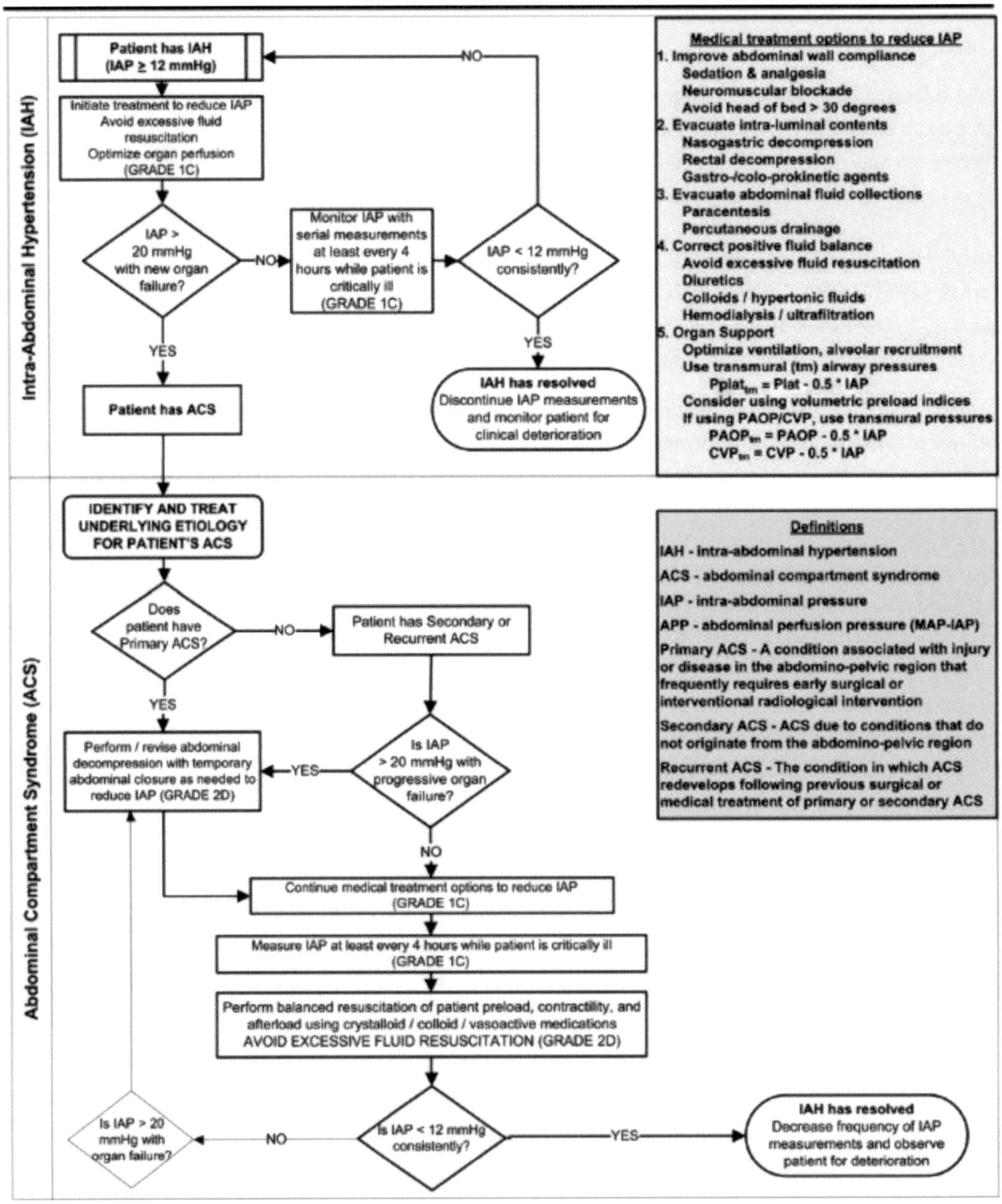

Figure 1. Intra-abdominal hypertension (IAH)/abdominal compartment syndrome (ACS) management algorithm. IAP, intra-abdominal pressure [16].

The main goals of decompressive laparotomy include reduction of the increased IAP in order to stop organ dysfunction, allow for a continued expansion of abdominal viscera during ongoing resuscitation, provide temporary abdominal coverage until the disease process resolves, prevent fascial retraction, and to allow a means for continued evacuation of fluid [2].

http://dx.doi.org/10.5772/intechopen.81428

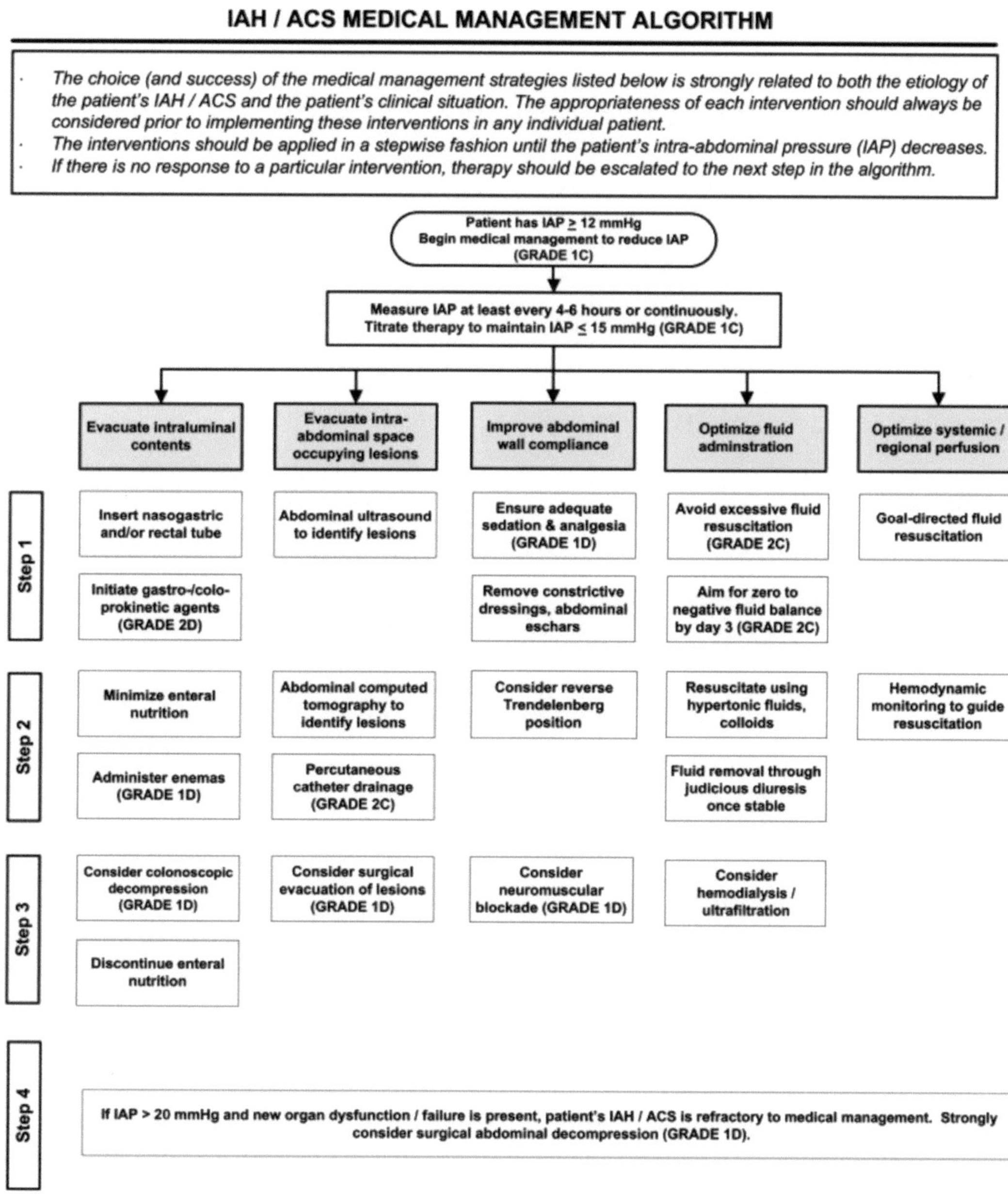

Figure 2. Intra-abdominal hypertension (IAH)/abdominal compartment syndrome (ACS) medical management algorithm. IAP, intra-abdominal pressure [16].

4.1. Key points

- IAH and ACS are commonly encountered among both surgical and nonsurgical critically ill patients.

- Abdominal perfusion pressure (APP), mean arterial pressure (MAP), intra-abdominal pressure (IAP).
- IAH can lead to tissue hypoperfusion, especially of the abdominal viscera, and organ dysfunction.
- Abdominal compartment syndrome develops as a result of alterations in perfusion related to IAH.
- All patients in the intensive care unit should have measurements of intra-abdominal pressure because the incidence of this entity remains sub-diagnosed and still unknown in some cases.
- The challenging situation to manage requires a multidisciplinary approach by the surgeon and the ICU team in a specific staged process.
- Although medical interventions are possible, the only solution for ACS is decreasing the pressure by decompressive laparotomy.

5. Management of the open abdomen

After the clinical scenarios that were just reviewed, *life-saving, decompressive laparotomy and temporary abdominal closure with future restoration of anatomic continuity of the abdominal wall* [20] *are frequently needed*. The chance of achieving one of the most important outcomes, the delayed primary fascial closure, depends on the severity of the underlying etiology [3]. While the management of an open abdomen has surely evolved over the last years, numerous strategies for temporary abdominal closure of an open abdomen have been described in the literature.

Besides prevention of evisceration, temporary abdominal closure can also facilitate subsequent access to the abdominal cavity and prevents retraction of the skin and fascia [3]. The ideal temporary abdominal closure should have some very specific qualities: it should be easy to apply and remove, it should allow rapid access to a surgical second look, it should drain secretions, it should ease primary closure and should have acceptable morbidity and mortality, it should allow easy nursing, and last but not least, it should be readily available and cheap [4] (**Table 2**).

Since the late 1970s and during the 1980s, abdominal dressings for an open abdomen were quite simple, and the treatment was centered only on the protection and control of the bowel that can be found outside the abdomen (nonabsorbable meshes were used, but these led to a high rate of intestinal fistulation) [4]. In the mid-1980s, a zipper was added to the mesh in order to make the process of re-exploration easier [21].

Throughout the years, the surgeons moved on from protection of the ileus to the preservation of the peritoneal space and the prevention of lateral retraction of the fascia, which are the most critical obstacles when dealing with the reconstruction of the abdominal wall at the end of the treatment [4].

For quick abdominal closure in damage control procedures, skin approximation with towel clips or running suture has been suggested in patients in extremis [2]. Another easy method is

1. Skin approximation with towel clips or running suture
2. Bogota bag
3. Synthetic meshes
4. Velcro or zipper-type synthetic materials (Wittmann patch, Starsurgical)
5. Negative-pressure dressing
a. Vacuum pack (Barker technique)
b. Vacuum-assisted closure (VAC Therapy, KCI)
c. Abthera™ system (KCI)

Table 2. Techniques for temporary abdominal wall closure [2].

the plastic silo, also known as the Bogotá bag, with a nonadherent plastic sheet, usually from a sterile 3 liter urology irrigation bag, sutured to the edges of the skin [4].

In 1995 the vacuum pack technique was described, where a perforated plastic sheet is used to cover the viscera and then sterile surgical towels are placed on the wound; a surgical drain is then connected to a continuous negative pressure that is placed on the towels, and everything is covered by an airtight seal; the dressing should be changed every 2–3 days in the operative room but could also be changed in the ICU [4, 21].

The vacuum pack was then developed with using a negative-pressure dressing system that includes a polyurethane foam covered with a protective fenestrated nonadherent layer tubing, a canister, and a computerized pump [2]. It has a few advantages, such as a reduced need for frequent dressing changes, increased vascularity of the wound, decreased bacterial counts, and an extended opportunity for definitive fascial closure [4].

In their systematic review and meta-analysis, Cirocchi et al. support the use of negative-pressure wound therapy in the temporary abdominal closure technique used to care for an open abdomen, concluding that negative-pressure wound therapy is associated with a better outcome than no negative-pressure wound therapy [22].

There is a new strategy that combines negative-pressure wound therapy with a mesh-mediated fascial traction tension. In a systematic review with 4358 patients, Atema et al. reported that negative-pressure wound therapy was the most frequently described temporary abdominal closure technique. The highest weighted fascial closure rate was found in series describing negative-pressure wound therapy with continuous mesh or suture-mediated fascial traction and dynamic retention sutures. Additionally, in a series applying negative-pressure wound therapy without fascial traction, a weighted fistula rate of 14.6% was seen, but when negative-pressure wound therapy was combined with continuous suture or mesh-mediated fascial traction, the fistula risk dropped to 5.7% [3].

Another implementation of the system was introduced by the Abthera™; it consists of a fenestrated plastic sheet with foam sponges that extend in a circular pattern, which is then placed over the viscera encompassing the paracolic gutters and the pelvis; foam sponges are placed on top of the protective layer. Furthermore, an adhesive drape covers the wound and extends over the skin. Suction tubing is attached to a portable suction device to create negative pressure [23].

The three main negative-pressure therapy modalities (Barker, VAC abdominal dressing system, Abthera™) have different mechanical properties, which may affect treatment outcomes. The most important difference between all of these modalities is the distribution pattern of the preset negative pressure [2]. Sammons applied a negative pressure of 125 mmHg to these three systems and measured the pressures in different areas of the dressing, concluding that pressure distribution of Abthera™ therapy was significantly superior to that of the Barker vacuum packing in all three measure zones and in medial and distal zones when comparing with the VAC system [24].

In the World Journal of Emergency Surgery Guidelines (2018), they recommend that negative-pressure wound therapy along with continuous fascial traction is the preferred method for temporary abdominal closure (Grade 1B). Temporary abdominal closure without negative-pressure wound therapy (e.g., mesh alone, Bogota bag) should NOT be used for the purpose of temporary abdominal closure, because of the low-delayed fascial closure rate and the significant intestinal fistula rate that often accompanies the method (Grade 1B) [8, 11].

The best and the right way to manage a patient with an open abdomen is still unclear: the technique is relatively new, and in the literature, the data and the casuistic reported are too varied and too heterogeneous to assess properly [4].

Early fascial and/or abdominal definitive closure should be the strategy for managing an open abdomen once any requirements for ongoing resuscitation have ceased, the source control has been definitively reached, there are no concerns regarding intestinal viability, no further surgical re-exploration is needed, and there are no concerns for abdominal compartment syndrome (Grade 1B) [8].

In many patients, early definitive fascial closure may not be possible because of the persistent bowel edema or intra-abdominal sepsis. In these cases, progressive closure should be attempted when there is a return to the operating room for a washout or dressing change, by placing a few interrupted sutures at the top and bottom of the fascia defect [2] with each new procedure.

Definitive closure of the abdominal wall has to be achieved as soon as possible. Different techniques can be applied in different settings: direct closure with dynamic traction techniques in early closure with little fascial gap, component separation, rotational flaps, the use of prosthetic or biologic mesh, etc.; nevertheless, a planned ventral hernia has to be considered if severe and persistent contamination of the peritoneal cavity is present [25].

5.1. Key points

- Life-saving decompressive laparotomy and temporary abdominal closure with later restoration of anatomic continuity of the abdominal wall are frequently needed.
- Besides prevention of evisceration, temporary abdominal closure can facilitate regaining access to the abdominal cavity and prevents retraction of the skin and fascia.

- We count with different techniques for temporary abdominal closure like skin approximation with towel clips or running suture, Bogota bag, synthetic meshes, velcro or zipper-type synthetic materials, or negative-pressure dressing.
- The best and the correct management of a patient with open abdomen is still unclear: the technique is relatively new, and in the literature, the data and the casuistic reported are too various and too heterogeneous to assess.
- Definitive closure of the abdominal wall has to be obtained as soon as possible. Different techniques can be applied for different settings.

6. Complications

Although the OA has addressed some serious and potentially lethal problems related to early closure of the abdomen, this technique is also *associated with significant complications, including wound infection, fluid and protein loss, a catabolic state, loss of abdominal wall domain, and development of enteroatmospheric fistula* [9].

The appearance of enteric contents from an abdominal incision is a devastating complication and can be emotionally distressing for both the patient and the surgeon. *Enteroatmospheric fistulas range from easily controlled low-output colocutaneous fistulas to high-output enteroatmospheric fistulas* that require a prolonged nutritional support, specialized wound care, and complex reoperative surgery [26]. The overall incidence of this complication is about 5%. However, in the chronically open abdomen, the incidence increases to about 15% [2].

Preemptive measures to prevent enteroatmospheric fistula and frozen abdomen are crucial (i.e., early abdominal wall closure, bowel coverage with plastic sheets, omentum or skin, no direct application of synthetic prosthesis over bowel loops, no direct application of negative-pressure wound therapy on the viscera, and deep burying of intestinal anastomoses under bowel loops) [11].

In some cases, numerous enteroatmospheric fistulas may develop, and the constant leak of enteric contents on the open abdomen aggravates the inflammation and encourages the formation of new fistulas [2]. Enteroatmospheric fistula management should be tailored according to patient condition, fistula output and position, and anatomical features (Grade 1C) [8, 11].

Enteric fistula management is composed of three phases: recognition and stabilization of the patient, anatomical definition and decision-making, and definitive operation [27].

Enteroatmospheric fistula is a life-threatening condition requiring longitudinal care for many months. A spectrum of vexing clinical problems ranging from hypovolemic shock to malnutrition to complex abdominal wall reconstruction challenges the skill of even highly experienced surgeons. *High-output fistulas and EAFs are best managed in centers providing comprehensive care of intestinal failure* [28].

6.1. Key points

- Open abdomen is associated with significant postsurgical complications, including wound infection, fluid and protein loss, a catabolic state, loss of abdominal wall domain, and development of enteroatmospheric fistula.
- Enteroatmospheric fistula can range from an easily controlled low-output colocutaneous fistula to a high-output enteroatmospheric fistula.
- Enteric fistula management is comprised of three phases: recognition and stabilization of the patient, anatomical definition and decision-making, and finally the definitive operation.
- High-output fistulas and EAFs are best managed in medical centers that provide comprehensive care of intestinal failure.

Author details

Juan José Santivañez Palomino[1*], Arturo Vergara[2] and Manuel Cadena[2]

*Address all correspondence to: juan.santivanez@urosario.edu.co

1 Department of Surgery, Fundación Santa Fe de Bogotá, Colombia

2 Department of Metabolic Support and General Surgery, Fundación Santa Fe de Bogota, FACS, Universidad Los Andes, Colombia

References

[1] Beckman M, Paul J, Weigelt JA, Neideen T. Role of the open abdomen in critically ill patients. Critical Care Clinics. 2016;**32**(2):255-264. DOI: 10.1016/j.ccc.2015.12.003

[2] Demetriades D, Salim A. Management of the open abdomen. Surgical Clinics of North America. 2014;**94**(1):131-153

[3] Atema JJ, Gans SL, Boermeester MA. Systematic review and meta-analysis of the open abdomen and temporary abdominal closure techniques in non-trauma patients. World Journal of Surgery. 2015;**39**(4):912-925

[4] Coccolini F et al. The open abdomen, indications, management and definitive closure. World Journal of Emergency Surgery. 2015;**10**(1):1-10. DOI: 10.1186/s13017-015-0026-5

[5] Ivatury R, Diebel L, Porter J. Damage control surgery: Intra-abdominal hypertension and the abdominal compartment syndrome. The Surgical Clinics of North America. 1997;**77**:783-800

[6] Lee JC, Peitzman AB. Damage control laparotomy. Current Opinion in Critical Care. 2006;**12**(4):346-350

[7] Teixeira P, Salim A, Inaba K. A prospective look at the current state of open abdomens. The American Surgeon. 2008;**74**(10):891-897

[8] Coccolini F, Roberts D, Ansaloni L, Ivatury R, Gamberini E, Kluger Y, et al. The open abdomen in trauma and non-trauma patients: WSES guidelines. World Journal of Emergency Surgery. 2018;**13**(7):1-16

[9] Demetriades D. Total management of the open abdomen. Surgical Clinics of North America. 2012;**9**:17-24

[10] Moore LJ, Moore FA. Epidemiology of sepsis in surgical patients. Surgical Clinics of North America. 2012;**92**(6):1425-1443. DOI: 10.1016/j.suc.2012.08.009

[11] Coccolini F, Montori G, Ceresoli M, Catena F, Moore EE, Ivatury R, et al. The role of open abdomen in non-trauma patient: WSES consensus paper. World Journal of Emergency Surgery. 2017;**12**(39):1-17

[12] Plantefeve G, Hellmann R, Pajot O, Thirion M, Bleichner G, Mentec H. Abdominal compartment syndrome and intraabdominal sepsis: Two of the same kind? Acta Clinica Belgica. 2007;**62**(Suppl 1):162-167

[13] Sartelli M et al. The role of the open abdomen procedure in managing severe abdominal sepsis: WSES position paper. World Journal of Emergency Surgery. 2015;**10**(1):1-11. DOI: 10.1186/s13017-015-0032-7

[14] Sartelli M, Catena F, Ansaloni L, Coccolini F, Corbella D, Moore EE, et al. Complicated intra-abdominal infections worldwide: The definitive data of the CIAOW study. World Journal of Emergency Surgery. 2014;**9**(37):1-10

[15] Bradley M, Dubose J, Scalea T, et al. Independent predictors of enteric fistula and abdominal sepsis after damage control laparotomy: Results from the pro- spective AAST open abdomen registry. JAMA Surgery. 2013;**148**:947

[16] Kirkpatrick AW, Roberts DJ, Ball CG, Regli A, Amours SD. Intra-abdominal hypertension and the abdominal compartment syndrome: Updated consensus definitions and clinical practice guidelines from the World Society of the Abdominal Compartment Syndrome World Society of the Abdominal. Intensive Care Medicine. Jul 2013;**39**(7):1190-1206

[17] Kaplan M, Banwell P, Orgill D. Guidelines for the management of the open abdomen. Wounds. 2005;**17**:1-24

[18] Papavramidis T et al. Abdominal compartment syndrome–Intra-abdominal hypertension: Defining, diagnosing, and managing. Journal of Emergencies, Trauma, and Shock. 2011;**4**(2):279-291

[19] Malbrain M et al. Results from the international conference of experts on intra-abdominal hypertension and abdominal compartment syndrome. I. definitions. Intensive Care Medicine. 2006;**32, 11**:1722-1732. DOI: 10.1007/s00134-006-0349-5

[20] Howdieshell T, Proctor C, Sternberg E, Cue J, Mondy J, Hawkins M. Temporary abdominal closure followed by definitive abdominal wall reconstruction of the open abdomen. American Journal of Surgery. 2004;**188**:301-306

[21] Quyn A et al. The open abdomen and temporary abdominal closure systems–Historical evolution and systematic review. Colorectal Disease. Aug 2012;**14**(8):e429-438

[22] Popivanov G, Chiara O, Tugnoli G. What is the effectiveness of the negative pressure wound therapy (NPWT) in patients treated with open abdomen technique? A systematic review and meta-analysis. The Journal of Trauma and Acute Care Surgery. Sep 2016;**81**(3):575-584

[23] Frazee RC, Abernathy SW, Jupiter DC, Hendricks JC, Davis M, Regner JL, et al. Are commercial negative pressure systems wortzh the cost in open abdomen management? Journal of the American College of Surgeons. 2013;**216**(4):730-735. DOI: 10.1016/j.jamcollsurg.2012.12.035

[24] Delgado A, Sammons A. In vitro pressure manifolding distribution evaluation of ABThera™ active abdominal therapy system, V.A.C. ® abdominal dressing system, and Barker's vacuum packing technique conducted under dynamic conditions. SAGE Open Medicine. 2016;**4**:205031211562498. DOI: 10.1177/2050312115624988

[25] Chiara O, Cimbanassi S, Biffl W, Leppaniemi A, Henry S, Scalea TM, et al. International consensus conference on open abdomen in trauma. The Journal of Trauma and Acute Care Surgery. Jan 2016;**80**(1):173-183

[26] Davis KG, Johnson EK. Controversies in the care of the enterocutaneous fistula. The Surgical Clinics of North America. 2013;**93**(1):231-250

[27] Schecter WP, Hirshberg A, Chang DS, Harris HW, Napolitano LM, Wexner SD, et al. Enteric fistulas: Principles of management. Journal of the American College of Surgeons. 2009;**209**(4):484-491. DOI: 10.1016/j.jamcollsurg.2009.05.025

[28] Schecter WP. Management of enterocutaneous fistulas. The Surgical Clinics of North America. 2011;**91**(3):481-491

Chapter 12

Facilitation of Wound Healing Following Laparoscopic and Conventional Abdominal Surgery with Dressings, Patches, Antibiotics, etc.

Rebekah Amarini, Sufan Chien and Girish J. Kotwal

Additional information is available at the end of the chapter

http://dx.doi.org/10.5772/intechopen.82614

Abstract

Wounds due to surgical incisions and due to injuries often do not heal and can result in complications like slow healing and infections. Several approaches to facilitate wound healing are constantly being developed. Here we discuss various wounds and multiple ways to treat wounds especially those resulting from abdominal surgery either due to conventional surgery or due to laparoscopic surgery. In future, there are various possibilities in the pipeline that could result in accelerated wound healing as well as tissue regeneration.

Keywords: wound, healing, surgery, laparoscopic, infection

1. Introduction

An estimated 313 million surgical procedures are performed worldwide annually [1]. The quality of incision selection and postoperative wound healing play significant critical roles in patient recovery and rehabilitation. Mortality and morbidity rates are affected by surgical wound complications. The importance of surgical incisions and wound care has been documented throughout history to primarily prevent wound infection has been from the time Alexander the Great was treated with saffron for injuries from a piercing spear. Over the years, several new ways of performing surgery and treating wound have advanced wound care. In the last century, endoscopic surgery has significantly reduced incision damage, and antibiotics were introduced to control infections and facilitate healing. Neosporin with its triple antibiotics has been commonly used, can be purchased over the counter, and can be used for minor

Diabetic wounds	Types of dressings	Process of cleaning and caring for wound
	• Daily saline • Dressings that provide a moist environment [5]	• Offload wound • Debridement if necessary of nonviable tissue to promote accelerated wound healing • Antibiotic therapy if indicated • Control blood glucose levels • Correction of peripheral arterial insufficiency • Diabetic footwear • Hyperbaric oxygen chamber • Skin grafting [6]
General surgical incisions Stitches, skin glue, staples, steri-strips	• Sterile dressing • Wet to dry dressing	• Keep incision clean and dry • Prophylactic antibiotics • Gauze pad or soft cloth to clean wound with normal saline or soapy water [7]
Laparoscopic incisions Subcuticular stitch, staples, skin glue	• Nonadherent dressing gauze to absorb light drainage • Transparent film	• Prophylactic antibiotics • Betadine prep • Post-op dressing can be removed in 48 h
Gunshot wounds	• Keep wound clean and dry • Stop bleeding with pressure/ tourniquet	• Possible surgery to remove bullet or bone [8] • Crushing tissue or stretching of tissue • Antibiotics
Wounds from sharp objects (knives, blades)	• Keep wound clean and dry • Clean dressing	• If through the sole of a shoe *Pseudomonas* can be the cause of infection • Possibly need tetanus shot

Table 1. Wound care table for different types of wounds.

cuts and wounds that do not require stitches. With antibiotic resistance manifesting itself in recent decades, other new ways have become essential. Current and future wound healing measures are in a constant state of flux, and when an agent proves useful, it can help many patients who have been affected. Carbohydrate-derived fulvic acid (CHD-FA) is a topical agent, which has been used to prevent drug-resistant bacterial and fungal infections, and contains anti-inflammatory properties for those who have suffered a traumatic wound [2]. Wounds can occur due to several different causes as summarized in **Table 1**. Several wound care options are currently available (**Table 2**) and could become available in the future (**Table 3**). A surgical incision is an aperture into the body to permit the work of the planned operation to proceed. The choice of incision for laparotomy depends on the area that needs to be exposed, the elective or emergency nature of the operation, and personal preference. There are two approaches used nowadays: traditional incision and minimally invasive. This book chapter provides a brief review of recent progress in surgical procedure and wound care of incisions during abdominal surgeries.

2. Traditional incision

Traditional abdominal surgery refers to operating through an open abdominal incision known as laparotomy. The goal is to provide adequate exposure for the anticipated procedure while taking into account the possibility that the planned procedure may change depending upon

Types of dressing	Primary or secondary dressing	Functions/indications	Pros	Cons	Frequency of dressing change
Hydrogels (e.g., IntraSite Gel, generic hydrogel)	Primary	• Give the wound a moist environment • Used for shallow dry ulcers • Autolytic debridement	• Hydrates wound, liquefies necrotic tissue on wound surface • Nonstick • Soothing effect	• Must have a secondary dressing • Not meant for significant exudate	• Change when other dressings are changed
Alginates • Calcium alginate (AlgiSite, Aquacel, Sorbsan) • Calcium alginate with silver (Aquacel Ag) • Calcium-sodium alginate (Kaltostat) • Carboxymethyl cellulose (CMC) silver oxysalt dressing • **Biosorb gelling fiber**	Primary	• Ulcers with copious exudate • Silver can be added to give antibacterial effect-infected ulcers/presence of a biofilm-oxidized silver reduces viable biofilm • High absorptive capacity can be used in packing • Form a gel like covering over the wound keeping it moist	• Significantly absorbent • Don't inhibit wound contraction • Can be used in infected pressure ulcers	• Must have a secondary dressing • May be too drying if wound isn't exudative • Fiber residue	• 1–2x a week • Silver–Weekly
Antimicrobial dressings • Gauze • Alginate • Foam	Primary	• 72 h of antibacterial properties • Use with negative pressure wound therapy • Used for packing wounds with dead space	• Doesn't require a secondary dressing • Inexpensive	• Doesn't eradicate bacteria in wound	Every 72 h
Transparent film • Generic transparent gauze • Tegaderm • Opsite	Primary or secondary	• Semipermeable membrane waterproof but permeable to water vapor and oxygen • Keep wound moisturized while preventing bacterial contamination • Provides autolytic debridement • Superficial/light exudative wounds • Often the preferred secondary dressing • Used to prevent friction injuries	• Transparent evaluation of wound without removal of dressing • Waterproof and gas permeable • Keep moist environment	• Skin damage if removed improperly • Limited absorptive properties • Shouldn't be used for infected ulcers • Roll up in coccyx region	Every 7–10 days

Types of dressing	Primary or secondary dressing	Functions/indications	Pros	Cons	Frequency of dressing change
Hydrocolloids • Generic hydrocolloids • Duoderm	Primary or secondary	• Used in epithelizing and granulation wounds Ulcers with light to moderate exudate [9] • Gel-forming covering keeps in moisture and protects wound • Hydrocolloid sheets help autolytic debridement by keeping wound exudate in contact with necrotic tissue (slough and eschar) • Paste and powders increase absorptive capacity	• Easy application, forms to wound well decreasing pain • Used to protect body areas at risk for friction injury or tape injury	• Never used for infected wounds • Not used for moderate to heavy exudative wounds • Reside and foul odor may arise from breakdown of product	Every 7 days
Foams • Generic foam • PolyMem • Foam with AMD	Primary	• Ulcers highly exudate • Highly absorbent of exudate which keeps it off the wound and decreases damage to surrounding tissue • Deep cavity wounds to prevent premature closure, absorbing exudate and maintaining a moist environment • Weeping ulcers • Diabetic foot ulcers [10]	• Absorbent characteristics • Comfortable and form well to wound • Used for painful /risk for shear injury pressure ulcers	• Require secondary dressing usually • Drying effect	• Varies • Silver- Up to 7 days
Debriding agents • Santyl (Health point) • Accuzyme (Health point)					
Other options **-Prp, PDGF, low-frequency ultrasound therapy (MIST, celleration) with composite dressings, and synthetic skin substitutes**					

Types of dressing	Primary or secondary dressing	Functions/indications	Pros	Cons	Frequency of dressing change
Negative pressure wound therapy (NPWT) • **Pico**	Computerized vacuum device applies negative pressure which decreases wound healing time				Changed every 72 h
Velcro adjustable wraps • **Ready wrap**	Limitations–training the patient and families to apply correctly with				
Larval debridement therapy	Limitations are asphyxiation of the larva mortality, escape	Offloading of the coccyx/sacral region provided the best chance for larval survival			
Near-infrared spectroscopy (NIRS)					
Dehydrated human amnion/ chorion membrane (dHACM) • **PURION**		Chronic wounds regenerate damaged tissue			
Dehydrated human umbilical cord allograft (dHUC) • PURION PLUS process		• Chronic wounds in difficult-to-heal areas • Provides connective tissue matrix to supplement damaged tissue			
Honey impregnated absorbent dressing (e.g., MANUKAhd)	Contains *Leptospermum scoparium* honey	• Maintains a moist environment • Moderate to heavy exudative wounds			
Trauma wounds • Polymeric membrane dressings (PMD) • PMD + silver	Standard protocol of care in the ED	• Resorbs blister exudate, reduces edema • Silver–Antibacterial			

Table 2. Types of dressings and patches that are currently available.

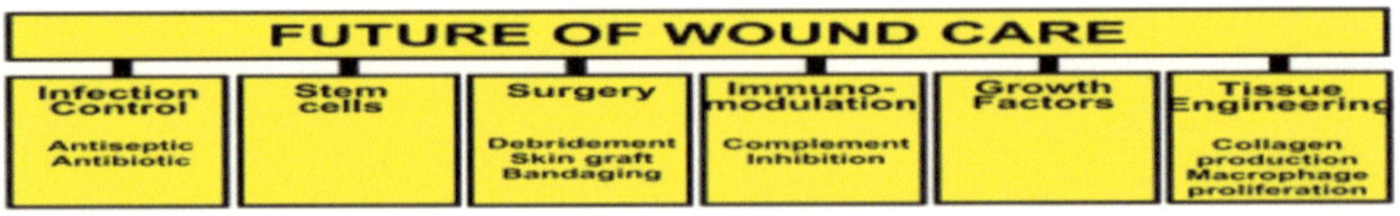

Table 3. Future options for wound care.

intraoperative findings or complications. Historically, the earliest surgeries were crude and were performed out of desperation. It wasn't until the 1900s that the risk of dying after surgery mainly due to infection was less than 50%. After the turn of the century, the likelihood of surviving surgery was greater than the chance of dying during or immediately after surgery. Early techniques were rudimentary, or even barbaric by today's standards, as anesthesia was not commonly used until the mid-to-late 1800s.

Today, surgery takes a wide variety of forms and is often performed using minimally invasive techniques. This has shortened recovery times, improved outcomes, and minimized complications for most patients. However, laparotomy is still used in some types of surgery, especially in organ transplantation (such as the liver, pancreas, and kidney), because it allows extensive dissection and anastomoses.

For traditional abdominal surgery, the incision should interfere minimally with abdominal wall function by preserving important abdominal structures and heal with adequate strength to reduce the risk of wound disruption and herniation. During surgery, wisely chosen incisions and correct methods of making and closing such wounds are factors of great importance. Any mistake, such as a badly placed incision, inept methods of suturing, or random selection of suture material, may result in serious complications such as unnecessary functional disruption, hematoma formation, ugly scar formation, wound dehiscence and herniation, or complete disruption of the wound [3].

The specific surgical incision will depend on the underlying pathology, site, patient factors, and the surgeon's preference and experience. The key principles of making surgical incisions are (1) for maximal wound strength with minimal scarring, incisions should try to follow Langer's lines where possible, and (2) where possible, muscles should be split and not cut. There are several types of laparotomy, such as longitudinal (vertical), transverse, and oblique, and each has various sizes and positions to fit different surgical goals.

3. Minimally invasive surgery

The recent development of endoscopic and laparoscopic technology has revolutionized traditional surgery concepts facilitating patient friendly access to even the most remote of abdominal organs [4]. Laparoscopic surgery requires small incisions to be made in the skin, which allows instruments to be passed into the abdominal cavity. Common instruments include the camera, cutting and dissecting scissors, and grippers. The port sites will vary depending on the

http://dx.doi.org/10.5772/intechopen.82614

surgery being performed, yet the umbilicus is nearly always used as a port site to allow the camera to pass through at this time; the technique is still under development, and further improvement such as artificial intelligence (AI) or real-time, dynamic AI system will speed up the procedure, enhance safety, and improve outcomes. Once the operation is over, surgical excisions can be closed by sutures, staples, steri-strips, tissue glue, or a combination of these agents. The wound should be covered in a protective dressing like gauze and attached with a paper adhesive tape and kept dry for a few days, before normal washing can resume. Pre- and postoperative prophylactic antibiotics can be administered for laparoscopic surgery but are debatable and not recommended by the WHO if the wound is not contaminated.

4. Routine care postsurgery

Wound care for an incision starts before making the initial cut and lasts until the end of the patients' healing process; it's important to maintain proper surgical field cleanliness and to prepare a patient with the right technique before performing any type of laparoscopic surgery [5]. Medical patients that are undergoing laparoscopic surgery should be given antibiotics usually a first-generation cephalosporin 30 minutes prior to the incision as well as prepped with betadine, a povidone iodine, or hexachlorophene before surgery. Giving antibiotics post-operatively depends on the type of the laparoscopic procedure done; the patient is normally given 1–3 postoperative doses, and if it's a colorectal surgery, then three doses is usually given due to the higher risk for infection.

When performing a laparoscopic surgery, various access approaches have been used. For the removal of the gallbladder or appendix, all the instruments may be inserted at a single incision using a Gel POINT (Applied Medical), SILSPORT (Medtronic), or Triport (Olympus) access platform. This approach is especially appropriate in a patient who is young and thin. It is more acceptable in female patients as it yields a great esthetic result, allows a wide range of motion during the surgery, and is a minimally invasive method [6, 7]. It is important to ensure if there is any suspicion of contamination or infection such as appendicitis, cholecystitis, and cystectomy that an end catch bag is used, to minimize the chance for an infection. A specimen retrieval bag, such as endocatch or endobag (Covidien), reliacatch (Medtronic), endopouch (Ethicon), and Conmed (eSutures), is used which avoids spillage and contamination of the infected specimen to minimize the chance for an infection. When closing a laparoscopic incision, there are options of using subcuticular stiches or staples. If the wound is small, a tissue adhesive skin glue such as Dermabond can be used to close the skin. The incision is then covered using Telfa, a nonadherent dressing gauze which conforms to the wound and absorbs light drainage; the gauze is then held in place with Tegaderm. Tegaderm is a semiocclusive transparent film, which self-adheres and allows insensible water loss and prevents the entry of bacteria and proteins; transparent films are known to have the fastest healing rates and lowest infection and are the most cost-effective [5]. The initial postoperative dressing can be removed in 48 h if the wound remains dry. No matter whether traditional or minimally invasive approach is used, surgical complications can occur after surgery. The most common complications include wound, infections, and dehiscence. Their management is presented here.

5. Postoperative wound infections

Surgical site infections are defined as infections that occur 30 days after surgery with no implant or within 1 year if an implant is placed and infection appears to be related to surgery. Surgical site infections (SSI) are seen in about 4% of clean wounds and 35% of contaminated wounds, so they are generally rare. However, certain risk factors predispose a patient to an SSI, which include diabetes, obesity, immunosuppression, cardiovascular disease, smoking, cancer, preventative surgery, malnutrition, and prior irradiation [8]. Obese patients are at increased risk especially if the incision is in the umbilical area due to fatty tissue not being well vascularized, the difficulty of cleaning it, and usually multiple incisions being made in obese patients. SSIs are associated with substantial morbidity and mortality. Patients with SSI are twice as likely to die, 60% more likely to be admitted to the intensive care unit, and more than five times more likely to be readmitted to the hospital after discharge.

Signs and symptoms of incisional infection vary significantly depending on the types, severity, and pathogens. The most frequent symptoms include fever, feeling of malaise, fluid drainage, increased wound pain, redness and swelling around the wound, and loss of function and movement. SSI may be caused either by endogenous or exogenous microorganisms. Most SSIs are caused by endogenous microorganisms present on the patient's skin at the site of surgical incision, and Gram-positive bacteria such as *Staphylococcus aureus* are the most common microorganisms. SSI may also be caused by organisms within the patient's body that are exposed during surgery, such as Gram-negative microorganisms in the gastrointestinal tract. Exogenous sources of microorganisms include surgical instruments, operating room surfaces, the air, and personnel. Usually all wound infections happen on day 5 after surgery, and it's safe to suspect a staph infection due to the commonality of it. Of the rarer types of infections, Group A strep is seen on day 2 and clostridium usually is seen on day 3. To diagnose surgical site infections, a clinician should look for redness, induration, warmth, pain, purulent wound drainage, separation, fever, and WBC count. If the wound is infected, the wound should be opened, explored, drained, irrigated, debridement, and dressed open then; when the infection has cleared and there is granulation tissue growth, the wound can be closed by secondary intervention [8]. Antibiotic therapy is only used for wound infections associated with cellulitis or edema. Superficial incisional infections that have been opened can usually be managed without antibiotics if there is no associated cellulitis [5].

When closing a wound, if there is a large incision, staples are usually used because they are less reactive than sutures and have a better end result; however, sutures are utilized when there might be tension on the skin to distribute it easily. Staples are also less likely to obscure wound drainage and impending separation than subcuticular sutures, and if part of the wound is infected with staples, only remove the selected staples without opening the entire skin incisions as it generally happens once a subcuticular stitch is cut [4]. The distance between the placements of staples is what determines how the wound will drain. The wound should stop draining in about 2–3 days; when it does, it should be left uncovered. If it continues to drain, it can be kept covered and the dressings changed daily until it stops draining.

Complications from surgery like bleeding beyond a certain period say 10 days from the incision site does not really happen after laparoscopic surgery. Any bleeding usually happens early; the trocar can tamponade during the surgery and can injure a vessel. The bleeding depends on where the incision site is. The subcuticular superficial arteries can bleed or the inferior epigastric vessel if there was a lateral incision made. Usually the nurse will inform the doctor that the dressings are saturated and a pressure dressing is placed until the bleeding stops.

Some other complications from surgery include seromas, hematomas, fascial dehiscence, hernias, evisceration, and nerve injury. Seromas and hematomas are not common with laparoscopic incisions and seen more with open surgery; when a seroma or hematoma has occurred, it can be aspirated, and if a seroma recurs, it should be aspirated until it's fully gone. The wound can also have dehiscence; the main reasons for wound dehiscence are failure of the suture to remain anchored to the fascia, suture damage, knot failure, and stiches applied too close together. In 95% of abdominal wall dehiscence, the sutures and knots are intact, but the suture has pulled through the necrotic fascia due to the sutures being too close to the edge of a wound or under too much tension. If fascial disruption is suspected, wound exploration should be done in the operating room; complete dehiscence is a surgical emergency and is associated with a 10% mortality rate [4]. Management of SSI depends on the severity of the infection. Minor and superficial infections may be treated with antibiotic therapy. If the infection is deep and severe with pus or fluid drainage, the wound should be opened, explored, drained, irrigated, debrided, and dressed open, and the dressing should be changed daily or more often if the drainage is severe. When the infection has cleared and there is granulation tissue growth, the wound can be closed by secondary intention [8]. Antibiotic therapy is only used for wound infections associated with cellulitis or edema. Superficial incisional infections that have been opened can usually be managed without antibiotics if there is no associated cellulitis [5].

6. Wound dehiscence

The quality of postoperative wound healing plays a significant role and is critical in patient recovery and rehabilitation because mortality and morbidity rates are affected by surgical wound dehiscence (SWD). SWD is defined as partial or total disruption of any or all layers of operative wounds—from simple skin dehiscence and hernia formation to the most severe and potentially lethal forms characterized by evisceration, gastrointestinal anastomotic leaks, pancreatic fistulas, and vascular pseudoaneurysms. The impact of SWD can be considerable: increased mortality, delayed hospital discharge, readmission, future surgery, delayed adjuvant treatment, suboptimal esthetic outcome, and impaired psychosocial well-being. SWD occurrence rates can vary significantly, from 0.65 to 2.1% in sternotomy to as high as 16.9–41.8% in pilonidal sinus surgery, and the cost for these wounds was $13.1 billion according to Medicare data from a 2014 report.

7. Bleeding and hematoma

Bleeding is a relatively rare complication if the wound is inspected carefully before closing. Bleeding usually happens early; the trocar can tamponade during the surgery and can injure a vessel. When the blood comes out from the wound, it can be seen. However, if the blood is inside the wound, it causes hematoma or seroma. Management depends on the site and severity of the bleeding. The hematoma should be decompressed and blood is removed. If a relatively larger vessel is involved and still shows active bleeding, a suture should be used to stop it, but this is rare. For minor bleeding, a pressure dressing is placed until the bleeding stops.

8. Concluding remarks

Risk factors for most young and healthy patients and surgical wound complications are rare when the surgery is done carefully. However, risk factors for developing wound complications exist in various patients, and surgical procedure itself can also play a major role in developing complications. This includes older age, diabetes, renal diseases, the use of tobacco products and steroids, compromised immune system, obesity, poor nutritional status, and bacterial infection or colonization at a remote body sites [9–12]. To reduce wound complications, the surgical team plays a critical role. This includes adequate preoperative preparation to improve patient's overall health, careful surgical site selection, accurate procedure with as little collateral damage as possible, careful wound closure, and postoperative management. A high-quality multidisciplinary team should be able to perform safe surgeries with little complications even in some health-compromised patients.

Acknowledgements

The authors thank Dr. Andrei Stieber, general surgeon at DeKalb Medical, for sharing his insights from his surgical practice in wound care.

Conflict of interests to declare

None.

Author details

Rebekah Amarini[1], Sufan Chien[2,3] and Girish J. Kotwal[2*]

*Address all correspondence to: gjkotw01@gmail.com

1 Hoboken University Medical Center, Carepoint Health System, Hoboken, NJ, USA

2 Noveratech Louisville, KY, USA

3 Department of Surgery, Price Institute of Surgical Research, University of Louisville School of Medicine, Louisville, KY, USA

References

[1] Weiser TG, Haynes AB, Molina G, Lipsitz SR, Esquivel MM, Uribe-Leitz T, et al. Estimate of the global volume of surgery in 2012: An assessment supporting improved health outcomes. Lancet. 2015;**27**(385 Suppl 2):S11. DOI: 10.1016/S0140-6736(15)60806-6

[2] Zhao Y, Paderu P, Delmas G, Dolgov E, Lee MH, Senter M, et al. Carbohydrate-derived fulvic acid is a highly promising topical agent to enhance healing of wounds infected with drug-resistant pathogens. Journal of Trauma and Acute Care Surgery. 2015;**79**(4 Suppl 2): S121-S129. DOI: 10.1097/TA.0000000000000737

[3] Carlson MA, Ludwig KA, Condon RE. Ventral hernia and other complications of 1,000 midline incisions. Southern Medical Journal. 1995;**88**(4):450-453

[4] Macintyre IM, Wilson RG. Laparoscopic cholecystectomy. The British Journal of Surgery. 1993;**80**(5):552-559

[5] Armstrong DG, Meyr A. Basic Principles of Wound Management. Up-to-date. 2016. Available from: https://www-uptodate-com.ezproxy.uthsc.edu/contents/basic-principles-of-wound management?source=search_result&search=basics%20wound%20management&selectedTitle=1~150

[6] Applied Medical Gel Point Access Platforms. Applied Medical Resources Corporation. 2016. Available from: http://www.appliedmedical.com/Products/GelPoint_Overview.aspx

[7] Asakuma M, Komeda K, Yamamoto M, et al. A concealed "natural orifice": Umbilicus anatomy for minimally invasive surgery. Surgical Innovation. 2018:1-4:1553350618797619. DOI: 10.1177/1553350618797619

[8] Mizell J. Complications of Abdominal Surgical Incisions. Up-to-date. 2016. Available from: https://www-uptodate-com.ezproxy.uthsc.edu/contents/complications-of-abdominal-surgical-incisions?source=search_result&search=complications%20of%20abdomnical%20surgical%20incisions&selectedTitle=1~150

[9] Brem H, Tomic-Canic M. Cellular and molecular basis of wound healing in diabetes. Journal of Clinical Investigation. 2007;**117**(5):1219-1222

[10] U.S. National Library of Medicine. Surgical Wound Care–Open. Bethesda, MD, USA: National Institutes of Health. 2018

[11] CCHCS. CCHCS Care Guide. Would and Skin Ulcer Management. 2012. Available from: http://www.cphcs.ca.gov/docs/careguides/Wound-and-Skin-Ulcer-Management-Care-Guide.pdf

[12] Park NJ, Allen L, Gu G, Driver V. Essential insights on treating chronic venous stasis ulcers. Podiatry Today. 2012;**25**(7):70-82. Available from: http://www.podiatrytoday.com/essential-insights-treating-chronic-venous-stasis-ulcers

Chapter 13

Multidisciplinary Approaches to the Stimulation of Wound Healing and Use of Dermal Substitutes in Chronic Phlebostatic Ulcers

Raffaele Capoano, Rita Businaro, Besar Kolce,
Andrea Biancucci, Silvia Izzo, Lidia De Felice and
Bruno Salvati

Additional information is available at the end of the chapter

http://dx.doi.org/10.5772/intechopen.81791

Abstract

Research focus: Skin injuries are evolving as an epidemic issue. Chronic skin lesion is a globally widespread disease, often referred to as a "wound difficult to heal" and one which has a strong impact on both overall health and quality of life. Genetic and clinical variables, such as diabetes, smoking and inflammatory/immunological pathologies, are among the important risk factors limiting the regenerative powers of many therapeutic applications. Therefore, optimisation of current clinical strategies is critical. **Experimental research:** Here we summarise the field's current state by focusing on the use of stem-cell therapeutic applications in wound healing, placing considerable emphasis on current clinical approaches being developed at Rome's *Sapienza* University. These involve protocols for the ex vivo expansion of adipose tissue-derived mesenchyme stem cells using a patented GMP-compliant platelet lysate, Mesengen™, and cellular and acellular dermal substitutes. A combination of multiple strategies, including genetic modifications of stem cells, biomimetic scaffolds or novel vehicles like nanoparticles, is also discussed as future approaches. **Case studies:** Here we present a report portraying our clinical experience of the treatment of chronic phlebostatic ulcers. The aim of the study reported here was to evaluate the effectiveness of treatment with dermal substitutes of cutaneous lesions originating from chronic venous insufficiency, therapy which took into consideration parameters such as the reduction of wound size and the improvement of quality of life. Chronic skin lesion, a globally widespread disease, is often referred to as a "difficult wound" and has a strong impact on both overall health and quality of life. The difficulties encountered when seeking to heal this ailment have led to a quest for and development of new therapeutic approaches, including dermal substitutes. We can subdivide these into acellular matrices, such as Integra and Hyalomatrix, and cell therapies such as platelet concentrate and mesenchyme cell concentrate. **Results:** In all the patients treated, elements of improvement were observed: the appearance on the wound bed of small islands of granulation tissue, superficialization of the bottom of the ulcer and a growth of marginal tissue. During the first 30 days, a reduction in more than 25% of the area of the lesion and a reduction in more than 50% at the end of the observation period were recorded in 10 of the patients who underwent preliminary surgical treatment out of the 13 subjects included in the study sample. On the whole, at the end of the observation period, we witnessed an average 57% decrease in the lesion in all the patients; furthermore, during the treatment period, there was a gradual reduction in pain, measured using the NRS numerical scale. An overall average reduction in pain of four points on the NRS numerical scale was achieved. At the end of the 8-week evaluation period, the majority of the patients reported an improvement in the quality of their lives, since, in addition to the reduction of spontaneous pain, there was a diminution of pruritus, secretions—often malodorous and capable of affecting social life negatively—with recovery of functional capacity and almost complete recovery of habitual daily activities. During the period of treatment, no superinfections of the wounds or secondary complications related to the use of the various products were detected. **Main conclusions:** The numerous technological opportunities provided by regenerative medicine—including advanced dressings and dermal substitutes—if applied correctly, in compliance with a multidisciplinary approach where necessary, seem to offer advantages not only in terms of clinical efficacy and patient life quality but also in terms, it would appear, of healthcare costs, an aspect which should not be either overlooked or underestimated.

Keywords: wound healing, skin lesion, regenerative medicine, dermal substitutes, phlebostatic ulcers

1. Introduction

The management of scarring in chronic wounds represents one of the most relevant clinical problems affecting healthcare in the United States and in Europe [1]. Scars can cause severe physical damage, resulting, predominantly, in damage to the skin.

This kind of lesion causes loss of cutaneous substance, varies in size and involves loss of underlying tissue as well; this kind of lesion is often defined as "difficult" because it fails to heal spontaneously or achieve speedy and complete recovery. Acute or chronic wounds of this type are due to multifactor pathogeneses, and their healing is impeded, as a rule, by persistent local or systemic factors which favour chronicisation.

Medical-surgical treatment of these so-called "difficult" lesions represents a constantly increasing social-health issue, a "silent epidemic" affecting large sectors of the world's population, one which, at present, concerns about 2,000,000 Italians; these numbers are destined to grow further due not only to diverse risk factors but also to the phenomenon of ageing [2, 3]. Subjects with pre-existing diseases are of particular concern, as treatment and resolution of injury frequently require long-term care. Healing is often compromised in similar individuals because of the presence of diabetes, the metabolic syndrome, chronic renal failure and ageing [4] since the ability to rapidly re-epithelialise and revascularise injured tissue is impaired. In some cases, the evolution of the lesion is correlated to the root-cause pathology, as, in particular, in the case of "immunohaematological" ulcers.

Both clinical and genetic features of individual patients must be considered when addressing wound healing, as well as variations in medical responses based on the type of chemical tools employed and the nature and extent of the injured area. In fact, large wounds, under either adverse local or systemic conditions, respond poorly to treatment and can frequently reopen.

It is calculated that about 10% of the population is likely to develop a chronic lesion during its lifetime, leading to discomfort (pain, reduced hygiene, sleep disturbance), loss of autonomy, need of assistance and frequent hospitalisation, with considerable deterioration of the quality of life (QoL) due, among other things, to embarrassment, social isolation, compromisation of employability, monetary costs, anxiety-depressive syndromes [5] as well as a mortality rate of 2.5% [6, 7]. A chronic dermal lesion means having to live with a persistent, enduring and treatment-resistant wound, which has a significant impact on the overall health and quality of life of patients, members of their families and caregivers.

Chronic venous insufficiency is responsible for 80% of the ulcers affecting the lower limbs, a sequela constituting one of the gravest complications encountered by CVIs [2].

As people grow older, venous ulcers begin to constitute a serious health problem, considering the fact that 4% of people aged over 65 suffer from them. This renders the whole issue highly topical while making possible therapeutic treatments within the ambit of regenerative medicine of considerable interest.

A number of strategies have been developed recently to treat dermal wounds resulting from chemical exposure. One of the most efficient methods used to reduce bacterial load and the incidence of sepsis is debridement of the wound [8]. Cleansing agents and topical antibiotics are also useful when seeking to reduce microbial growth and invasive infection [9].

Current literature contains numerous studies [10–12], which underline the diffusion of medication considered "advanced" and capable of producing improved clinical and economic outcomes associated with the healing of similar lesions. The notion "advanced" implies not only the use of particular products and medications, surpassing the therapeutic concept of keeping the ulcer in a "dry" environment and leaving medication on the lesion for lengthy periods of time, but also means changing wound management substantially. Advanced methodologies seem to lead to a diminution of the number of medication sessions required compared to those prescribed by traditional approaches and, theoretically speaking, a reduction in overall healing time, which also spells a reduction in costs. We have expressed ourselves in dubitative terms here because many factors of a logistic and not simply clinical nature, capable of impacting negatively or positively on the treatment opted for, are involved and can contribute to the success or failure of the therapy. One of the factors—common to acute and chronic lesions and, therefore, regardless of aetiopathogenesis—which is capable of having a positive impact on regenerative therapy is appropriate "wound bed preparation" (WBP). "Wound bed preparation" involves a detailed, coordinated and sometimes multidisciplinary management of the lesion aimed at removing all the factors, which may hamper tissue regeneration, while favouring endogenous healing, promoting cellular proliferation and the reparatory processes "triggered" by the products applied. This concept, no longer considered recent, has significantly affected the management of chronic cutaneous wounds and the results obtained.

In order to outline the principles of WBP more precisely, the English acronym TIME (tissue, infection or inflammation, moisture imbalance, epidermal margin) is used. TIME breaks up what is actually a single therapeutic process into parts, indicating the fundamental aspects to be dealt with during preparation of the wound bed.

In lesion management, WBP permits definitive elimination of all the elements that may hinder the development of granulation tissue, thus laying the foundations for effective use of innovative therapeutic tools. The purpose of advanced dressing is to create an environment ideal for proliferative cicatrisation processes, for the isolation of the wound from traumatic and infectious agents, while improving the state of the bottom of the wound and promoting maximum possible tropism of the margins and the periwound skin.

Additionally, treatment of the wound with autologous leukocytes seeded in a proangiogenic matrix and enriched with a platelet concentrate preparation has been reported to induce the release of growth factors, cytokines and chemokines, thus increasing the in situ recruitment of endothelial precursor cells and promoting the resolution of microbial infections [13]. Despite these improvements, treatment of dermal wounds has not always produced positive outcomes. Major drawbacks include the fact that the skin is a highly complex organ and is, therefore, difficult to reconstruct after injury. In actual fact, the physiological re-epithelialisation phase is a multistep process involving several cell types and molecular mechanisms, and the presence of a favourable environment for bacterial colonisation is highly undesirable [14, 15]. As a consequence, most current treatments have been palliative only, aiming mainly at accelerating healing time and limiting additional clinical complications caused by fortuitous bacterial infection. Therefore, alternative strategies are required to balance the treatment of patients, economic costs and the safety of civilians.

The main aim of regenerative medicine is to repair organs and tissues that have been damaged by pathological events and/or trauma and/or ageing in order to restore or improve their biological functions. It is a multidisciplinary field undergoing rapid growth and involving the medical, humanistic and engineering sciences, a field which endeavours to develop functional cells and substitute tissues or organs with a view to repairing, replacing or improving the biological functions lost due to congenital anomalies, trauma and illness or as a result of ageing. The increase in average life expectancy has led, actually, to the need to protract the time people spend in active employment and has made the physical and mental efficiency of older subjects mandatory, but it also implies an inevitable rise in incidences of neoplasms and pathologies that cannot always be cured by the therapies available at present. From this stems the need to develop therapies capable of replacing or regenerating organs damaged by pathological processes or traumas. Referring specifically to the present text, regenerative medicine can solve the problem of chronic vascular ulcers. Some lesions can benefit particularly from regenerative, cellulated and acellulated materials as well as biochemical supports (scaffolds) used to "trigger" granulation, repair tissue and, therefore, cover wounds.

Scaffolds, according to the definition of tissue engineering provided by the National Science, are materials that can best attend to the restoration, maintenance and improvement of the function of tissues, playing a unique role in their repair and above all, in their regeneration [16–18]. Scaffolds provide an appropriate platform for the essential provision of various factors associated with cell survival, proliferation and differentiation [19]. They can consist in synthetic or absorbable polymeric materials present in nature which may be biological, degradable or nondegradable.

The four main approaches to scaffolding include the use of ECM-secreting cell sheets; preconstituted porous scaffolds of synthetic, natural and biodegradable biomaterials; decellularised ECM scaffolds and cells enveloped in hydrogel [20].

In the field of surface-tissue regeneration, numerous grafts based on acellular dermal and epidermal scaffolds have been tested, using natural and synthetic polymers, or a combination of both, described as "effective substitutes for wound healing".

Another important area where regenerative medicine is applied is that of cell therapy, which is based on the autologous cell suspension (SCAut) technique, that is, the exploitation of cells taken from the patients themselves.

A new chapter in the history of regenerative medicine, though still very controversial and limited to specifically clinical application, is that of tissue bioengineering, that is, the use of totipotent, pluripotent and unipotent cells, potentially capable of originating, respectively, any kind of tissue, a wide range of tissues and a sole cell line; the cells chosen for cropping can come from autologous, homologous and heterologous samples. The isolation, culture and maturation of stem cells are recurred to with a view to replacing damaged tissue. Among the first mechanical and chemical processing techniques used is the in vitro cultivation of the epidermis using the "feeder-layer" methodology proposed by Rheinwald J.G. and Green H. in 1977 and the grafting of laminates of expanded in vitro keratinocytes or keratinocyte suspensions onto de-epidermised human dermis (DED) introduced by Cuono C.B. in 1987. The potential use of different types of stem cells for regenerative skin-lesion repair has recently received considerable attention [21]. "Difficult" or "stubborn" chronic wounds, characterised by extensive loss of substance and an enduring clinical history of healing and recurrence, represent one of the fields where the bioengineering of tissue may be applied and one of the discipline's main areas of challenge.

The cell lines which arouse the greatest interest at the moment are those taken from the embryo, the foetus and the umbilical cord as well as a number of adult cells like adipose-tissue-derived mesenchymal stem cells.

Several protocols have been established aimed at ensuring the resolution of wound issues by targeting different phases of the healing process, namely, control of inflammation in a suitable microenvironment, enhancement of stem-cell engraftment after implantation, efficient and terminal transdifferentiation of progenitors towards dermal lineages and the reconstruction of the vasculature system surrounding the wound [22, 23]. Mesenchymal stem cells (MSCs) have recently been proposed as a promising solution capable of enhancing the re-epithelialisation phase [24]. Studies using mouse models have shown that the intradermal injection of human MSCs or adipose-tissue-derived stromal cells (ASCs) accelerates skin-wound healing in nude mice [1]. Similarly, results of clinical trials have demonstrated the benefits derived from the employment of both autologous or heterologous MSCs, especially in chronic wounds [25–28]. Defined as adult multipotent cells, MSCs can be easily obtained from multiple sources, including adipose tissue deposits localised in different areas of the body and gathered during major and/or aesthetic surgical procedures [29, 30]. Multiple mechanisms underlying the potential ability of both populations to influence wound repair positively have been proposed; these include modulation of inflammatory states, stimulation of angiogenesis, cell proliferation and fibroblast activity, activation and enhanced migration of keratinocytes to sites of injury in a paracrine fashion, possible direct transdifferentiation of MSCs towards dermal lineage (including fibroblasts and keratinocytes) and, finally, the recruitment of host cells [25, 31, 32]. After in vivo administration, the immune tolerance generated by ASCs, defined as the ability to modulate the immune-surveillance system in the recipient, has been largely reported as their chief biological property, thus highlighting one important advantage their use brings [33, 34]. Moreover, cross communication between ASCs and inflammatory cells at the site of an injury is a major contributory factor. Soluble factors released by MSCs and ASCs, such as vascular endothelial growth factor, interleukin-6 or transforming growth factors, are known to regulate local cellular responses during cutaneous injury [24]. It has been noted that MSCs may also exert antibacterial effects at the site of a wound both by secreting an antimicrobial protein, IL-37, directly and by influencing immune-system phagocytosis positively [24, 35]. The proliferative and transdifferentiative potential of MSCs has been highlighted also in tissue-engineering-based applications, specifically with regard to skin graft reconstruction, where MSCs are employed either alone, as a feeder layer for keratinocytes or seeded in combination with gelatine-, collagen-/chitosan- or fibrin polymer-based scaffolds [36–38]. Of note among suitable substrates, synthetic polymers have been shown to possess considerable ability to absorb and transport fluids as well as provide protection against bacterial exposure [39]. Other methods used to deliver MSCs to the wound site include injection and local or systemic administration of a range of conveyers such as scaffolds, matrices and human amniotic membrane grafts [40–43].

2. Novel strategies developed at Rome's *Sapienza* University

Despite considerable improvements in the employment of ASCs and MSCs in skin-regenerative procedures, their current use is limited because of the presence of foetal bovine serum (FBS) in the cultures during their ex vivo expansion. According to the European Union's Good Manufacturing Practice (GMP) guidelines, the employment of FBS is to be discouraged, as it is a potential source of zoonoses [29, 44, 45]. In the light of this, platelet lysate (PL), a haemoderivative enriched with soluble mitogenic factors [29, 44, 46], represents a superior alternative to FBS. Reported to enhance the biological stem-cell properties of ASCs, such as proliferation, clonogenic capacity and migration [28, 46, 47], PL has been also been recently shown to be capable of promoting ASC's pluripotency and being committed to specific phenotypes [46–49]. Interestingly, PL, manufactured in injectable form or gel [8, 9, 13, 14], embedded in scaffolds or incorporated in nanoparticles, also represents a widely investigated clinical strategy deemed to accelerate wound healing in chronic ocular and diabetic dermal ulcers. Because of the large amounts of cytokines and growth factors contained in PL, it presents multiple and significant advantages if applied locally to skin wounds when seeking enhancement of angiogenesis and fibroblast migration, restoration of collagen synthesis and reduction of oxidative stress [46]. In addition, it has been demonstrated that PL is capable of re-establishing skin integrity efficiently [50].

Recently, a GMP-compliant PL (Mesengen™, Pub. No. WO/2013/042095) has been developed as an adjuvant for culturing human ASCs, endothelial progenitor cells and fibroblasts [29, 46, 51, 52].

The Mesengen™ generation method has been standardised and optimised so as to determine the amounts of cytokines and growth factors in the preparation. Importantly, potential fungi, viruses and bacteria known to contaminate human haemoderivatives are avoided by rapidly inactivating the Mesengen™ by means of a combination of a photochemical agent and UV radiation. A summary of the basic steps in the preparation of PL is provided in **Figure 1**. It is worth noting that researchers at *Sapienza* have exploited the biological and molecular properties of Mesengen™ by concurrently establishing a standardised protocol (**Figure 2**) to isolate and expand ex vivo ASCs from alternative fat deposits like the mediastinum (**Figure 3**) [29, 47]. Recent studies on Mesengen™ carried out by our team have also elucidated its ability to influence the commitment of ASCs by inducing epigenetic modifications [47] as well as positively altering the in vitro microenvironment by decreasing oxidative stress [46]. These studies highlight the ability of PL to boost the biological and functional properties of mesenchymal-like cell populations. Therefore, it is plausible that the combination of Mesengen™ and ASCs or other progenitor-cell populations might be employed successfully to target wound repair and regeneration. Furthermore, PL has been reported to maintain its properties either as a liquid formulation or frozen, highlighting an important clinical advantage. In the future, this approach might be considered complementary to routine strategies developed at Rome's *Sapienza* University, where a centre of excellence for

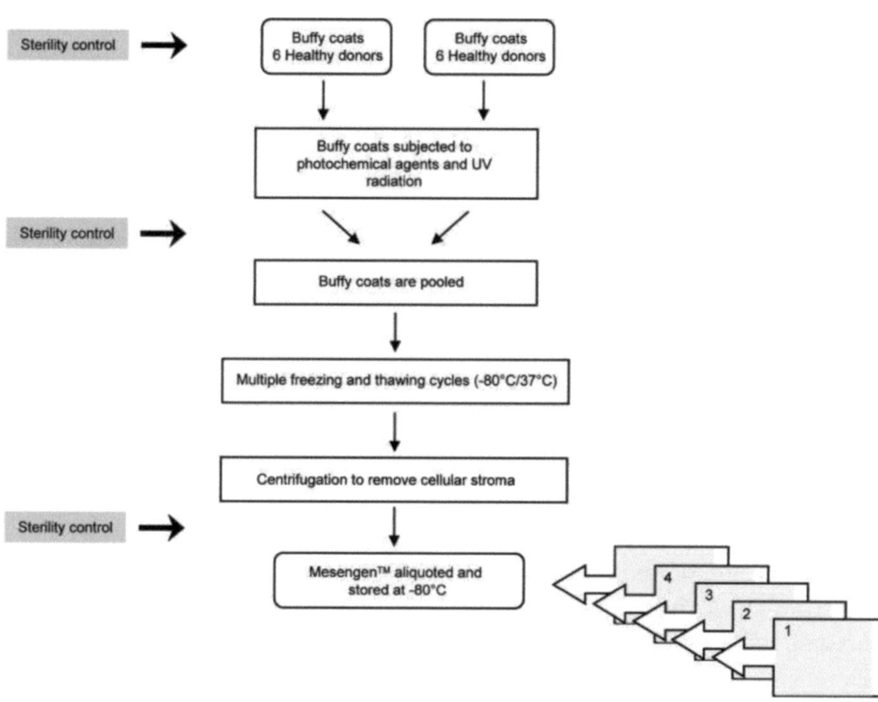

Figure 1. Overview of the major steps in the manufacturing of platelet lysate (Mesengen™).

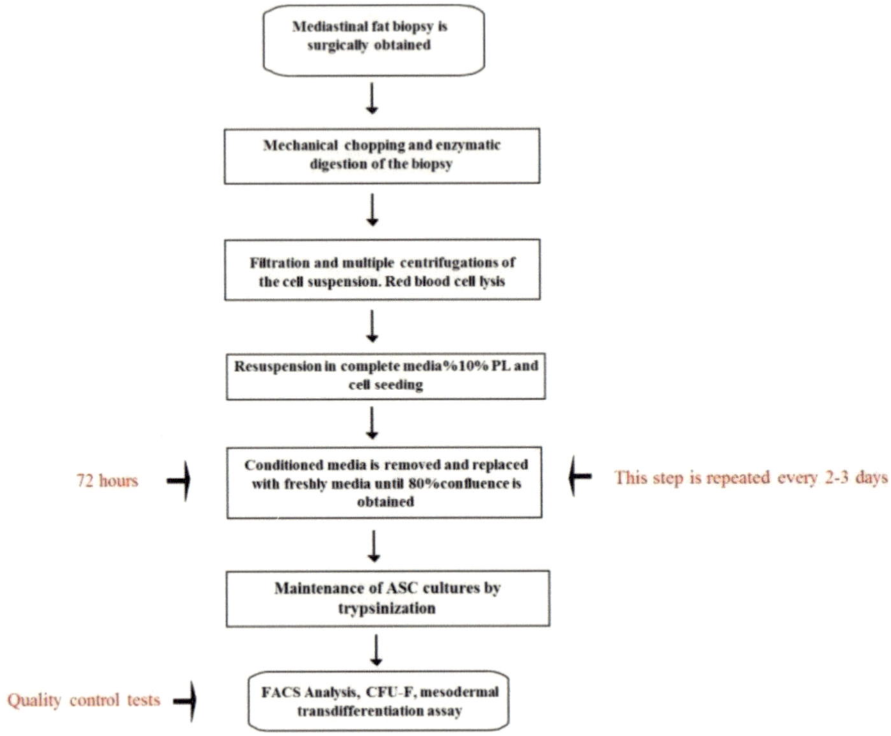

Figure 2. Flow diagram showing the optimization and standardisation phases to isolate and expand in vitro ASCs derived from the mediastinal fat depots.

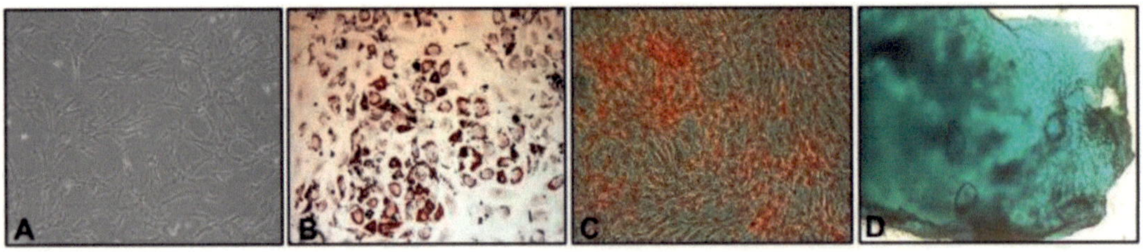

Figure 3. Optical image of ASCs at passage 3 cultured in PL and displaying the typically spindle-shaped morphology (A). Note that platelet lysate is able to preserve the mesodermal transdifferentiation of ASCs towards the adipogenic (B), osteogenic (C) and chondrogenic (D) lineages. Magnification 5×.

in vitro culturing of skin substitutes exists already, providing the treatment of a wide range of dermal disorders, such as burns, chronic ulcers, giant congenital melanocytic nevi and even the reconstruction of epithelial mucosa [53–58]. Specifically, the epithelial "organoid" developed by our research group is based on a combination of transplanted autologous cells seeded in biomimetic scaffolds. This methodology has been successfully established, is clinically available at several hospitals collaborating with *Sapienza* and has already been shown to significantly reduce hospitalisation time and costs [59].

Our group's experience of advanced dressings and dermal substitutes over the years during treatment of patients with acute and chronic ulcers of multifactorial origin (arteriopathic, phlebopathic, immunological and traumatic) produced a study based on chronic arteriopathic patients, the results of which were published in the article "Wounds Difficult to Heal: An Effective Treatment Strategy" [60]. There we highlighted the fact that recognition of the aetiology of a skin lesion and the correction of the pathophysiological conditions that determine and support it are the assumption and "step" fundamental to the success of local treatment. It also emerged that a "standard", univocal treatment applicable to all and every kind of wound does not exist. Appropriate local treatment involves a combination of multiple medications, products and devices demanding respect of their timing and guarantees regarding their ongoing management.

In a very recent study we focused, instead, on the treatment of chronic phlebostatic ulcers. This study was conducted at the Department of Surgical Sciences of Rome's *Sapienza* University between October 2016 and March 2018.

The purpose of that study was to assess the efficacy of using dermic substitutes when treating patients suffering from chronic skin ailments due to and sustained by venous insufficiency.

This examination took parameters like the following into consideration: reduction of the size of the wound and improvement of quality of life (QoL) as expressed subjectively, on the basis of a number of elective factors.

2.1. Materials and methodology

The study sample involved 13 patients suffering from chronic venous insufficiency (CVI) and postthrombotic syndrome, 5 of whom were also affected by pronounced varicosity, with incontinence of the saphenous-femoral junction and protracted reflux of the great saphenous vein (GSV). Ten of the patients, before proceeding to treatment with dermal substitutes, had been treated surgically for phlebopathy: six had undergone "stripping" of the GSV (of the "short" in two cases); two patients underwent crossectomy due to recurrence accompanied by inguinal-crural cavernoma; in five of the patients, the "feeder" veins were identified and linked, two of them as treatment in isolation (the other three in association with treatment for varices); and in the remaining three cases, the only management, besides local intervention, was elastic compression.

Eight other patients, initially included in the study, were excluded later on because of the impossibility of proceeding with the therapy in the manner set down by the team's protocol.

The patients were chosen according to the following criteria:

- They had to be aged 50 or over.
- They had to present with chronic venous insufficiency, accompanied or not by varicosity of the great saphenous vein.
- Their ulcers had to have an area no greater than 20 cm^2.

The presence of undermined margins was an indication of treatment with infiltrations of platelet concentrate (PC) or mesenchymal ("regenerate") cells.

The presence of wound contamination was a criterion dictating temporary exclusion although patients were readmitted to the study once this condition was resolved.

All the patients provided informed consent, having evaluated compliance with the proviso requiring their participation for the entire duration of the treatment.

The criteria for exclusion were:

- Exposure of bone or nerve, ligament or aponeurotic tissue
- The presence of immunohaematological disease
- Neoplasms and chemoradiotherapy treatment
- The use of anti-inflammatory drugs, immunosuppressant and cytostatic drugs and oral anticoagulants for severe comorbidity (chronic renal failure requiring dialysis, congestive cardiomyopathies, liver failure) and concomitant arteriopathies (mixed genesis of the ulcer)
- Poor/low self-sufficiency and/or lack of family or caregiving support, a factor mandatory for participation in the study

All the patients were assessed preliminarily by an ecocolor Doppler examination and other tests useful for inclusion/exclusion in the study. The ultrasound check sought confirmation of proximal saphenous-femoral valve incontinence and/or of saphenous perforators; in cases with referred stripping, it looked for the presence of accessory saphenoids or lapses of the cross (cavernoma) and, as far as deep circulation was concerned, the patency and absence of reflux with severe incontinence. These data, together with an objective examination, were the criteria adopted for preliminary surgical treatment and for the choice of local treatment recurring to one or more of the four dermal substitutes foreseen by the study, in some cases in sequence and/or in combination.

All the patients underwent local "wound bed preparation", requiring different lengths of time for different patients. WBP was followed by the applications of dermal substitutes. The dermal substances used were autologous or homologous platelet concentrates (PC); "micro-grafts" of autologous mesenchymal origin ("Rigenera Activa" System); "HyaloMatrix" PA Tissue Reconstruction Matrix (Fidia), on a hyaluronic acid base; and "Integra" Dermal Regeneration Template (LifeSciences Corp.), on a collagen base.

For the preparation and application of platelet concentrate, both from whole autologous and homologous blood, a specific protocol is followed: in the former case, the donor's personal data are recorded in the Blood Transfusion Service's management system (Emonet) which assigns an identification number to the donation; the blood collected is contained in a bag containing ACD (citrate glucose) anticoagulant, and the CP is produced by recurring to two centrifugation cycles: the first of these at a low rpm rate (210 g × 10 minutes) to obtain platelet-rich plasma and eliminate the red blood cells and leucocytes and the second at a higher rpm rate (2000 g × 15 minutes) to concentrate the platelets by eliminating the depleted plasma.

The platelet concentrate should be 1 × 10^6/ml ± 20%. All the preparations thus obtained are checked for the biological validation required by law; a blood count is carried out as well as a microbiological test to verify their sterile state.

To keep the CP, sterile containers are used, each dose is rendered identifiable by its donation code; the type of the blood component and the expiry date of the product are also provided. All production and packaging procedures are carried out in aseptic conditions, in a sterile-welded closed circuit or under a laminar flow hood during the phases when it is necessary to open the circuit. The pouches containing the CP are deposited in protective cases with labels bearing the same data as those indicated on each dose and stored in a freezer at −80°C.

In cases where the patient's clinical and/or haematological conditions, the size of the ulcer and the number of medications to be carried out do not permit harvesting of autologous blood, umbilical cord or fractional blood from an adult donor is used.

To produce CP from umbilical-cord blood, cord blood units deemed unsuitable for the haematopoietic stem-cell transplant bank are availed of. Cord units are considered suitable for the production of CP if they meet the foreseen regulatory requirements and are endorsed by specific informed consent as prescribed for their use. The production method used is the same as that described for CP obtained from whole autologous blood. For the treatment units compatible with the blood group of the candidate for treatment are used.

For the production of homologous fractional-blood CP, the blood component is prepared by collecting one or more units of single buffy-coat platelets and a bag of freshly frozen plasma, fractioned with blood donations free of transmissible viral diseases. The final platelet concentration should always be 1 × 10^6/ml ± 20%. The CP thus obtained is stored in the manner described above.

On the day of the treatment, the platelet concentrate is defrosted and activated by adding 10% calcium gluconate (0.3 ml of Ca per ml of CP): in practice, 10 ml of the CP are placed on a sterile plate and mixed with 3 ml of calcium gluconate. The solution, stirred gently and left to rest for 10′–15′, forms the platelet gel to be placed on a sterile gauze and placed directly on the ulcer, making sure that it covers the entire area of the lesion.

CP gel was used on seven patients, in compliance with our protocol of one application every 4 days for a maximum of 8 weeks (for a total of 14 dressings), in three cases homologous CP (with low Hb values found upon haemochromocytometric examination), and in four cases, autologous CPs (blood sampling of 410 cc) were considered sufficient for the applications foreseen.

In six patients, the "regenerate" system was used, with one application every 4–5 days, for a maximum of four applications, over a total of about 20 days; in three of these cases, the treatment was used in association with and subsequent to CP, because it had not been possible to prolong the application of CP for the entire 8-week period (in the case of two patients) or because, at the end of the maximum number of 14 applications of the platelet concentrate, a completely unsatisfactory result was obtained (in the case of one patient); in the other three cases, after treatment with Rigenera (for a maximum of four applications over a total period of 3 weeks), Thiersch thin dermo-epidermal grafts were carried out.

The "Hyalomatrix PA" dermal substitute was applied to one patient and the "Integra" dermal substitute to two patients. This choice was made when the patients presented a particularly "lively" tissue granulation phase and the size of the lesion was close to the 20-cm^2 limit (the size of the product used being 5 × 5 cm). These patients were medicated every 3–4 days, according to the modalities set down in the technical data sheet, until the product was absorbed. On the basis of our protocol, all 13 patients were medicated every 3–7 days, monitored and observed for a total period of 8 weeks.

At the beginning of the study and at the end of the 8-week treatment period, in order to assess its efficacy, the following parameters were considered and used to define the results:

a. The extent of the reduction of the size of the ulcer

b. Patients' subjective perception of pain according to the NRS numerical scale, a scale of values from 0 to 10, where 0 corresponds to absence of pain and 10 to the maximum level of pain perceived

c. Quality of life, this too based on patients' subjective judgement, with reference to night-time rest, itching, pain, need for painkillers, wet impregnation of the wound, bad smell and hygiene of the wound.

All these are elements that strongly impact upon life relationships and recovery of habitual daily activities, including work. A numerical value was attributed to each parameter, used together with all the others and employed to calculate overall average values.

Our study's 13-patient sample, as shown in **Table 1**, included 6 females and 7 males, whose ages ranged between 65 and 77 (for a mean age of 71); at the beginning of the treatment, the maximum average diameter of the wounds was 5 cm, a range of between 3 and 6.5 cm.

2.2. Results

During the 8 weeks of treatment, some signs of improvement were observed in all patients: appearance in the wound bed of small islands of granulation tissue, superficialization of the bottom of the ulcer and growth of margin tissue. During the first 30 days, a reduction in over 25% of the area of the wound was observed; a reduction in more than 50% was observed in the 10 patients who underwent preliminary surgical treatment. In the remaining three cases, that is, the patients subjected to elastic-compressive bandaging only, there was an average reduction in 45% by the end of the 8 week.

The first four patients treated with CP, obtained on average a 57.5% reduction of the wound's maximum diameter. The three patients treated with a combination of CP and Rigenera achieved

Diameters of the ulcers during the treatment				
	Beginning (cm)	**End (cm)**	**Reduction (%)**	**P-value**
Average value	5.0	2.1	56.9	0.001
Standard deviation	1.1	0.6	7.2	

Table 1. Variations of the diameters of the lesions from the beginning to the end of the treatment.

Pain (numerical rating scale)				
	Time 0	**4 weeks**	**8 weeks**	**P-value**
Average value	6.9	4.3	3.2	0.001
Standard deviation	1.3	1.3	1.2	

Table 2. Variations of the "pain" from the beginning to the end of the treatment.

	Aggravated (A)	Unmodified (B)	Slightly ameliorated (C)	Clearly ameliorated (D)
Nocturnal rest	0 pts.	3 pts.	3 pts.	7 pts.
Itch	0 pts.	3 pts.	2 pts.	8 pts.
Pain	0 pts.	0 pts.	4 pts.	9 pts.
Need of analgesics	0 pts.	0 pts.	3 pts.	10 pts.
Mobilisation	0 pts.	3 pts.	3 pts.	7 pts.
Foul odour	0 pts.	2 pts.	2 pts.	9 pts.
Restart of daily activities	0 pts.	2 pts.	4 pts.	7 pts.
Social and relational life	0 pts.	1 pts.	3 pts.	9 pts.
Total (average values)	0	1.75	3	8.25

Table 3. Variations in QoL, stated by the patients.

a 60% reduction, a result just marginally better than the previous one; but one needs to keep in mind that these presented graver lesions are harder to manage than those of other patients. The three other cases, treated with Rigenera and a Thiersch graft, achieved a 55% reduction in the ulcer's greatest diameter. The two patients treated with the "Integra" dermic substitute obtained a 52.5% diminution of the wound's maximum diameter. Finally, the patient treated with the "Hyalomatrix" skin substitute achieved a 60% reduction. On the whole, by the end of the observation period, the average reduction of the lesion for 13 patients was 57%.

All the patients during the period of treatment reported a gradual reduction in pain, from an initial average of 7 on the NRS scale (range 9–5) to an average of 3 (range 6–2) at the end of the period (see graph 1). On the whole, the average reduction of perceived pain dropped by 4 points on the NRS numerical scale.

At the end of the 8-week treatment period, an average of 8.25 out of 13 patients reported improvements in their quality of life, a spontaneous reduction in pain, a lessening of itchiness and secretion, lower incidence of bad odour with a recovery of functional capacity and almost complete resumption of habitual everyday activities. The results are summarised in **Tables 1–3**.

It needs to be pointed out that during the treatment period no superinfections of the wounds requiring interruption of the therapy arose nor did other secondary complications associated with the use of the products occur.

3. Perspectives and conclusions

Despite advances in wound-healing treatment, dermal tissue still remains a difficult organ to regenerate. Our work in the future will probably consist in multistep approaches rather than in single repair strategies, which have proven to be only partially efficacious. Future strategies will, most likely, combine stem-cell properties, next-generation scaffolds or vehicles (i.e. nanoparticles) and growth factors or supplements, like PL. Improvements in our understanding of skin biology and the physiological processes of wound repair should permit us to interpret healing microenvironments better. To achieve our final goal, we will be required to design more personalised therapies, taking into account genetic variability, wound types as well as patients' clinical and metabolic features.

It is not possible, in actual fact, to reach definitive conclusions given the variability of the factors capable of influencing the outcome of therapy and the difficulty of rendering populations of patients treated totally homogeneous. Furthermore, this aspect also emerges from the field's latest literature [60–62], being the only source available at present (since there are no definitive guidelines available). In addition, this kind of patient is not always willing to follow the lengthy periods of treatment often deemed necessary or comply with the temporal parameters the cure requires. Due to certain events like intercurrent pathologies, hospitalisation or logistic problems, exclusion from a study sample may become inevitable. For these reasons we consider the results obtained here as preliminary.

- Having said this, we are in a position to assert that skin substitutes are capable of determining a clinical improvement of chronic ulcers caused by pathologies of the vein when, after use of traditional medication, or accurate advanced debridement, the condition of the ulcer is such that regeneration of tissue is feasible. Indeed, timing seems essential for prescriptions as well: both precocious and tardy dressing may nullify the effectiveness of a treatment, jeopardising the outcome.
- The integrated use of different compounds can prove useful, especially in relation to the long periods often needed to obtain complete healing. Every single treatment may determine partial, even substantial, improvement but may fail to cure the lesion completely: there is no "ideal" medication for all ulcers, just as there is no "ideal" medication applicable to all the developmental stages of an ulcer.
- The specific treatment of comorbidities and restoration of a satisfactory level of nutrition are of great importance when pursuing positive outcomes of any local therapy, though chances of complete success are related mainly to a correct diagnosis regarding the origin of the ulcer and, above all, the removal, surgical if necessary, of factors impeding recovery: "The beginning of healing lies in knowledge of the ailment" (*Epicurus, 341–270 BCE*).
- Dermal substitutes have become, therefore, part of the modern concept of the multidisciplinary approach to the treatment of chronic skin lesions, in particular, the management of wounds that are less likely to heal availing of standard therapy. They represent a valid therapeutic "step", whether used alone or in combination, also considering the potential clinical benefits demonstrated and the low percentage of complications related to their use.

http://dx.doi.org/10.5772/intechopen.81791

- The use of these substitutes *does* cause a reduction in the size of ulcers, improving, above all, the quality of life of patients. One notices, in particular, a reduction in levels of pain and resumption of habitual everyday activities.
- The choice of the best therapy, from among the different options available, also depends on the physician's ability to perceive the one most suitable for the type and characteristics of the patient and the availability of his/her caregivers.

In conclusion, the numerous technological opportunities made available by regenerative medicine, including advanced dressings and dermal substitutes, if used correctly and following a multidisciplinary approach if necessary, seem to offer advantages in terms of clinical efficacy, patients' quality of life and, last but not least, also in terms of healthcare costs.

Acknowledgements

This work was supported by Ateneo ("Sapienza" University of Rome).

Conflicts of interest

The authors declare no conflicts of interest.

Author details

Raffaele Capoano[1]*, Rita Businaro[2], Besar Kolce[1], Andrea Biancucci[1], Silvia Izzo[1], Lidia De Felice[3] and Bruno Salvati[1]

*Address all correspondence to: raffaele.capoano@uniroma1.it

1 Department of Surgical Sciences, "Sapienza" University of Rome, Italy

2 Department of Medico-Surgical Sciences and Biotechnologies, "Sapienza" University of Rome, Italy

3 Department of Molecular Medicine, "Sapienza" University of Rome, Italy

References

[1] Rodriguez J, Boucher F, Lequeux C, et al. Intradermal injection of human adipose-derived stem cells accelerates skin wound healing in nude mice. Stem Cell Research & Therapy. 2015;**6**:241

[2] Hellström A, Nilsson C, Nilsson A, Fagerström C. Leg ulcers in older people: A national study addressing variation in diagnosis, pain and sleep disturbance. BMC Geriatrics. 2016;**16**:25

[3] Fried LP, Tangen CM, Walston J, Newman AB, Hirsch C, Gottdiener J, et al. Frailty in older adults: Evidence for a phenotype. Journal of Gerontology. Series A, Biological Sciences and Medical Sciences. 2001;**56**(3):M146-M156

[4] Scuderi N, Ceccarelli S, Onesti MG, et al. Human adipose-derived stromal cells for cell-based therapies in the treatment of systemic sclerosis. Cell Transplantation. 2013; **22**:779-795

[5] Maddox D. Effects of venous leg ulceration on patients' quality of life. Nursing Standard. 2012;**26**(38):42-49

[6] Suthar M, Gupta S, Bukhari S, Ponemone VJ. Treatment of chronic non-healing ulcers using autologous platelet rich plasma: A case series. Biomedical Science. 2017;**24**(1):16

[7] Agale SV. Chronic leg ulcers: Epidemiology, aetiopathogenesis, and management. Ulcers. 2013; Art ID 413604. DOI: 10.1155/2013/413604

[8] Sandri G, Bonferoni MC, Rossi S, et al. Platelet lysate embedded scaffolds for skin regeneration. Expert Opinion on Drug Delivery. 2015;**12**:525-545

[9] Fontana F, Mori M, Riva F, et al. Platelet lysate-modified porous silicon microparticles for enhanced cell proliferation in wound healing applications. ACS Applied Materials & Interfaces. 2016;**8**:988-996

[10] Treadwell T, Sabolinski ML, Skornicki M, Parsons NB. Comparative effectiveness of a bioengineered living cellular construct and cryopreserved cadaveric skin allograft for the treatment of venous leg ulcers in a real-world setting. Advances in Wound Care (New Rochelle). 2018;**7**(3):69-76

[11] Mostow EN, Haraway GD, Dalsing M, Hodde JP, King D. OASIS Venus Ulcer Study Group. Effectiveness of an extracellular matrix graft (OASIS Wound Matrix) in the treatment of chronic leg ulcers: A randomized clinical trial. Journal of Vascular Surgery. 2005;**41**(5):837-843

[12] Edwards H, Finlayson K, Courtney M, Graves N, Gibb M, Parker C. Health service pathways for patients with chronic leg ulcers: Identifying effective pathways for facilitation of evidence based wound care. BMC Health Services Research. 2013;**13**:86

[13] Fabi S, Sundaram H. The potential of topical and injectable growth factors and cytokines for skin rejuvenation. Facial Plastic Surgery. 2014;**30**:157-171

[14] Sun BK, Siprashvili Z, Khavari PA. Advances in skin grafting and treatment of cutaneous wounds. Science. 2014;**346**:941-945

[15] Eming SA, Martin P, Tomic-Canic M. Wound repair and regeneration: Mechanisms, signaling, and translation. Science Translational Medicine. 2014;**6**:265,sr6

[16] Chaudhari AA, Vig K, Baganizi DR, Sahu R, Dixit S, Dennis V, et al. Future prospects for scaffolding methods and biomaterials in skin tissue engineering: A review. International Journal of Molecular Sciences. 2016;**17**(12):1974

[17] Nyame TT, Chiang HA, Leavitt T, Ozambela M, Orgill DP. Tissue-engineered skin substitutes. Plastic and Reconstructive Surgery. 2015;**136**:1379-1388

[18] Suresh DH, Suryanarayan S, Sarvainamurthy S, et al. Treatment of a non-healing diabetic foot ulcer with platelet rich plasma. Journal of Cutaneous and Aesthetic Surgery. 2014;**7**(4):229-231

[19] AS1 M, DJ2 M. Regenerative medicine: Current therapies and future directions. Proceedings of the National Academy of Sciences of the United States of America. 2015; **112**(47):14452-14459

[20] Eming SA, Krieg T, Davidson JM. Inflammation in wound repair: Molecular and cellular mechanisms. The Journal of Investigative Dermatology. 2007;**127**(3):514-525

[21] Ojeh N, Pastar I, Tomic-Canic M, et al. Stem cells in skin regeneration, wound healing, and their clinical applications. International Journal of Molecular Sciences. 2015;**16**: 25476-25501

[22] Caramella CM, Sandri G, Rossi S, et al. New therapeutic platforms for the treatment of epithelial and cutaneous lesions. Current Drug Delivery. 2013;**10**:18-31

[23] Kasuya A, Tokura Y. Attempts to accelerate wound healing. Journal of Dermatological Science. 2014;**76**:169-172

[24] Li X, Hamada T, Ohata C. Potential mesenchymal stem cell therapy for skin diseases. Experimental Dermatology. 2013;**22**:515-516

[25] Wu Y, Chen L, Scott PG, et al. Mesenchymal stem cells enhance wound healing through differentiation and angiogenesis. Stem Cells. 2007;**25**:2648-2659

[26] Isakson M, de Blacam C, Whelan D, et al. Mesenchymal stem cells and cutaneous wound healing: Current evidence and future potential. Stem Cells International. 2015;**2015**: 831095

[27] Kruglikov IL, Scherer PE. Dermal adipocytes: From irrelevance to metabolic targets? Trends in Endocrinology and Metabolism. 2016;**27**:1-10

[28] Chen D, Hao H, Fu X, Han XW. Insight into reepithelialization: How do mesenchymal stem cells perform? Stem Cells International. 2016;**2016**:6120173

[29] Siciliano C, Ibrahim M, Scafetta G, et al. Optimization of the isolation and expansion method of human mediastinal-adipose tissue derived mesenchymal stem cells with virally inactivated GMP-grade platelet lysate. Cytotechnology. 2015;**67**:165-174

[30] Bastianelli D, Siciliano C, Puca R, et al. Influence of Egr-1 in cardiac tissue-derived mesenchymal stem cells in response to glucose variations. BioMed Research International. 2014;**2014**:254793

[31] Sasaki M, Abe R, Fujita Y, et al. Mesenchymal stem cells are recruited into wounded skin and contribute to wound repair by transdifferentiation into multiple skin cell type. Journal of Immunology. 2008;**180**:2581-2587

[32] Ozpur MA, Guneren E, Canter HI, et al. Generation of skin tissue using adipose tissue-derived stem cells. Plastic and Reconstructive Surgery. 2016;**137**:134-143

[33] Vériter S, Wivine A, Aouassar N, et al. Human adipose-derived mesenchymal stem cells in cell therapy: Safety and feasibility in different "hospital exemption" clinical applications. PLoS One. 2015;**10**:e0139566

[34] Condé-Green A, Marano AA, Lee ES, et al. Fat grafting and adipose-derived regenerative cells in burn wound healing and scarring: A systematic review of the literature. Plastic and Reconstructive Surgery. 2016;**137**:302-312

[35] Krasnodembskaya A, Song Y, Fang X, et al. Antibacterial effect of human mesenchymal stem cells is mediated in part from secretion of the antimicrobial peptide LL-37. Stem Cells. 2010;**28**:2229-2238

[36] Fierro FA, O'Neal AJ, Beegle JR, et al. Hypoxic pre-conditioning increases the infiltration of endothelial cells into scaffolds for dermal regeneration pre-seeded with mesenchymal stem cells. Frontiers in Cell and Development Biology. 2015;**3**:68

[37] Wahl EA, Fierro FA, Peavy TR, et al. In vitro evaluation of scaffolds for the delivery of mesenchymal stem cells to wounds. BioMed Research International. 2015;**2015**:108571

[38] Rodrigues C, De Assis AM, Moura DJ, et al. New therapy of skin repair combining adipose-derived mesenchymal stem cells with sodium carboxymethylcellulose scaffold in a pre-clinical rat model. PLoS One. 2 May 2014;**9**(5):e96241

[39] Gomathysankar S, Halim AS, Yaacob NS. Proliferation of keratinocytes induced by adipose derived stem cells on a chitosan scaffold and its role in wound healing, a review. Archives of Plastic Surgery. 2014;**41**:452-457

[40] Gould LJ. Topical collagen-based biomaterials for chronic wounds: Rationale and clinical application. Advances in Wound Care (New Rochelle). 2016;**5**:19-31

[41] Oyarzun-Ampuero F, Vidal A, Concha M, et al. Secretory profiles and wound healing effects of human amniotic fluid-derived mesenchymal stem cells. Stem Cells and Development. 2010;(6):887-902

[42] Sánchez-Sánchez R, Brena-Molina A, Martínez-López V, et al. Generation of two biological wound dressings as a potential delivery system of human adipose-derived mesenchymal stem cells. ASAIO Journal. 2015;**61**:718-725

[43] Chimenti I, Gaetani R, Forte E, et al. Serum and supplement optimization for EU GMP-compliance in cardiospheres cell culture. Journal of Cellular and Molecular Medicine. 2014;**18**:624-634

[44] Committee for Medicinal Products for Human Use (CHMP). Guideline on the Use of Bovine Serum in the Manufacture of Human Biological Medicinal Products. 2013 EMA/CHMP/BWP/457920/2012 rev 1

[45] Carducci A, Scafetta G, Siciliano C, et al. GMP-grade platelet lysate enhances proliferation and migration of tenon fibroblasts. Frontiers in Bioscience (Elite Edition). 2016;**8**:84-99

[46] Siciliano C, Chimenti I, Bordin A, et al. The potential of GMP-compliant platelet lysate to induce a permissive state for cardiovascular transdifferentiation in human mediastinal adipose tissue-derived mesenchymal stem cells. BioMed Research International. 2015;**2015**:162439

[47] Keating A. Mesenchymal stromal cells. Current Opinion in Hematology. 2006;**13**:419-425

[48] Zuk PA, Zhu M, Mizuno H, et al. Multilineage cells from human adipose tissue: Implications for cell-based therapies. Tissue Engineering. 2001;**7**:211-228

[49] Lima AC, Mano JF, Concheiro A, Alvarez-Lorenzo C. Fast and mild strategy, using superhydrophobic surfaces, to produce collagen/platelet lysate gel beads for skin regeneration. Stem Cell Reviews. 2015;**11**:161-179

[50] Tasev D, van Wijhe MH, Weijers EM, et al. Long-term expansion in platelet lysate increases growth of peripheral blood-derived endothelial-colony forming cells and their growth factor-induced sprouting capacity. PLoS One. 2015;**10**:e0129935

[51] Mirabet V, Solves P, Miñana MD, et al. Human platelet lysate enhances the proliferative activity of cultured human fibroblast-like cells from different tissues. Cell and Tissue Banking. 2008;**9**:1-10

[52] Onesti G, Carella S, Ceccarelli S, et al. The use of human adipose-derived stem cells in the treatment of physiological and pathological vulvar dystrophies. Stem Cells International. 2016;**2016**:2561461

[53] Benedetti Panici P, Maffucci D, Ceccarelli S, et al. Autologous in vitro cultured vaginal tissue for vaginoplasty in women with Mayer-Rokitansky-Küster-Hauser syndrome: Anatomic and functional results. Journal of Minimally Invasive Gynecology. 2015;**22**:205-211

[54] Nodale C, Vescarelli E, D'Amici S, et al. Characterization of human vaginal mucosa cells for autologous in vitro cultured vaginal tissue transplantation in patients with MRKH syndrome. BioMed Research International. 2014;**2014**:201518

[55] Nodale C, Ceccarelli S, Giuliano M, et al. Gene expression profile of patients with MayerRokitansky-Küster-Hauser syndrome: New insights into the potential role of developmental pathways. PLoS One. 2014;**9**:e91010

[56] Fioramonti P, Onesti MG, Marchese C, et al. Autologous cultured melanocytes in vitiligo treatment comparison of two techniques to prepare the recipient site: Erbium-doped yttrium aluminum garnet laser versus dermabrasion. Dermatologic Surgery. 2012;**38**:809-812

[57] Mancino R, Aiello F, Ceccarelli S, et al. Autologous conjunctival epithelium transplantation and scleral patch graft for postlensectomy wound leakage in Marfan syndrome. European Journal of Ophthalmology. 2012;**22**:830-833

[58] Gurtner GC, Werner S, Barrandon Y, et al. Wound repair and regeneration. Nature. 2008;**453**:314-321

[59] Businaro R, Corsi M, Di Raimo T, Marasco S, Laskin DL, Salvati B, et al. Multidisciplinary approaches to stimulate wound healing. Annals of the New York Academy of Sciences. 2016;**1378**(1):137-142

[60] Oliveira MG, Abbade LPF, Miot HA, Ferreira RR, Deffune E. Pilot study of homologous platelet gel in venous ulcers. Anais Brasileiros de Dermatologia. 2017;**92**(4):499-504

[61] Frykberg RG, Driver VR, Carman D, Lucero B, Borris-Hale C, Fylling CP, et al. Chronic wounds treated with a physiologically relevant concentration of platelet-rich plasma gel: A prospective case series. Ostomy/Wound Management. 2010;**56**:36-44

[62] Capoano R, Businaro R, Tesori MC, Donello C, Lombardo F, Lo Vasco VR, et al. Wounds difficult to heal: An effective treatment strategy. Current Vascular Pharmacology. 2017; **15**(6):582-588

Chapter 14

The Impact of Biofilm Formation on Wound Healing

Rafael A. Mendoza, Ji-Cheng Hsieh and
Robert D. Galiano

Additional information is available at the end of the chapter

http://dx.doi.org/10.5772/intechopen.85020

Abstract

Chronic wounds represent an important challenge for wound care and are universally colonized by bacteria. These bacteria can form biofilm as a survival mechanism that confers the ability to resist environmental stressors and antimicrobials due to a variety of reasons, including low metabolic activity. Additionally, the exopolymeric substance (EPS) contained in biofilm acts as a mechanical barrier to immune system cells, leading to collateral damage in the surrounding tissue as well as chronic inflammation, which eventually will delay healing of the wound. This chapter will discuss current knowledge on biofilm formation, its presence in acute and chronic wounds, how biofilm affects antibiotic resistance and tolerance, as well as the wound healing process. We will also discuss proposed methods to eliminate biofilm and improve wound healing despite its presence, including basic science and clinical studies regarding these matters.

Keywords: biofilm, chronic wounds, delayed healing, exopolymeric substance, slime, extracellular matrix

1. Introduction

Intact skin provides a protective barrier to bacterial invasion. Any wound comprises a break in this epidermal barrier, allowing microbial invasion into deeper layers.

Along with hypoxia/poor perfusion, ischemia-reperfusion injury, and inadequate offloading or compression therapy, microbial infection is one of the most significant causes of delay in healing [1–3].

Over the last few years, bacterial biofilms in general and their role in chronic wounds have been the subject of intense research. Biofilms have been reported to be present in 60% [4] to

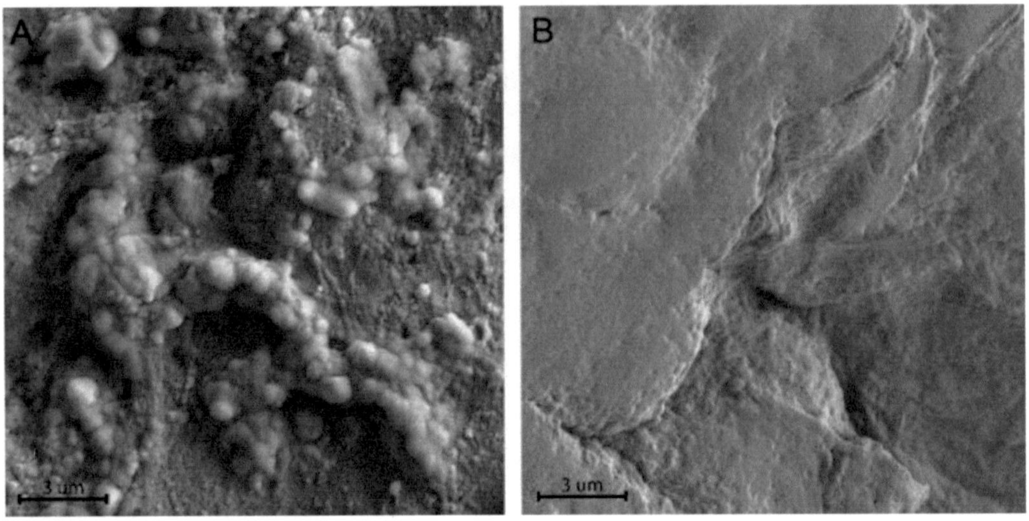

Figure 1. Representative scanning electron microscopy of wounds on mice dorsal skin. (A) Inoculated wound with *S. aureus* showed aggregates encased in EPS matrix. (B) Non-inoculated wound without EPS (image from Nguyen et al. [10], with permission).

80% [5] of chronic wounds, and a recent meta-analysis confirms their presence in 78.2% of chronic wounds [2]. Therefore, biofilms have been categorized as an important factor in most chronic non-healing skin wounds [6].

Non-healing or poorly healing wounds affect close to 25 million people in the US [7], more than 7% of its population, while reports from the UK [8] predict that 1–2% of the population in developed countries will experience a chronic wound in their lifetime. Posnett et al. [9] reports the financial burden to the healthcare system of caring for chronic wounds in the UK, totaling US$ 3.4–4.6 billion a year, close to 3% of the healthcare budget. The US, a larger and more complex system, observed $35.3 billion in spending of Medicare funds on wound care alone in 2014, of which 16.7 billion was spent on infections and 9.4 billion on chronic ulcers [9] (**Figure 1**).

The implications of a biofilm-covered wound are not limited to delayed healing and financial burden. Biofilms pose a risk for persistent wound infections, especially when medical hardware is inserted into the body [11]. Biofilms can also develop into an overt infection, contribute to antimicrobial resistance, and increase the risk for adverse or tissue toxic effects caused by topical agents [12].

2. Background

Wound healing can be deranged by multiple causes, including local hypoxia or poor perfusion, repetitive ischemia-reperfusion injury, inadequate offloading or compressive therapy, and bacterial infection. Bacterial infection, playing a great role among these causes, has been

Planktonic vs. biofilm phenotype		
Trait	**Planktonic**	**Biofilm**
Virulence	Acute, aggressive course	Chronic disease
Host inflammatory response	High, sudden	Mild, persistent
Risk for antibiotic resistance	Moderate	High
Spread	Disseminating	Sessile
Extracellular polymetric substance (EPS)	No	Yes
Metabolic activity	High	Low
Species count	Monospecies, polyspecies	Polyspecies

Table 1. Planktonic and biofilm phenotypes comparison in regards to various bacterial traits and behaviors.

associated with both acute and chronic wounds *via* different rates and mechanisms. An infection with a more predominantly planktonic phenotype is more aggressive, with rapidly dividing cells invading host tissues and stimulating a strong inflammatory response typical of an acute infection. Several microorganisms can adopt a different, sessile phenotype, called a biofilm, that allows them to attach to biotic or abiotic surfaces, form aggregates, and regulate the production of an extracellular polymeric substance (EPS), contributing to their ability to survive [13, 14] (**Table 1**).

This aggregate or cluster, once called "*slime*," constitutes the biofilm, a complex tertiary structure of sessile communities of one or more species of bacteria embedded within a matrix of EPS. The EPS is composed mainly by water, polysaccharides, DNA and other substances secreted by the embedded bacteria, but also by substances scavenged from the host. It is important to appreciate that all the building blocks of a wound biofilm are ultimately derived from the wound bed and skin. Cell lysis and subsequent local decomposition of the EPS matrix is advantageous for the biofilm population, creating new pores and channels that improve nutrient access, and the intracellular level of the second messenger cyclic di-GMP are involved in regulating biofilm formation and the production of matrix components [15].

For many years, biofilm has been known to exist on dental plaque and industrial water processing and even considered the predominant state of bacteria within the human body [16]. Later on, its presence was reported on endocardium, urinary tract mucosa, nasal and sinus epithelium and pulmonary tissue, and more recently biofilms have been found in healed surgical wounds, sutures, implants and IV catheters which can be contaminated at time of insertion or as a result of hematologic seeding from a colonized tissue. The relationship between biofilm and host will depend on the location and the bacterial composition of the biofilm; for instance, in the gastrointestinal mucosa, biofilm has a commensal behavior, while in wounds or respiratory tract mucosa, a pathogenic behavior. This difference is thought to be due to the host's capacity to coexist or eradicate biofilm [6, 12, 17, 18].

3. Composition of biofilm

Several functions have been attributed to biofilm: genetic material reservoir, nutrient source, matrix stabilization, adhesion, and bacterial communication. Most of these functions will depend on the particular substances present in the biofilm, which depend exclusively on the species and even the strain of the bacteria. For instance, *P. aeruginosa* produces a biofilm with a higher density EPS, with a well-defined matrix interspersed within clusters of bacterial cells and has the particularity to be predominant over other species in a polybacterial microbiome. In general, the interaction of these substances and how the bacteria inside the biofilm manage to utilize these substances will affect the morphology of the biofilm with common effects: immobilizing biofilm cells and allowing the existence of a very diverse habitat favoring biodiversity, where every member can contribute with their own EPS [15] (**Figure 2**).

3.1. Polysaccharides

Polysaccharides comprise a major fraction of the EPS matrix and are responsible for the biofilm's mechanical properties. Interestingly, it seems to be mainly the exopolysaccharides in multivalent inorganic ions with EPS can greatly influence the mechanical properties of

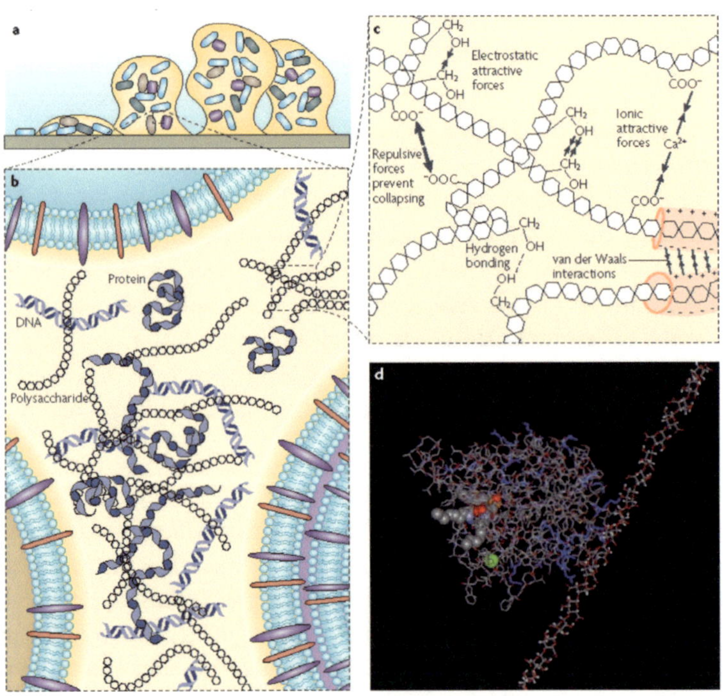

Figure 2. The extracellular polymeric substances matrix at different dimensions. (a) A model of a bacterial biofilm attached to a solid surface. (b) The major matrix components—polysaccharides, proteins and DNA—in a non-homogeneous pattern. (c) Physicochemical interactions and the entanglement of biopolymers that give stability to the EPS matrix. (d) A molecular modelling simulation of the interaction between alginate (right) and lipase (left) of *P. aeruginosa* (image from Flemming and Wingender [15], with permission).

http://dx.doi.org/10.5772/intechopen.85020

biofilms. For instance, presence of Ca^{2+} in biofilm formed by mucoid strains of *P. aeruginosa* experienced an enhancement in their mechanical stability. In *S. epidermidis*, poly-*N*-acetylglucosamine (PNAG) makes a considerable contribution to biofilm integrity [15].

As seen in *P. aeruginosa* and *S. epidermidis*, polysaccharide compositions are very diverse, even between strains of a single species. *P. aeruginosa*, for instance, produces at least three distinct exopolysaccharides that have a direct effect on its biofilm architecture: alginate, *Pel* and *Psl*. Mucoid strains of *P. aeruginosa* contain alginate, an exopolysaccharide for biofilm formation that, although non-essential, has a notable effect on biofilm architecture. Alginate takes part at the beginning of biofilm formation and is responsible for the mechanical stability of mature biofilms. Alginate from this strain has a particular clinical relevance, being comprised of uronic acids, in that it can be used as an EPS marker, since this type of acid is not found inside the bacterial cells. In non-mucoid strains, *Pel* and *Psl* participate in the first stages of biofilm formation, while *Psl* alone is involved in adherence to surfaces [15].

3.2. Proteins

Biofilms also contain a diversity of enzymes, lending a complex organization and capability of adaptation. Enzymes will break down biopolymers into low molecular mass products, degrade the structural EPS to promote detachment, act as virulence factors, and even degrade EPS components during starvation. Cell surface-associated proteins and extracellular carbohydrate-binding proteins (*lectins*) are also a key component in the biofilm, involved in the formation and stabilization of the matrix network [15].

Among these proteins we can find the glucan-binding proteins present in dental plaque caused by *S. mutans*, the galactose-specific lectin *lecA* and fucose-specific lectin *lecb* of *P. aeruginosa*, which have been associated with biofilm formation. Biofilm associated surface protein (*bap*) from *S. aureus* and the bap-like proteins, which promote biofilm formation in several species while also playing a role in bacterial infectious processes. Biofilms also contain amyloids, involved in adhesion to inanimate surfaces and host cells and invasion of host cells; additionally, they can function as cytotoxins for bacterial and plant cells [15].

3.3. Extracellular DNA

eDNA is an integral part of the matrix and biofilm mode of life. *B. cereus* uses DNA as an adhesion molecule, and in *P. aeruginosa*, eDNA serves as an intercellular connector, with DNase inhibiting biofilm formation specifically in *P. aeruginosa*. In *S. aureus*, eDNA serves the same structural role of PNAG in *S. epidermidis* eDNA, although seen initially as residual material from lysed cells, is also actively excreted. Although primarily occurring in waste-water biofilms, biofilms from various origins have been found to contain eDNA of varying levels and importance, even between closely related species. For example, eDNA plays a critical structural role in the biofilm matrix of *S. aureus* but only serves as a minor component of *S. epidermidis* biofilms. eDNA is localized differently between biofilms; in *P. aeruginosa*, for example, forms a grid-like structure. Additionally, eDNA has antimicrobial activity, having the ability to chelate cations that stabilize lipopolysaccharide and the bacterial outer membrane, provoking cell lysis [15].

EPS composition	
Component	**Function(s)**
Polysaccharides	Mechanical strength, adherence
Proteins	Mechanical strength, adherence, detachment, virulence
eDNA	Mechanical strength, adherence, antimicrobial, genetic transfer
Water	Source of ions and compounds in solution
Biosurfactants	Adherence, detachment

Table 2. Composition of biofilm exopolymeric substance (EPS) and associated functions.

3.4 Water and biosurfactants

Water is by far the largest component of the matrix, and water management is so critical that bacteria actively respond to desiccation by producing EPS. Molecular composition of the water component is critical as well, and the EPS matrix acts as a molecular sieve, sequestering cations, anions, nonpolar compounds and particles from the water phase. By comparison, biosurfactants have antibacterial and antifungal properties and are important for bacterial attachment and detachment from oil droplets. *Rhamnolipids*, which can act as surfactants, have been found in the EPS matrix of *P. aeruginosa* [15] (**Table 2**).

4. Pathophysiology

4.1. Biofilm development

Biofilms utilize a variety of mechanisms in order to establish themselves. When exposed to adverse conditions, planktonic bacteria facilitate survival by forming biofilms. This occurs through *"phase variation"* and *"adaptive mutation,"* genetic alterations that include point mutations, recombination, and transpositions, with the goal of producing individuals more capable of producing biofilms. *V. cholera*, *S. typhi*, and *E. coli* all exhibit stress-induced genetic alteration by adaptive mechanisms that produce a biofilm-capable phenotype, producing distinct, wrinkled individuals. *V. cholera* produces a more chlorine-resistant subtype called rugose, while *S. typhi* and *E. coli* change to an *"rdar"* phenotype, or red, dry, and rough [19].

4.2. Biofilms and chronic disease

By establishing biofilms, bacterial species not only increase their antibiotic resistance 1000-fold, they produce optimal conditions for chronic infections. By sacrificing aggressive movement throughout the body for confinement within a protective extracellular matrix, bacterial species effectively hide antigens, reduce the effectiveness of antibiotics, and blunt the immune response, promoting chronic disease: endocarditis, chronic kidney stones, and CF infections [19, 20].

Biofilms play a significant role in the development of chronic cutaneous wounds, with up to 80% of chronic wounds having been found to contain a biofilm compared to 6% of acute wounds [2, 4, 5, 21].

Biofilms cause chronic infections through mechanisms that are either innate or interact closely with the host immune system: genetic changes, surface and excreted molecular messengers, physical barriers, and escape behaviors. Although the bacteria may not disseminate throughout the body, pathogenicity is retained and arguably increased, as bacterial concentration within the biofilm increases and individuals tend to leave the biofilm, either through purposeful dissolution of EPS or through stresses on the biofilm itself by the fluid encasing the biofilm [19].

When bacteria cluster in a biofilm, movement of advantageous genetic traits, such as antibiotic resistance, throughout the constituents of the biofilm is expedited through transformation, horizontal gene transfer, or phage infection, making each individual bacterium even more virulent when it leaves the biofilm. *P. aeruginosa* biofilms, for example, exhibit a high concentration of DNA within their EPS. This also promotes significant genetic variability within a biofilm, increasing the chances that one of the many individuals will survive an environmental insult [19]. This includes antibiotics, leading to concern that excessive and inappropriate antibiotic use against biofilms expedites the development of antibiotic resistant strains [12].

4.3. Wound healing inhibition

Biofilms involve a complex relationship between bacteria virulence factors, survival mechanisms, and the host immune response [22]. Different species all exhibit particular biofilm characteristics that inhibit wound healing. EPS by itself represents a physical barrier against inflammatory cell phagocytosis, and has the potential to inhibit the complement cascade and antibiotic penetration into the wound [23]. Acellular extract from *S. aureus* biofilms inhibits the movement of keratinocytes and promotes apoptosis, leading to impaired cutaneous wound healing. This extract did not differ in pH or calcium levels; its effect on keratinocytes was due to direct cytotoxic substances secreted from or present on *S. aureus* bacterium: alpha-toxin and cell surface-expressed fibronectin-binding proteins [21].

P. aeruginosa biofilms similarly inhibit neutrophil movement but may spare their capacity for oxidative burst, and exhibit a capacity for ejecting individual bacterium from the biofilm [24]. Another potential mechanism for *P. aeruginosa* biofilm resistance to neutrophils is the rapid necrosis induced by the production of *rhamnolipids* [23]. Additionally, significant delay in wound healing, re-epithelization and collagen deposition have been reported without significant difference in PMN infiltration or granulation tissue [6]. The ultimate result is neutrophil aggregation near the biofilm, with oxidative burst products accumulating and causing neutrophil death, while individuals within the biofilm leave to create new colonies away from the initial site [24, 25].

Biofilms in general promote a host inflammatory response that poorly penetrates the biofilm itself, causing surrounding cell damage instead [18]. Host inflammatory signal expression also characterizes the biofilm infection; in general, those with impaired host immune responses, such as those with diabetes or arterial insufficiency, tend to have more significant wounds [22].

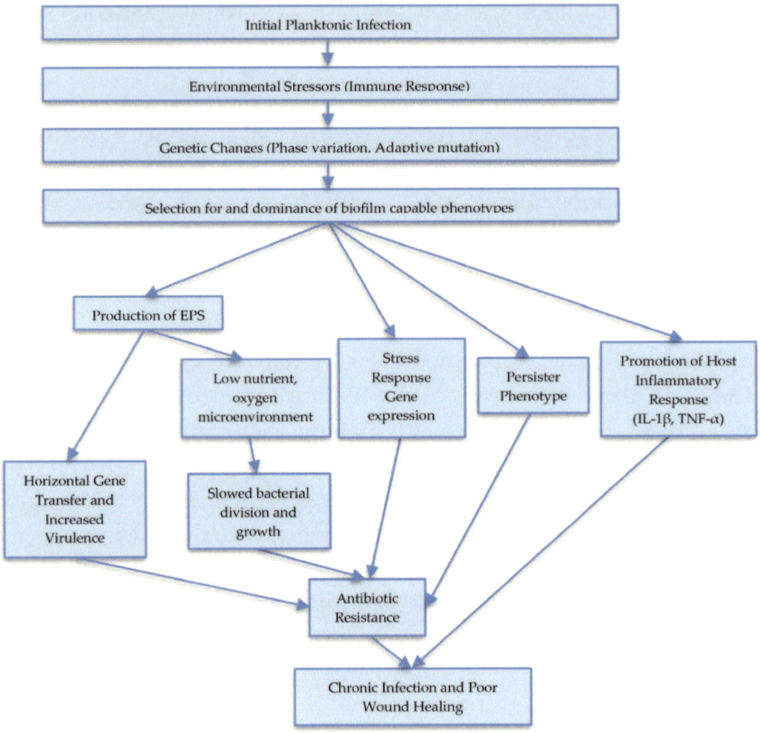

Figure 3. Biofilm pathophysiology. Common pathways followed by bacteria to chronic infection and wound healing impairment.

S. aureus biofilms promote a distinct profile of *IL-1β* and *TNF-α* expression indicative of a mild but chronic inflammatory response [17]. While mild inflammation is helpful towards eradicating the infection by attracting an immune response and increasing collagen synthesis and granulation tissue formation, persistently high amounts of *IL-1β* and *TNF-α* decrease growth factors and increase metalloproteases, delaying resolution of the infection and wound healing [20].

P. aeruginosa in particular exhibits the highest virulence compared to *S. aureus* and *K. pneumoniae* due to this reason; *P. aeruginosa* biofilms exhibit the lowest bacterial counts but cause the highest elevation in *IL-1β* and *TNF-α* compared to the other two strains [23]. MRSA biofilms modulate the immune response by stimulating macrophages towards an M2 instead of M1 response, inhibiting inflammation and promoting fibrosis [26]. Chronic diseases caused by biofilms, in essence, are due to a complex equilibrium between bacterial defenses and the host immune response (**Figure 3**).

5. Antibiotic resistance mechanisms

Biofilms are notoriously resistant to antibiotics, making them frustrating to treat, particularly in implanted devices, where usually the most viable solution is replacing the device entirely [27, 28].

Most literature cites the exopolymeric substance (EPS), serving as a physical barrier, as a cause of antibiotic resistance, and this is seen in some species; *P. aeruginosa* EPS contains negatively-charged alginate that easily slows the diffusion of positively-charged aminoglycosides [22, 23, 27].

However, some specific pairs of antibiotics and species do exhibit unrestricted diffusion: ciprofloxacin and ampicillin through *K. pneumoniae*, rifampin through *S. epidermidis*, ciprofloxacin through *P. aeruginosa*, and tetracycline through *E. coli*, illustrating that although the EPS does contribute, there are many more factors, related to or independent from the EPS, that contribute in sum to resistance [27].

While the EPS does indeed slow diffusion of antibiotic, eventually enough antibiotic will accumulate and kill the offending pathogen; this result has been observed in *P. aeruginosa* with tobramycin, despite the alginate produced. An important role, then, of the EPS is not blocking the antibiotic, but slowing its effect and allowing the bacteria within the biofilm to prepare. Antibiotics, for example, can stimulate the production of additional EPS in *S. epidermidis*, *E. coli*, and *P. aeruginosa* [27].

More specifically, a variety of antibiotics stimulated polysaccharide intracellular adhesion production in *S. epidermidis*, and beta-lactam antibiotics upregulated *cps* gene expression in *E. coli*, promoting the production of colonic acid; both are critical for biofilm formation in their respective species. As for *P. aeruginosa*, imipenem stimulated alginate production and the *arr* gene was found to influence biofilm resistance to aminoglycosides [27].

Within the biofilm, constituent bacteria construct a hypoxic and nutrient-deprived microenvironment that slows bacterial division and, as a result, blunts the effect of antibiotics.

Factors for chronic disease and antibiotic resistance in biofilms

Factor	Function	Examples
EPS	Block host detection of bacterial antigens, inflammatory response, and effect of antibiotics	Alginate in mucoid *P. aeruginosa*
Molecular messengers/host immune modulation	Establishes chronic infection and inhibits host inflammatory response and wound healing	*S. aureus* biofilms impair keratinocytes; *P. aeruginosa* biofilms impair neutrophils
Genetic changes	Genetic diversity, exchange of virulence factors and antibiotic resistance genes	Horizontal gene transfer, eDNA, phage infection, transformation
Escape behaviors	Promote establishment of new colonies away from site under antimicrobial or immune system attack	*S. viridans* seeding from dental plaque to endocardium
Persister phenotype	Increased resistance to antibiotics	*E. coli* persister genes glpD, glpABC, plsD
Stress response genes	Increased resistance to antibiotics	*E. coli* rpoS gene
Environmental alterations	Reduction of bacterial division and susceptibility to antibiotics targeting division	Low oxygen, nutritional state microenvironment within the biofilm

Table 3. Mechanisms by which biofilms lead to chronic disease, with associated functions and examples.

For example, *E. coli* increases *cydAB* and *b2997-hybABC* genes expression. Along with this micro-environment, bacteria establish a stationary-phase state and express stress response genes; *E. coli* increases *rpoS* expression, while *P. aeruginosa* increases *groES*, *dnaK*, catalase, *katA*, and *katB* [27].

Biofilm bacteria also increase the population of slow-growing "persisters," particularly hardy individual bacterium that can resist antibiotics. In *E. coli*, *glpD*, *glpABC*, *plsD*, are critically involved in persister development, as well as chromosomal toxin/antitoxin genes *relE* and *hipBA*. Finally, there are also specific biofilm-only products, such as *ndvB* in *P. aeruginosa*, that specifically target certain antibiotics, in this case tobramycin [27] (**Table 3**).

6. Diagnosis

Bacterium often do not present purely in a planktonic or biofilm state; infections often contain a mixture of both. Basic criteria of the present of a biofilm are proposed by Parsek and Singh [19] and include the following: (1) bacteria are attached to a particular surface, (2) when examined, bacteria are organized into groups surrounded by EPS, (3) the infection is isolated to a particular area, and (4) the infection is difficult to treat with antibiotics despite significant eradication when in planktonic form.

Current diagnosis of wound infections is based on the bacterial side of the infection, rather than the host side; culturable CFUs is the most basic diagnostic tool but limits the diagnosis to only culturable bacteria [29]. Additionally, as biofilms are an observed mode of growth for bacteria in living hosts, it is difficult to sample a suspected host and have the bacteria establish the same biofilm on culture [19].

Furthermore, a significant amount of biofilms contain multiple species, an average of 5.4 and a maximum of 106 [18, 25]. PCR surpasses this limitation and allows clinicians to detect unculturable species, but the severity of the infection cannot be assessed in a multi-species infection [29]. There has also been success in determining biofilm formation by *P. aeruginosa* in CF patients by measuring the ratio between two quorum sensing messengers [19]. Autoinducers indicating virulence factor expression is another proposed diagnostic measurement [18].

Newer proposed tests measure the host side of the infection beyond clinical assessment, where the appearance of inflammatory signs can be unreliable and change over time. New upcoming methods of diagnosing and assessing the severity of chronic wounds revolve around measuring host inflammatory markers [29].

However, tests must be designed around each individual species' unique course and profile of inflammatory markers, as well as the unique relationship between the inflammatory marker levels and virulence; for example, *P. aeruginosa* exhibits the lowest bacterial counts but the highest $IL\text{-}1\beta$ and $TNF\text{-}\alpha$ response, as compared to *S. aureus* and *K. pneumoniae* [22, 23].

7. Management of biofilm

Even though there is not a standard debridement type, frequent sharp and mechanical debridement have been suggested as the standard treatment for biofilm infection. Nevertheless, up to 30% [30] of biofilm infected wounds continued unresolved after these, and therefore other options are being considered, such as biological, enzymatic and autolytic [12, 30–33]. Mechanical debridement involves the application of wound dressings that expedite wound healing and resolve the biofilm infection [12]. For example, silver-based dressing is effective against *P. aeruginosa* biofilms [16]. Additionally, antimicrobial coatings, on inserted devices, for example, can hinder biofilm formation [27]. Sharp debridement, by contrast, involves scraping away at the wound with a sharp instrument to remove necrotic tissue [12]. Beyond debridement, many other treatment modalities for biofilms are being explored, including molecular solutions, energy-based interventions, and new topical medications.

Given the complex interactions between biofilm bacterium, the physical extracellular matrix, secreted signals and toxins, and the host immune response, there are understandably many molecular solutions for disrupting the biofilm and promoting resolution of chronic wounds. Among these, we have the following:

- Furanone, a substance structurally similar to a class of quorum sensing signal produced by the marine alga *Delisea pulchra*, has been successfully used to treat *V. harvey*, *B. subtilis*, and *P. aeruginosa* biofilms. Furanone acts by disrupting quorum sensing using this similarity [27].
- Patulin, a molecule found in *Penicillium* extracts has the ability to disrupt quorum-sensing, and also was proven to be effective against *P. aeruginosa* biofilm pulmonary infection in a mouse model, acting synergistically with tobramycin [27].
- Farnesol, produced by *C. albicans* is effective against *S. aureus* biofilms by compromising its membrane integrity, additionally, it increases the effect of Gentamycin on *MRSA* and methicillin sensitive *S. aureus* [27].
- Ursolic acid, a natural plant extract, also disrupts *P. aeruginosa*, *V. harvey*, and *E. coli* biofilms *via* a mechanism that is not completely dilucidated, involves several bacterial metabolic activities except quorum-sensing [27].
- Staphylococcal accessory regulator (*sarA*) has been identified as a key regulator for biofilm formation, and therefore is, in effect, a potential therapeutic target. sarA mutant strains of *S. aureus* and *S. epidermidis* experienced limited biofilm formation and increased susceptibility to daptomycin [28].
- For MRSA in particular, due to its particular trait of promoting a fibrotic M2 response, rather than a strongly inflammatory M1 response, inserting M1 macrophages or stimulating such a response using *EP67* can prevent MRSA biofilms entirely and also resolves MRSA biofilms better than antibiotics or administration of neutrophils. *EP67* is a CD88 agonist that converts an M2 response by increasing the amount of inflammatory cytokines produced and increases the potency of macrophage movement into the biofilm [26].

- Ribonucleic acid III inhibiting peptide (RIP) is a promising new intervention for biofilms, as it inhibits the quorum sensing necessary for biofilms to form [34]. RIP treatment accelerates wound healing in *S. aureus* and *S. epidermidis* biofilms to equal that of uninfected wounds. RIP also exhibits increased effect when combined with antibiotics in the treatment of *S. epidermidis* infections in devices [27].
- D-amino acids is a specific mix containing D-tyrosine, D-leucine, D-tryptophan and D-methionine that form a factor that was first found to prevent biofilm formation in *B. subtilis*, and later on tested on *P. aeruginosa* and *S. aureus*. In *S. aureus*, another combination (D-phenylalanine, D-proline, D-tyrosine) was found to be more effective and, more importantly, that its action is targeted to the growth stage of biofilm formation [23, 35, 36].

However, treatment cannot only consist of quorum sensing inhibitors or interventions that specifically target the biofilm, as bacteria can still survive and grow in planktonic form; daptomycin is the antibiotic of choice most effective against biofilm-forming bacteria [28].

Energy-based therapeutic options, such as ultrasound, are another viable option for treating biofilms; for *P. aeruginosa* biofilms, daily or every other day low frequency ultrasound is effective in reducing inflammation and improving wound healing [16, 37]. Additional research has also investigated the application of different topical medications on biofilm resolution and wound healing; for example, wound healing from *S. aureus* biofilms benefits from exposed desiccation or the application of honey or molasses on the wound site compared to saline, exhibiting greater granulation tissue and decreased inflammation, primarily due to the action of air or osmotic agents in drying the wound [38].

8. Conclusions

Contrasting with free-floating, acutely infectious planktonic forms of bacteria, a biofilm is an aggregated colony of bacteria, usually of multiple species, that produces a protective EPS and establishes a microenvironment within that is conductive to survival and ultimately leads to chronic infection in the form of kidney stones, pulmonary infections, endocarditis, and cutaneous non-healing wounds.

When exposed to environmental stressors, bacterial undergo genetic changes that promote biofilm formation. Biofilms are made up of multiple elements—polysaccharides, proteins, extracellular DNA, and water/biosurfactants—all which have unique structural and functional traits that establishes the biofilm and its properties. Biofilms are a primary cause of chronic cutaneous wounds, due to the secretion of signals that inhibit a proper host immune response. While each species' biofilm is different in its particular properties, make-up, and response to antibiotics, biofilms are, in general, notoriously difficult to treat using antibiotics due to the EPS blocking the diffusion of antibiotics and allowing the production of a microenvironment conductive to gene transfer, metabolic slowing, selection for hardier individuals, and the development of escape behaviors that create new biofilms elsewhere in the body.

http://dx.doi.org/10.5772/intechopen.85020

Biofilms are clinically diagnosed with four basic criteria—attached, organized, local, and antibiotic resistant. Assessment with older culture methods has been proven inefficient. Modern methods such as PCR and detection of molecular inflammatory markers and secreted bacterial products are more useful methods of diagnosis. While the standard treatment is frequent and aggressive debridement, there are multiple modalities for the treatment of biofilms—biologic, enzymatic, autolytic, and mechanical—with newer molecular treatments in combination with traditional antibiotic therapy showing promising results.

Conflict of interest

The authors declare no conflict of interest.

Thanks

The authors would like to thank our families and the Division of Plastic & Reconstructive Surgery staff for their unconditional support and help.

Author details

Rafael A. Mendoza, Ji-Cheng Hsieh and Robert D. Galiano*

*Address all correspondence to: rgaliano@nm.org

Division of Plastic and Reconstructive Surgery, Department of Surgery, Northwestern University, Chicago, IL, USA

References

[1] Sen CK. Wound healing essentials: Let there be oxygen. Wound Repair and Regeneration. 2009;**17**(1):1-18

[2] Malone M, Bjarnsholt T, McBain AJ, James GA, Stoodley P, Leaper D, et al. The prevalence of biofilms in chronic wounds: A systematic review and meta-analysis of published data. Journal of Wound Care. 2017;**26**(1):20-25

[3] Armstrong DG, Boulton AJM, Bus SA. Diabetic foot ulcers and their recurrence. The New England Journal of Medicine. 2017;**376**(24):2367-2375

[4] James GA, Swogger E, Wolcott R, Pulcini E, Secor P, Sestrich J, et al. Biofilms in chronic wounds. Wound Repair and Regeneration. 2008;**16**(1):37-44

[5] Romling U, Balsalobre C. Biofilm infections, their resilience to therapy and innovative treatment strategies. Journal of Internal Medicine. 2012;**272**(6):541-561

[6] Brandenburg KS, Calderon DF, Kierski PR, Czuprynski CJ, McAnulty JF. Novel murine model for delayed wound healing using a biological wound dressing with *Pseudomonas aeruginosa* biofilms. Microbial Pathogenesis. 2018;**122**:30-38

[7] Mostafalu P, Tamayol A, Rahimi R, Ochoa M, Khalilpour A, Kiaee G, et al. Smart bandage for monitoring and treatment of chronic wounds. Small. 2018:e1703509

[8] Jarbrink K, Ni G, Sonnergren H, Schmidtchen A, Pang C, Bajpai R, et al. Prevalence and incidence of chronic wounds and related complications: A protocol for a systematic review. Systematic Reviews. 2016;**5**(1):152

[9] Gupta S, Andersen C, Black J, de Leon J, Fife C, Lantis Ii JC, et al. Management of chronic wounds: Diagnosis, preparation, treatment, and follow-up. Wounds. 2017;**29**(9):S19-S36

[10] Nguyen KT, Seth AK, Hong SJ, Geringer MR, Xie P, Leung KP, et al. Deficient cytokine expression and neutrophil oxidative burst contribute to impaired cutaneous wound healing in diabetic, biofilm-containing chronic wounds. Wound Repair and Regeneration. 2013;**21**(6):833-841

[11] Akers KS, Mende K, Cheatle KA, Zera WC, Yu X, Beckius ML, et al. Biofilms and persistent wound infections in United States military trauma patients: A case-control analysis. BMC Infectious Diseases. 2014;**14**:190

[12] Bianchi T, Wolcott RD, Peghetti A, Leaper D, Cutting K, Polignano R, et al. Recommendations for the management of biofilm: A consensus document. Journal of Wound Care. 2016;**25**(6):305-317

[13] Blanchette KA, Wenke JC. Current therapies in treatment and prevention of fracture wound biofilms: Why a multifaceted approach is essential for resolving persistent infections. Journal of Bone and Joint Infection. 2018;**3**(2):50-67

[14] Tahir S, Malone M, Hu H, Deva A, Vickery K. The effect of negative pressure wound therapy with and without instillation on mature biofilms in vitro. Materials (Basel). 2018;**11**(5)

[15] Flemming HC, Wingender J. The biofilm matrix. Nature Reviews Microbiology. 2010;**8**(9):623-633

[16] Seth AK, Nguyen KT, Geringer MR, Hong SJ, Leung KP, Mustoe TA, et al. Noncontact, low-frequency ultrasound as an effective therapy against *Pseudomonas aeruginosa*-infected biofilm wounds. Wound Repair and Regeneration. 2013;**21**(2):266-274

[17] Gurjala AN, Geringer MR, Seth AK, Hong SJ, Smeltzer MS, Galiano RD, et al. Development of a novel, highly quantitative in vivo model for the study of biofilm-impaired cutaneous wound healing. Wound Repair and Regeneration. 2011;**19**(3):400-410

[18] Seth AK, Geringer MR, Hong SJ, Leung KP, Mustoe TA, Galiano RD. In vivo modeling of biofilm-infected wounds: A review. The Journal of Surgical Research. 2012;**178**(1):330-338

[19] Parsek MR, Singh PK. Bacterial biofilms: An emerging link to disease pathogenesis. Annual Review of Microbiology. 2003;**57**:677-701

[20] Edwards R, Harding KG. Bacteria and wound healing. Current Opinion in Infectious Diseases. 2004;**17**(2):91-96

[21] Kirker KR, Secor PR, James GA, Fleckman P, Olerud JE, Stewart PS. Loss of viability and induction of apoptosis in human keratinocytes exposed to *Staphylococcus aureus* biofilms in vitro. Wound Repair and Regeneration. 2009;**17**(5):690-699

[22] Seth AK, Geringer MR, Gurjala AN, Abercrombie JA, Chen P, You T, et al. Understanding the host inflammatory response to wound infection: An in vivo study of *Klebsiella pneumoniae* in a rabbit ear wound model. Wound Repair and Regeneration. 2012;**20**(2):214-225

[23] Seth AK, Geringer MR, Galiano RD, Leung KP, Mustoe TA, Hong SJ. Quantitative comparison and analysis of species-specific wound biofilm virulence using an in vivo, rabbit-ear model. Journal of the American College of Surgeons. 2012;**215**(3):388-399

[24] Jesaitis AJ, Franklin MJ, Berglund D, Sasaki M, Lord CI, Bleazard JB, et al. Compromised host defense on *Pseudomonas aeruginosa* biofilms: Characterization of neutrophil and biofilm interactions. Journal of Immunology. 2003;**171**(8):4329-4339

[25] Seth AK, Geringer MR, Hong SJ, Leung KP, Galiano RD, Mustoe TA. Comparative analysis of single-species and polybacterial wound biofilms using a quantitative, in vivo, rabbit ear model. PLoS One. 2012;**7**(8):e42897

[26] Hanke ML, Heim CE, Angle A, Sanderson SD, Kielian T. Targeting macrophage activation for the prevention and treatment of *Staphylococcus aureus* biofilm infections. Journal of Immunology. 2013;**190**(5):2159-2168

[27] Anderson GG, O'Toole GA. Innate and induced resistance mechanisms of bacterial biofilms. Current Topics in Microbiology and Immunology. 2008;**322**:85-105

[28] Weiss EC, Zielinska A, Beenken KE, Spencer HJ, Daily SJ, Smeltzer MS. Impact of sarA on daptomycin susceptibility of *Staphylococcus aureus* biofilms in vivo. Antimicrobial Agents and Chemotherapy. 2009;**53**(10):4096-4102

[29] Leung KP, D'Arpa P, Seth AK, Geringer MR, Jett M, Xu W, et al. Dermal wound transcriptomic responses to infection with *Pseudomonas aeruginosa* versus *Klebsiella pneumoniae* in a rabbit ear wound model. BMC Clinical Pathology. 2014;**14**:20

[30] Hurlow JJ, Humphreys GJ, Bowling FL, McBain AJ. Diabetic foot infection: A critical complication. International Wound Journal. 2018

[31] Hoppe IC, Granick MS. Debridement of chronic wounds: A qualitative systematic review of randomized controlled trials. Clinics in Plastic Surgery. 2012;**39**(3):221-228

[32] Smith F, Dryburgh N, Donaldson J, Mitchell M. Debridement for surgical wounds. Cochrane Database of Systematic Reviews. 2013;**9**:CD006214

[33] Wilcox JR, Carter MJ, Covington S. Frequency of debridements and time to heal: A retrospective cohort study of 312 744 wounds. JAMA Dermatology. 2013;**149**(9):1050-1058

[34] Fang RC, Galiano RD. Adjunctive therapies in the treatment of osteomyelitis. Seminars in Plastic Surgery. 2009;**23**(2):141-147

[35] Hochbaum AI, Kolodkin-Gal I, Foulston L, Kolter R, Aizenberg J, Losick R. Inhibitory effects of D-amino acids on *Staphylococcus aureus* biofilm development. Journal of Bacteriology. 2011;**193**(20):5616-5622

[36] Kolodkin-Gal I, Romero D, Cao S, Clardy J, Kolter R, Losick R. D-amino acids trigger biofilm disassembly. Science. 2010;**328**(5978):627-629

[37] Seth AK, Zhong A, Nguyen KT, Hong SJ, Leung KP, Galiano RD, et al. Impact of a novel, antimicrobial dressing on in vivo, *Pseudomonas aeruginosa* wound biofilm: Quantitative comparative analysis using a rabbit ear model. Wound Repair and Regeneration. 2014;**22**(6):712-719

[38] Park E, Long SA, Seth AK, Geringer M, Xu W, Chavez-Munoz C, et al. The use of desiccation to treat *Staphylococcus aureus* biofilm-infected wounds. Wound Repair and Regeneration. 2016;**24**(2):394-401